RADIOLOGY
RECALL

RECALL SERIES EDITOR

LORNE H. BLACKBOURNE, M.D.
General Surgeon
Fayetteville, North Carolina

RADIOLOGY RECALL

SENIOR EDITORS

SPENCER B. GAY, M.D.
Associate Professor of Radiology
University of Virginia
Charlottesville, Virginia

RICHARD J. WOODCOCK, Jr., M.D.
Chief Resident in Radiology
University of Virginia
Charlottesville, Virginia

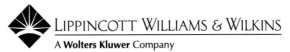

LIPPINCOTT WILLIAMS & WILKINS
A **Wolters Kluwer** Company
Philadelphia · Baltimore · New York · London
Buenos Aires · Hong Kong · Sydney · Tokyo

Editor: Elizabeth Nieginski
Development Editor: Melanie Cann
Editorial Intern: Elizabeth Dillon
Managing Editor: Marette D. Magargle-Smith
Marketing Manager: Jennifer Conrad

Library of Congress Cataloging-in-Publication Data

Radiology recall / senior editors, Spencer B. Gay, Richard J. Woodcock, Jr.
    p. ; cm. — (Recall series)
   Includes index.
   ISBN 0-683-30663-4
   1. Radiography, Medical—Examinations, questions, etc. 2. Diagnostic imaging—Examinations, questions, etc. 3. Echocardiography—Examinations, questions, etc.
I. Gay, SpencerB. II. Woodcock, Richard J. III. Series
   [DNLM: 1. Diagnostic Imaging—Examination Questions. WN 18.2R129 1999]
RC78.15.R325 1999
616.07′54′076—dc21   99-040820

4 5 6 7 8 9 10

CONTRIBUTORS

Suresh K. Agarwal, Ph.D.
Professor of Radiology
University of Virginia
Director, Radiological Physics
    Division
Charlottesville, Virginia

J. Fritz Angle, M.D.
Associate Professor of Radiology
University of Virginia
Charlottesville, Virginia

James R. Brookeman, Ph.D.
Professor of Radiology
Director of Magnetic Resonance
    Research
University of Virginia
Charlottesville, Virginia

Gia A. DeAngelis, M.D.
Associate Professor of Radiology
University of Virginia
Charlottesville, Virginia

Paul M. Dee, M.D.
Professor of Radiology
University of Virginia
Charlottesville, Virginia

Jonas H. Goldstein, M.D.
Fellow, Interventional Radiology
Emory University Hospital
Atlanta, Georgia

Gary D. Hartwell, Ds.C.
Assistant Professor of Radiological
    Physics
University of Virginia
Charlottesville, Virginia

Jennifer A. Harvey, M.D.
Assistant Professor of Radiology
Director of Breast Imaging
University of Virginia
Charlottesville, Virginia

Joan McIlhenny, M.D.
Associate Professor of Radiology and
    Pediatrics
Co-Director of Pediatric Radiology
University of Virginia
Charlottesville, Virginia

Ruth Moran, M.D.
Assistant Professor of Radiology
Director of Ultrasound
University of Virginia
Charlottesville, Virginia

Jayashree Parekh, M.D.
Assistant Professor of Radiology
University of Virginia
Charlottesville, Virginia

C. Douglas Phillips, M.D.
Associate Professor of Radiology
University of Virginia
Charlottesville, Virginia

Hubert A. Shaffer, Jr., M.D.
Professor of Radiology
Co-Director, Division of
    Thoracoabdominal Radiology
University of Virginia
Charlottesville, Virginia

Charles D. Teates, M.D.
Professor of Radiology
Director, Division of Nuclear
    Medicine
University of Virginia
Charlottesville, Virginia

Preface

Radiology Recall is intended for students and residents with a love for medicine and an interest in the technology that permits us to see inside the body.
   Radiology Recall has several qualities that readers will find useful:

- **Interactive approach.** This book, as part of the popular Recall series, is different from most other radiology texts in that it takes an interactive approach to the material. Based on the questions that one would ask a trainee at the view box, *Radiology Recall* enables the reader to test and reinforce his or her knowledge of radiographic and cross-sectional anatomy and pathology. In addition, *Radiology Recall* provides the reader with ways to methodically and thoroughly evaluate imaging studies.
- **Practical organization.** Chapters 1 and 2 contain introductory material—a list of abbreviations commonly encountered in radiology and a discussion of the imaging techniques and physics involved in creating images. The rest of the material in the book is organized by organ system. This approach facilitates thinking in terms of organ system pathology and reflects the way that radiologists usually interact with referring colleagues. In addition, the organ system approach mimics the format of the oral board examination in Radiology.
- **Extensive use of illustrations.** Radiology is a visual specialty that requires the physician to grasp certain key spatial relationships. I tend to remember facts best by visualizing them. For this reason, I chose to include more than 300 illustrations in *Radiology Recall,* most in the form of line drawings. Some of these illustrations are redrawn from the same ones that taught me the concepts presented here. Some illustrations, such as the patterns of lobar collapse on a chest radiograph, should actually be drawn by the student for practice until the concept and pattern are mastered.
- **Comprehensive coverage of material.** An effort has been made to discuss the subject of radiology and imaging of the entire body comprehensively, but without going into excessive detail. For example, I have included material on echocardiography, which is not traditionally in the purview of radiologists. However, this is the way the heart is optimally imaged, and I felt that the inclusion of this material was necessary in order to provide the reader with a concise yet complete overview of cardiac imaging.

   Very little of the material in *Radiology Recall* is new work. Rather, *Radiology Recall* seeks to organize and present the existing body of information in such a way as to make the path easier for the student interested in imaging. Ultimately, this book has the potential to improve interspecialty communication and to make better surgeons, family practitioners, internists, and radiologists. My hope is that this book makes learning radiology straightforward, fun, and relatively easy.

Acknowledgments

Although this book has encompassed nearly every minute of my time not committed to patient care or family over the last two years, it would not have happened without the help of my friends and colleagues here at the University of Virginia. My coauthor and chapter authors have been great resources, usually doing more than was asked. The chapters were also generously reviewed by faculty at the University of Virginia to ensure that the information they contained was as current and as accurate as possible. I must also credit my mother, who practiced medicine for fifty years and loved learning.

A special thanks to my secretary, Ms. Shirley Yowell, who worked very hard on this project. She typed much of this manuscript, kept the material organized, and remained extremely pleasant throughout the lengthy process.

Contents

Figure Credits

Chapter 2

Page 7, Basic principle of radiologic imaging. Sprawls P Jr: *Physical Principles of Medical Imaging*, 2e. Madison, WI, Medical Physics Publishing, 1995, p 18.

Page 16, Components of an x-ray tube. Huda W, Slone RM: *Review of Radiologic Physics*. Baltimore, Williams & Wilkins, 1995, p 22.

Page 18, Five factors that affect the patient dose. Sprawls P Jr: *Physical Principles of Medical Imaging*, 2e. Madison, WI, Medical Physics Publishing, 1995, p 478.

Page 21, Window width. Barbaric ZL: *Principles of Genitourinary Radiology*, 2e. New York, Thieme Medical Publishers, 1994, p 9.

Page 27, Relation of signal intensity to the TR and TE in a spin-echo sequence. Sprawls P Jr: *Physical Principles of Medical Imaging*, 2e. Madison, WI, Medical Physics Publishing, 1995, p 464.

Page 35, Flow at a stenosis. Kisslo J: *Doppler Color Flow Imaging*. New York, Churchill Livingstone, 1988, pp 914, 915.

Page 36, Blood flow to organs versus systemic arterial flow. Huda W, Slone RM: *Radiologic Review of Physics*. Baltimore, Williams & Wilkins, 1995, p 163.

Page 37, Gamma camera system. Sprawls P Jr: *Physical Principles of Medical Imaging*, 2e. Madison, WI, Medical Physics Publishing, 1995, p 530.

Chapter 3

Page 58, Hilar structures. Naidich DP, Zerhouni EA, Siegelman SS: *Computed Tomography and Magnetic Resonance of the Thorax*, 2e. New York, Raven Press, 1991, p 236.

Page 59, Mediastinal structures. Naidich DP, Zerhouni EA, Siegelman SS: *Computed Tomography and Magnetic Resonance of the Thorax*, 2e. New York, Raven Press, 1991, p 238.

Chapter 4

Page 121, Location of the coronary arteries. Kubicka RA, Smith C: How to interpret coronary arteriograms. *Radiographics* 6(4):661–701, 1986.

Page 124, Branches of the right coronary artery. Chen JTT: *Essentials of Cardiac Imaging*, 2e. Philadelphia, Lippincott-Raven, 1997, p 179.

Page 125, Branches of the left coronary artery. Chen JTT: *Essentials of Cardiac Imaging*, 2e. Philadelphia, Lippincott-Raven, 1997, p 180.

Page 126, Arterial supply of the myocardium. Thrall JH, Ziessman HA: *Nuclear Medicine: The Requisites (Requisites Series)*. St. Louis, Mosby-Year Book, 1995, p 63.

Page 127, Approach to cardiac valvular anatomy. Netter F: *Ciba Collection of Medical Illustrations. Volume 5. Heart.* Summit, NJ, Ciba-Geigy, 1969, pp 22, 25.

Page 131, Left ventricular enlargement. Higgins CB: *Essentials of Cardiac Radiology and Imaging*. Philadelphia, Lippincott-Raven, 1991, p 13.

Page 136, Two-dimensional echocardiography orthogonal imaging planes. Elliott LD: *Cardiac Imaging in Infants, Children, and Adults*. Philadelphia, JB Lippincott, 1991, p 33.

Page 137, Two-dimensional echocardiography transducer positions and planes. Elliott LD: *Cardiac Imaging in Infants, Children, and Adults*. Philadelphia, JB Lippincott, 1991, p 33.

Page 137, Parasternal long-axis plane. Reprinted with the permission of Simon & Schuster Inc. from *Echocardiographic Diagnosis* by Ivan A. D'Cruz. Copyright © 1983 Ivan A. D'Cruz.

Page 139, Parasternal short-axis plane, level of the aorta. Reprinted with the permission of Simon & Schuster Inc. from *Echocardiographic Diagnosis* by Ivan A. D'Cruz. Copyright © 1983 Ivan A. D'Cruz.

Page 139, Parasternal short-axis plane, level of the mitral valve. Reprinted with the permission of Simon & Schuster Inc. from *Echocardiographic Diagnosis* by Ivan A. D'Cruz. Copyright © 1983 Ivan A. D'Cruz.

Page 139, Parasternal short-axis plane, mid-papillary level. Reprinted with the permission of Simon & Schuster Inc. from *Echocardiographic Diagnosis* by Ivan A. D'Cruz. Copyright © 1983 Ivan A. D'Cruz.

Page 140, Apical four-chamber plane. Reprinted with the permission of Simon & Schuster Inc. from *Echocardiographic Diagnosis* by Ivan A. D'Cruz. Copyright © 1983 Ivan A. D'Cruz.

Page 141, Apical two-chamber plane. Reprinted with the permission of Simon & Schuster Inc. from *Echocardiographic Diagnosis* by Ivan A. D'Cruz. Copyright © 1983 Ivan A. D'Cruz.

Page 143, Suprasternal long-axis plane. Weyman AE: *Cross-Sectional Echocardiography*. Philadelphia, Lea & Febiger, 1982, p 132.

Page 143, Suprasternal short-axis plane. Weyman AE: *Cross-Sectional Echocardiography*. Philadelphia, Lea & Febiger, 1982, p 133.

Page 157, Left ventricular segments. Higgins CB: *Essentials of Cardiac Radiology and Imaging.* Philadelphia, Lippincott-Raven, 1991, p 111.

Page 160, Opening of the mitral valve. Salcedo E: *Atlas of Echocardiography,* 2e. Philadelphia, WB Saunders, 1985, p 53.

Page 176, Ventricular septal defect. Gedgaudas W, Moller JH, Castaneda-Zuniga WR, et al: *Cardiovascular Radiology.* Philadelphia, WB Saunders, 1985, p 68.

Chapter 5

Page 190, General structure of the arterial wall. Junqueira LC, Carneiro J, Kelley RO: *Basic Histology,* 8e. Norwalk, CT, Appleton & Lange, 1995, p 203.

Page 193, Branches of the celiac artery. Sauerland EK: *Grant's Dissector,* 11e. Baltimore, Williams & Wilkins, 1994, p 63.

Page 193, Branches of the superior mesenteric artery. Snell RS: *Clinical Anatomy for Medical Students,* 5e. Philadelphia, Lippincott-Raven, 1995, p 198.

Page 194, Branches of the inferior mesenteric artery. Snell RS: *Clinical Anatomy for Medical Students,* 5e. Philadelphia, Lippincott-Raven, 1995, p 203.

Page 195, Arterial supply of the stomach. Sauerland EK: *Grant's Dissector,* 11e. Baltimore, Williams & Wilkins, 1994, p 63.

Page 196, Portal venous anatomy. Sutton D: *Textbook of Radiology and Imaging,* 4e. New York, Churchill Livingstone, 1997, p 753.

Page 201, Femoral vessels and nerves. Sauerland EK: *Grant's Dissector,* 11e. Baltimore, Williams & Wilkins, 1994, p 132.

Page 218, Percutaneous transluminal angioplasty. Sutton D: *Textbook of Radiology and Imaging,* 4e. New York, Churchill Livingstone, 1997, p 698.

Page 234, Aortic dissection. Weissleder R, Rieumont MJ, Wittenberg J: *Primer of Diagnostic Imaging,* 2e. St. Louis, Mosby-Year Book, 1997, p 616.

Chapter 6

Page 260, Posterior ligament complex. Greenspan A: *Orthopedic Radiology,* 2e. Philadelphia, Lippincott-Raven, 1992, p 10.37.

Page 263, Rotator cuff. Zlatkin MB: *MRI of the Shoulder.* New York, Raven Press, 1991, p 921.

Page 263, Subacromial bursa. Berquist TR: *MRI of the Musculoskeletal System,* 3e. Philadelphia, Lippincott-Raven, 1996, p 558.

Page 265, Carpal bones. April EW: *NMS Clinical Anatomy,* 3e. Baltimore, Williams & Wilkins, 1997, p 104.

Page 267, Pelvic columns. Greenspan A: *Orthopedic Radiology*, 2e. Philadelphia, Lippincott-Raven, 1992, p 7.13.

Page 268, Knee joint. Gay SB: Knee MRI. *Journal of Postgraduate Radiology* 11(4):201, 1991.

Page 270, Superior view of the knee. Gay SB: Knee MRI. *Journal of Postgraduate Radiology* 11(4):200, 1991.

Page 272, Ligaments of the ankle. Berquist TR: *MRI of the Musculoskeletal System*, 3e. Philadelphia, Lippincott-Raven, 1996, p 451.

Page 273, Bones of the foot. Greenspan A: *Orthopedic Radiology*, 2e. Philadelphia, Lippincott-Raven, 1992, p 9.2.

Page 291, Avulsion fracture. Blackbourne LH: *Surgical Recall*, 2e. Baltimore, Williams & Wilkins, 1998, p 647.

Page 297, LeFort type I. Blackbourne LH: *Surgical Recall*, 2e. Baltimore, Williams & Wilkins, 1998, p 567.

Page 298, LeFort type II. Blackbourne LH: *Surgical Recall*, 2e. Baltimore, Williams & Wilkins, 1998, p 567.

Page 298, LeFort type III. Blackbourne LH: *Surgical Recall*, 2e. Baltimore, Williams & Wilkins, 1998, p 568.

Page 301, Cervical spine landmarks. Greenspan A: *Orthopedic Radiology*, 2e. Philadelphia, Lippincott-Raven, 1992, p 10.5

Page 302, Jefferson's fracture. Greenspan A: *Orthopedic Radiology*, 2e. Philadelphia, Lippincott-Raven, 1992, p 10.18.

Page 303, Odontoid fractures. Greenspan A: *Orthopedic Radiology*, 2e. Philadelphia, Lippincott-Raven, 1992, p 10.20.

Page 305, Flexion teardrop injury. Greenspan A: *Orthopedic Radiology*, 2e. Philadelphia, Lippincott-Raven, 1992, p 10.24.

Page 309, Scotty dog. Greenspan A: *Orthopedic Radiology*, 2e. Philadelphia, Lippincott-Raven, 1992, p 10.31.

Page 311, Pseudospondylolisthesis versus true spondylolisthesis. Greenspan A: *Orthopedic Radiology*, 2e. Philadelphia, Lippincott-Raven, 1992, p 10.42.

Page 323, Bennett's fracture. Reprinted with permission from Kilcoyne RF, Farrer EL: *Handbook of Radiologic Orthopedic Terminology.* Copyright CRC Press, Boca Raton, Florida.

Page 331, Meniscal injuries. Greenspan A: *Orthopedic Radiology*, 2e. Philadelphia, Lippincott-Raven, 1992, p 8.27.

Page 333, Terrible triad of O'Donoghue. Greenspan A: *Orthopedic Radiology*, 2e. Philadelphia, Lippincott-Raven, 1992, p 8.32.

Page 337, Lateral margin avulsion of the distal tibia. Greenspan A: *Orthopedic Radiology*, 2e. Philadelphia, Lippincott-Raven, 1992, p 9.21.

Page 337, Triplane fracture. Greenspan A: *Orthopedic Radiology*, 2e. Philadelphia, Lippincott-Raven, 1992, p 9.22.

Page 338, Dupuytren's fracture (two variants). Greenspan A: *Orthopedic Radiology*, 2e. Philadelphia, Lippincott-Raven, 1992, p 9.23.

Page 339, Maisonneuve fracture. Greenspan A: *Orthopedic Radiology*, 2e. Philadelphia, Lippincott-Raven, 1992, p 9.24.

Page 342, Heberden's nodes and Bouchard's nodes. Greenspan A: *Orthopedic Radiology*, 2e. Philadelphia, Lippincott-Raven, 1992, p 11.16.

Page 343, Classic findings in osteoarthritis. Greenspan A: *Orthopedic Radiology*, 2e. Philadelphia, Lippincott-Raven, 1992, p 11.15.

Page 344, Neuropathic arthritis. Greenspan A: *Orthopedic Radiology*, 2e. Philadelphia, Lippincott-Raven, 1992, p 11.15.

Page 346, Rheumatoid arthritis. Greenspan A: *Orthopedic Radiology*, 2e. Philadelphia, Lippincott-Raven, 1992, p 11.24, 11.23.

Page 347, Septic arthritis. Greenspan A: *Orthopedic Radiology*, 2e. Philadelphia, Lippincott-Raven, 1992, p 11.15.

Page 351, Psoriatic arthritis. Greenspan A: *Orthopedic Radiology*, 2e. Philadelphia, Lippincott-Raven, 1992, p 11.16.

Page 362, Periosteal reactions. Greenspan A: *Orthopedic Radiology*, 2e. Philadelphia, Lippincott-Raven, 1992, p 15.22.

Page 363, Benign versus malignant tumors. Greenspan A: *Orthopedic Radiology*, 2e. Philadelphia, Lippincott-Raven, 1992, p 15.26.

Chapter 7

Page 386, Postoperative views of the stomach. Jarrell BE, Carabasi RA III: *NMS Surgery*, 3e. Baltimore, Williams & Wilkins, 1996, pp 191, 276.

Page 389, Nine liver subsegments. Weissleder R, Rieumont MJ, Wittenberg J: *Primer of Diagnostic Imaging*, 2e. St. Louis, Mosby-Year Book, 1997, p 192.

Page 390, Hepatic anatomy. Zeman RK, Burrell MI: *Gallbladder and Bile Duct Imaging*. New York, Churchill Livingstone, 1987, p 4.

Page 391, Axial views of the liver. Zeman RK, Burrell MI: *Gallbladder and Bile Duct Imaging*. New York, Churchill Livingstone, 1987, pp 4, 8, 11, 15.

Page 392, Extrahepatic biliary and pancreatic duct system. Toledo-Pereyra LH: *The Pancreas: Principles of Medical and Surgical Practice*. New York, Churchill Livingstone, 1985, pp 31–50.

Page 422, Gastric volvulus. Kirks DR: *Practical Pediatric Imaging. Diagnostic Radiology of Infants and Children,* 3e. Philadelphia, Lippincott-Raven, 1997.

Chapter 8

Page 515, Periaortic lymph nodes. Gay SB, Armistead JP, Weber ME, et al: Left infrarenal region: anatomic variants, pathologic conditions, and diagnostic pitfalls. *Radiographics* 11(4):560, 1991.

Chapter 10

Page 573, Placenta previa. Kobayashi M: *Illustrated Manual of Ultrasonography in Obstetrics and Gynecology.* Tokyo, Igaku-Shoin, 1980, p 263.

Page 574, Abruptio placentae. Kobayashi M: *Illustrated Manual of Ultrasonography in Obstetrics and Gynecology.* Tokyo, Igaku-Shoin, 1980, p 246.

Chapter 11

Page 595, Neonatal umbilical circulation. Reproduced with permission from *Pediatrics,* Vol 31, page 146–51, 1963.

Page 608, Patent ductus arteriosus. Gedgaudas E, Moller JH, Castaneda-Zuniga WR, et al: *Cardiovascular Radiology.* Philadelphia, WB Saunders, 1985, p 78.

Page 610, Tetralogy of Fallot. Gedgaudas E, Moller JH, Castaneda-Zuniga WR, et al: *Cardiovascular Radiology.* Philadelphia, WB Saunders, 1985, p 148.

Page 611, Transposition of the great vessels. Gedgaudas E, Moller JH, Castaneda-Zuniga WR, et al: *Cardiovascular Radiology.* Philadelphia, WB Saunders, 1985, p 102.

Page 612, Ebstein's anomaly. Gedgaudas E, Moller JH, Castaneda-Zuniga WR, et al: *Cardiovascular Radiology.* Philadelphia, WB Saunders, 1985, p 163.

Page 614, Hypoplastic left heart syndrome. Gedgaudas E, Moller JH, Castaneda-Zuniga WR, et al: *Cardiovascular Radiology.* Philadelphia, WB Saunders, 1985, p 169.

Page 616, Pulmonary sling. Kirks DR: *Practical Pediatric Imaging. Diagnostic Radiology of Infants and Children,* 3e. Philadelphia, Lippincott-Raven, 1997.

Page 620, Malrotation. Gay SB, Kunberger LE, McGraw JK, et al: The transverse portion of the duodenum: A key to unlocking the retroperitoneum. *Applied Radiology* 26(1):17, 1997.

Page 621, Problems caused by malrotation. Kirks DR: *Practical Pediatric Imaging. Diagnostic Radiology of Infants and Children,* 3e. Philadelphia, Lippincott-Raven, 1997.

Page 638, Salter-Harris classification. Blackbourne LH: *Surgical Recall,* 2e. Baltimore, Williams & Wilkins, 1998, pp 665–67.

Page 645, Radiographic features of developmental dysplasia of the hip (DDH). Dahnert W: *Radiology Review Manual,* 4e. Baltimore, Williams & Wilkins, 1998, p 52.

Page 662, Images routinely obtained on ultrasound. Rumack CM, Johnson ML: *Perinatal and Infant Brain Imaging.* St. Louis, Mosby-Year Book, 1984 and Rumack CM, Manco-Johnson ML: Neonatal brain ultrasonography. In Sarti DA: *Diagnostic Ultrasound: Text and Cases,* 2e. St. Louis, Mosby-Year Book, 1987.

Chapter 12

Page 684, Branches of the external carotid artery. Weissleder R, Rieumont MJ, Wittenberg J: *Primer of Diagnostic Imaging,* 2e. St. Louis, Mosby-Year Book, 1997, p 457.

Page 685, Branches of the intracranial internal carotid artery. Weissleder R, Rieumont MJ, Wittenberg J: *Primer of Diagnostic Imaging,* 2e. St. Louis, Mosby-Year Book, 1997, p 459.

Page 686, Branches of the vertebral artery. Weissleder R, Rieumont MJ, Wittenberg J: *Primer of Diagnostic Imaging,* 2e. St. Louis, Mosby-Year Book, 1997, p 458.

Page 686, Circle of Willis. Weissleder R, Rieumont MJ, Wittenberg J: *Primer of Diagnostic Imaging,* 2e. St. Louis, Mosby-Year Book, 1997, p 458.

1   Introduction

Spencer B. Gay

THE IMPORTANCE OF A BASIC UNDERSTANDING OF RADIOLOGY

Radiology is the study of imaging in medicine. Most of radiology practice is accomplished through basic knowledge of anatomy and radiology, careful observation, and effective interaction with other physicians and patients. While it is not essential for every physician to learn how to read a chest radiograph, a basic understanding of radiology facilitates communication between clinicians and radiologists. It also provides the clinician with the knowledge of how imaging can be used as a tool for gaining insight into pathology within the body. This is especially important these days, because nearly every patient has an imaging study while in the hospital and usually, the diagnosis is made in Radiology.

For those desiring a basic understanding of radiology, there are three steps that must be taken. First, you must familiarize yourself with radiographic and cross-sectional anatomy. Second, you must learn how to look systematically for findings on an imaging study—an active search for structures and findings is more productive than simply gazing at an image in hopes that the finding will present itself. Third, you must learn to correlate the findings with the clinical picture in order to generate a diagnosis or list of possible diagnoses.

Taking a team approach to health care enables each member on the team to share his or her expertise, ultimately guiding the patient toward health. For the non-radiologist, a key part of knowing how to use imaging relates to the radiology request and report. When requesting a radiology examination, it is important to pose a clinical question or state a goal for the study. This serves to maximize the usefulness of the radiology report. The radiology report contains a description of the findings of the study plus procedural details, followed by a conclusion that summarizes the findings and gives the most likely diagnosis. (Like medicine in general, radiology is an inexact science.) The referring physician who is well-versed in radiology principles will understand this conclusion in the clinical framework, permitting effective patient care based on imaging and clinical judgement.

COMMON ABBREVIATIONS

AAA	Abdominal aortic aneurysm
ABC	Aneurysmal bone cyst
ABI	Ankle to brachial index

ABPA	Acute bronchopulmonary aspergillosis
ACE	Angiotensin-converting enzyme
ACS	American Cancer Society
ADH	Antidiuretic hormone
AFP	α-Fetoprotein
AICA	Anterior inferior cerebellar artery
ALARA	As Low As Reasonably Achievable
ALS	Amyotrophic lateral sclerosis
AP	Anterior-posterior
APGAR	Appearance (color), Pulse (heart rate), Grimace (reflex irritability), Activity (muscle tone), and Respiration
ARDS	Adult respiratory distress syndrome
AS	Ankylosing spondylitis
ASD	Atrial septal defect
AV	Arteriovenous (fistula)
AVM	Arteriovenous malformation
β-hCG	β-Human chorionic gonadotropin
BIRADS	Breast Imaging Reporting and Dictation System
BOOP	Bronchiolitis obliterans, organizing pneumonia
BPD	Bronchopulmonary dysplasia
BPH	Benign prostatic hypertrophy
BPP	Biophysical profile
Bq	Bequerels
BSE	Breast self-examination
BUN	Blood urea nitrogen
CAD	Coronary artery disease
CBD	Common bile duct
CC	Craniocaudal (view)
CCK	Cholecystokinin
CF	Cystic fibrosis
CHD	Congenital heart disease
CHF	Congestive heart failure
Ci	Curies
CMV	Cytomegalovirus
CNS	Central nervous system
COP	Cryptogenic organizing pneumonia
COPD	Chronic obstructive pulmonary disease
CPPD	Calcium pyrophosphate deposition disease
CRL	Crown-rump length
CRT	Cathode ray tube
CSF	Cerebrospinal fluid
CSP	Corrected sinusoidal pressure
CT	Computed tomography
CTA	Computed tomography angiogram

CVP	Central venous pressure
CXR	Chest x-ray (radiograph)
DCBE	Double contrast barium enema
DCIS	Ductal carcinoma *in situ*
2DE	Two-dimensional echocardiography
DDH	Developmental dysplasia of the hip
DES	Diethylstilbestrol
DEXA	Dual energy x-ray absorptiometry
DCIS	Ductal carcinoma in situ
DIC	Disseminated intravascular coagulation
DISI	Dorsal intercalary segment instability
DJD	Degenerative joint disease
DMSA	Dimercaptosuccinic acid
DTPA	Diethylenetriamine penta-acetic acid
DSA	Digital subtraction angiography
DVT	Deep venous thrombosis
EBCT	Electron beam computed tomography
ECG	Electrocardiogram
ED	Emergency department
EDV	End-diastolic volume
EF	Ejection fraction
EGA	Estimated gestational age
EGD	Esophagogastroduodenoscopy
EM	Electromagnetic
ERCP	Endoscopic retrograde cholangiopancreatography
ESR	Erythrocyte sedimentation rate
ESV	End-systolic volume
ESWL	Extracorporeal shock wave lithotripsy
EV	Endovaginal
FDA	Food and Drug Administration
FLAIR	Fluid-attenuated inversion recovery (images)
FMD	Fibromuscular dysplasia
FNA	Fine needle aspiration
FNH	Focal nodular hyperplasia
FOV	Field of view
GAGs	Glycosaminoglycans
GBM	Glioblastoma multiforme
Gd-DTPA	Gadolinium-diethylenetriamine penta-acetic acid
GERD	Gastroesophageal reflux disease
GFR	Glomerular filtration rate
GH	Glucoheptonate
GRE	Gradient-recalled echo
HCC	Hepatocellular carcinoma
HIDA	Hepato-iminodiacetic acid (scan)
HIV	Human immunodeficiency virus

HRCT	High-resolution computed tomography
HRT	Hormone replacement therapy
HSG	Hysterosalpingogram
HSV	Herpes simplex virus
HU	Hounsfield units
I-123	Iodine 123
I-131	Iodine 131
ICU	Intensive care unit
ID	Inner diameter
IDA	Iminoacidiacetic acid
IMA	Inferior mesenteric artery
IR	Inversion recovery
IUGR	Intrauterine growth retardation
IUP	Intrauterine pregnancy
IV	Intravenous
IVC	Inferior vena cava
IVP	Intravenous pyelogram
JPA	Juvenile pilocystic astrocytoma
JRA	Juvenile rheumatoid arthritis
KUB	Kidneys, ureters, bladder
kV	Kilovoltage
kVp	Peak kilovoltage
Lp/mm	Line pairs/millimeter
LAC	Linear attenuation coefficient
LAO	Left anterior oblique (view)
LCIS	Lobular carcinoma *in situ*
LLL	Left lower lobe
LMP	Last menstrual period
LRV	Left renal vein
LUL	Left upper lobe
MAA	Macroaggregated albumin
MAG3	Mercaptylacetyltriglycine
mAs	Milliamperage-seconds
mCi	Millicurie
MCKD	Multicystic kidney disease
MDP	Methyldiphosphonate
MEN-I	Multiple endocrine neoplasia, type I
MHZ	Megahertz
MIBG	Meta iodobenzylguanidine
MLCN	Multilocular cystic nephroma
MLO	Mediolateral oblique (view)
MO	Myositis ossificans
MRA	Magnetic resonance angiogram
MRCP	Magnetic resonance cholangiopancreatography
MRI	Magnetic resonance imaging
MRV	Magnetic resonance venogram

MUGA	Multiple-gated equilibrium radionucleotide cineangiography
MVC	Motor vehicle crash
NOMI	Non-occlusive mesenteric ischemia
NTD	Neural tube defect
NOF	Nonossifying fibroma
OCD	Osteochondritis desiccans
OCI	Osteitis condensans ilii
OD	Outer diameter
PA	Posterior-anterior
PAN	Polyarteritis nodosa
PAPVR	Partial anomalous pulmonary venous return
PCA	Posterior cerebral artery
PCKD	Polycystic kidney disease
PCOM	Posterior communicating artery
PCP	*Pneumocystis carinii* pneumonia
PDA	Patent ductus arteriosus
PE	Pulmonary embolus
PICA	Posterior inferior cerebellar artery
PICC	Peripherally introduced central catheter
PID	Pelvic inflammatory disease
PIE	Pulmonary interstitial emphysema
PIOPED	Prospective Investigation Of Pulmonary Embolism Diagnosis
PSA	Prostate-specific antigen
PSC	Primary sclerosing cholangitis
PT	Prothrombin time
PTA	Percutaneous transluminal angioplasty
PTC	Percutaneous transhepatic cholangiography
PTH	Parathyroid hormone
PTT	Partial thromboplastin time
PVD	Peripheral vascular disease
PVNS	Pigmented villonodular synovitis
RAO	Right anterior oblique (view)
RBC	Red blood cell
RCC	Renal cell carcinoma
RDS	Respiratory distress syndrome
RLL	Right lower lobe
RLQ	Right lower quadrant
RML	Right middle lobe
RSD	Reflex sympathetic dystrophy
RSV	Respiratory syncytial virus
rTPA	Recombinant tissue plasminogen activator
RUL	Right upper lobe

RUQ	Right upper quadrant
SAH	Subarachnoid hemorrhage
SBFT	Small bowel follow-through (study)
SC	Sulfur colloid
SCFE	Slipped capital femoral epiphysis
SIADH	Syndrome of inappropriate antidiuretic hormone secretion
SID	Source-to-image distance
SLAP	Superior labrum anterior posterior
SLE	Systemic lupus erythematosus
SMA	Superior mesenteric artery
SMV	Superior mesenteric vein
S:N	Signal-to-background noise ratio
SPECT	Single photon emission computer tomography
STIR	Short-tau inversion recovery
SVC	Superior vena cava
TAPVR	Total anomalous pulmonary venous return
Tc-99m	Technetium 99m
TE	Time to echo
TEE	Transesophageal echocardiography
TIPS	Transjugular intrahepatic portosystemic shunt
Tl^{201}	Thallium 201
TOF	Time-of-flight
TR	Repetition time
TTE	Transthoracic echocardiography
TTN	Transient tachypnea of the newborn
UPJ	Uteropelvic junction
UTI	Urinary tract infection
UVJ	Uterovesical junction
VCUG	Voiding cystourethrography
VISI	Volar intercalary segment instability
V̇/Q̇	Ventilation-perfusion
VSD	Ventricular septal defect
WBC	White blood cell
XCCL	Exaggerated CC lateral
XGPN	Xanthogranulomatous pyelonephritis

2

Imaging Techniques

Mark B. Williams
John J. Smith

GENERAL PRINCIPLES

What is the basic principle of radiologic imaging?

A source emits energy (e.g., x-rays, ultrasound), which interacts with the patient and is detected by a receptor, forming an image. The image is then interpreted by a radiologist in order to make a clinical diagnosis.

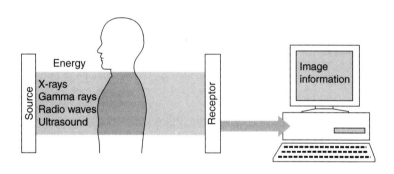

What is the difference between ultrasound and x-ray?

Ultrasound is high-frequency sound waves; x-rays are electromagnetic (EM) waves.

Name 4 imaging modalities that use EM waves to produce an image.

Plain radiography, computed tomography (CT), nuclear medicine, magnetic resonance imaging (MRI)

Order the following types of energy by wavelength (λ) size (smallest to largest): gamma ray, radio wave, x-ray, light

Gamma ray, x-ray, light, radio wave

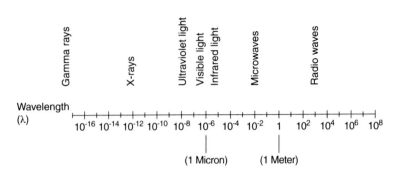

| What is the relationship between wavelength size and energy? | The shorter the wavelength, the higher the energy |

RADIATION EXPOSURE (RADIOBIOLOGY)

What effect can EM radiation have on molecules?	Ionization
What is the relationship between energy and ionization?	In general, higher energy increases ionization.
Why is ionization significant?	Ionization is responsible for the biologic effects of radiation on DNA and tissues.
What are the major potential biological effects of EM radiation?	Carcinogenesis and genetic effects (caused by gonadal irradiation)
Which organ is the most radiosensitive?	The thyroid gland
List the 5 tumors that are most likely to occur after exposure to ionizing radiation.	Leukemia, thyroid tumors, breast tumors, lung tumors, skin tumors
What is the limit for radiation to a patient undergoing an imaging procedure?	There is no absolute limit. The rule is to follow the **ALARA principle** (i.e., to use a dose that is **A**s **L**ow **A**s **R**easonably **A**chievable).
What is primary radiation exposure?	Exposure to the site being examined

What is secondary radiation exposure?

Exposure to sites not being examined, also known as "scatter"

List 5 ways of reducing primary radiation.

1. Perform only the clinically relevant studies
2. Reduce the need for repeated studies
3. Reduce the number of films taken
4. Choose appropriate films and screens
5. Use an appropriate projection

List 5 ways of reducing secondary radiation.

1. Reduce primary radiation
2. Ensure tight collimation
3. Immobilize the patient properly
4. Position the patient carefully
5. Shield sensitive areas

How is exposure to the radiologist controlled in fluoroscopy?

Exposure of the radiologist to radiation is controlled by:

Increasing the examiner's distance from the beam

Decreasing the fluoroscopy time

Shielding (lead apron and thyroid shields; leaded glasses for those with high exposures)

How does the amoun of radiation change as you move away from the x-ray source?

It is reduced according to the inverse square law:

$$\frac{1}{distance^2}$$

What is a rad?

A measure of absorbed dose

How does the radiation dose from a head CT scan compare with that of a chest radiograph (CXR)?

The radiation associated with a head CT scan is much greater than that associated with a CXR (4000 versus 12 millirads).

How would the dose associated with 1 minute of fluoroscopy compare with that of a head CT scan?

About the same

Do multiple short exposures have the same effect as a single dose that occurs over the same total exposure time?

No. The total dose required to produce carcinogenesis when multiple short exposures are taken could be about twice that required to produce carcinogenesis as a result of a single dose.

Name 3 natural sources of radiation that are unavoidable.	Cosmic radiation, radiation from the earth, radon
How does exposure to natural radiation compare with medical exposure?	The annual exposure of a person living at sea level to natural radiation is about 10 times the amount of 30 posterior-anterior (PA) CXRs. Spending 1 year at altitudes greater than sea level (e.g., in Denver) delivers about twice the natural radiation associated with living at sea level.
Is the radiation risk from mammography greater than the diagnostic benefit?	No. Even if a woman had a screening mammogram every year between the ages of 35 and 75 years, the benefit of reduced mortality would still be 25 times greater than the increased risk from irradiation.
When is the carcinogenic effect of breast irradiation the greatest?	In young women
Is there evidence of a significantly increased risk of cancer as a result of mammography after the age of 40 years?	No.
Are men or women at greater risk for genetic effects as a result of gonadal irradiation?	Men (2:1)
What recommendation should be made to women who have had significant scatter radiation as a result of a radiograph?	Delay conception for at least 3 cycles
Men?	Delay conception for 2 cell renewal times (about 130 days)
Is gonadal shielding indicated for all children undergoing radiologic evaluation?	No. Gonadal shielding is not necessary if the gonads are more than 5 cm away from the edge of the field. Most of the radiation comes from internal scatter, so shielding will not reduce it.

What is the most important factor in determining the risk to a fetus for damage following radiation exposure?

The stage of gestation

When is the most critical period?

Days 16–45 (i.e., during the period of organogenesis)

What type of anomaly is most commonly caused by irradiation at this stage?

Neurologic damage

Does *in utero* radiation increase the incidence of childhood cancer?

Yes, especially that of leukemia

Is there a risk to the fetus from a fetal ultrasound?

No.

MEDICAL IMAGING

What routine planes are used in medical imaging?

Axial, coronal, and sagittal

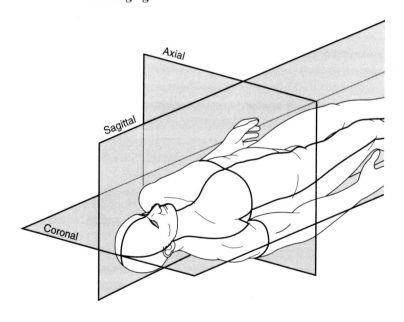

By convention, how are the following viewed:

Axial images? As if seen from below, with the patient's left on your right:

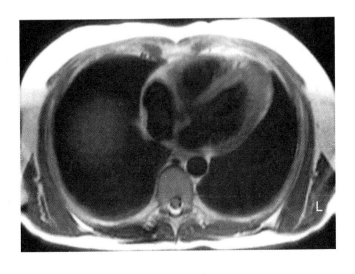

Coronal images? Like a CXR (from the anterior aspect, with the patient's left on your right):

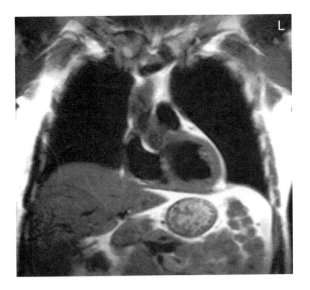

Sagittal images?

From the left, with the patient's anterior (A) on your left:

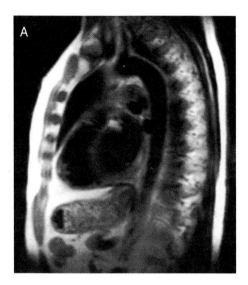

What is a pixel?

The smallest unit of an image matrix. Each pixel is assigned a shade of gray for display and together they form the image.

What is a voxel?

A pixel with depth (e.g., slice thickness in CT)

What is the field of view?

The width of the image for a digital image

What is the matrix size?

The number of pixels in each dimension (e.g., 256×256 or 256×512)

How is the in-plane pixel size (d) related to the field of view (FOV) and the digital matrix size (N)?

$d = FOV/N$

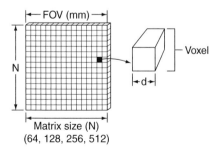

How does increasing the matrix size change the image? (FOV constant)

Smaller pixels = improved spatial resolution, but less data is contained in each pixel (decreased signal/noise ratio)

How does increasing the field of view change the image? (matrix constant)

Larger pixels = more data in each pixel (increased signal/noise ratio), but poorer spatial resolution

How many different shades of gray (levels) may be displayed in an image?

It depends on how much digital (binary) space is used. Each bit (i.e., binary space) may be either on or off. Combinations of bits produce gray scale.

How many gray levels does an 8-bit image display?

2^8, or 256

A 12-bit image?

2^{12}, or 4096

What are the advantages and disadvantages of having more gray levels?

More gray levels improve contrast resolution, but contain more data, and thereby require more computer memory and bandwidth and take longer to transmit.

What are the 2 types of resolution?

Contrast resolution and spatial resolution

How are they measured?

Contrast resolution is the ability to distinguish shades of gray. Spatial resolution may be measured in line pairs/ millimeter (lp/mm); that is, the ability to separate an increasing smaller structures in an image.

Does a higher 1p/mm mean higher or lower resolution?

Higher (i.e., better) resolution

What is the approximate resolution of:

X-ray films?

5–15 1p/mm

A fluoroscopic image?	1–5 lp/mm
Ultrasonograms?	2 lp/mm
CT scans?	5 lp/mm
MRI scans?	2 lp/mm
Nuclear medicine?	< 1 lp/mm
Mammography?	As many as 25 lp/mm
Why is such a high resolution required for mammography?	It is critical to be able to display the small microcalcifications associated with breast cancer.

RADIOGRAPHY

CONVENTIONAL RADIOGRAPHY

How are x-rays produced?	In an x-ray tube, electrons are generated and are accelerated toward a high-voltage anode, which has a target that generates x-rays.
What are the major parts involved in electron generation?	Power source, transformer, and the filament
What does the transformer do in an x-ray generator?	It increases or decreases the voltage for the x-ray tube.
What does the filament do?	Current from the power source flows through a tungsten-wire filament, which emits electrons by a process called thermionic emission.
What are the 2 major components of an x-ray tube?	A cathode (filament side, negative charge) and anode (target side, positive charge)

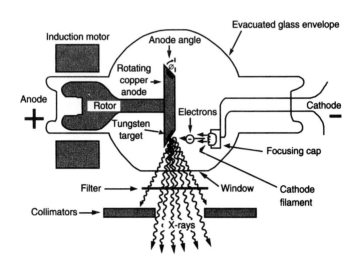

What forms the anode?

A target, usually tungsten, embedded within another solid, usually copper

Which part of the x-ray tube actually emits x-rays?

The portion of the anode exposed to the electron beam (i.e., the target or focal spot)

Do most of the electrons emitted make x-rays?

No. Almost all produce heat. Only about 1% make x-rays.

How does an x-ray tube limit heat build-up?

The anode rotates so that a different region of the target absorbs electrons all of the time. In addition, the tube radiates heat and loses heat by conduction.

Describe the energy of an x-ray beam.

It is a spectrum of energies, with a maximum equal to the peak kilovoltage (kVp) set by the technologist.

What happens to the x-ray beam when it meets the patient?

Two main interactions occur, Compton scatter and the photoelectric effect.

Which process improves contrast?

The photoelectric effect. Each tissue produces a characteristic absorption.

What does Compton scatter do?

It decreases contrast.

Which occurs most often?

This depends on the kilovoltage (beam energy, kV) and tissue type, but generally Compton scatter predominates, especially as the kV increases.

What occurs when an x-ray interacts with the film cassette?

The x-ray is absorbed by a screen, which emits light to expose the film. Exposed film is then developed to create an image.

What are the screen and film made of?

The screen is made of a phosphor, a substance that absorbs energy and emits light. The film is coated with silver bromide, which is sensitive to light.

How does increased exposure affect the film?

Darker film

What factors affect the resultant exposure and image contrast in the x-ray?

Current (milliamperage), beam energy (kV) and exposure time(s)

What factor most effects contrast on x-rays?

kV

What factor most affects exposure on x-rays?

mAs

What effects will increasing the kV have on the film?

Increased kV increases penetration and exposure while decreasing contrast.

What effect will increasing the milliamperage seconds (mAs) have on the film?

Increased mAs increases the exposure, causing more film darkening.

For a given tube voltage and current, name 5 factors that affect the patient dose in radiography.

1. Source-to-patient distance
2. Patient thickness
3. Exposure time
4. Use of a collimator
5. Use of an x-ray scatter reduction grid

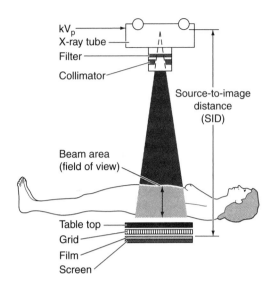

Holding all else fixed, how will changing the following items affect the film darkening in radiography?

Increased mAs	Increased film darkening
Increased screen thickness	Increased film darkening
Increased SID	Decreased film darkening
Increased patient thickness	Decreased film darkening

What is a collimator? A device consisting of 2 lead sheets that narrows the x-ray beam as the beam passes between them

Where is a collimator placed? Between the x-ray tube and the patient

Why are collimators used? Collimators reduce the patient dose by reducing the exposed field to only the area clinically needed. They also reduce scatter, thus improving contrast.

What is an x-ray scatter reduction grid? A device consisting of a grid of lead strips with space between them that is placed between the patient and the film.

Why are grids used? They reduce scatter, thus improving contrast.

What is the disadvantage of using a grid?

It increases dose, because some of the non-scatter x-rays passing through the patient that would have formed the image are also blocked.

What is the definition of the grid ratio?

$$\text{Grid ratio} = \frac{\text{Height of the lead strips}}{\text{Distance between the lead strips}}$$

FLUOROSCOPY

What is fluoroscopy?

X-ray beams are produced continuously and passed through the patient, and they fall on a fluorescent screen. An image intensifier brightens the image and produces a real-time image. A camera captures this image and it is displayed on a cathode ray tube (CRT) screen (i.e., a television screen).

How is a fluoroscopic image different from that of a plain x-ray?

Black and white are usually inverted from plain film. The fluoroscopic image is continuously updated.

Why is an image intensifier used?

The image intensifier intensifies the light, allowing a lower dose of radiation to be used.

COMPUTED TOMOGRAPHY (CT)

How does CT scanning work?

A thin beam of x-rays passes through the body in the axial plane chosen for study as the x-ray tube moves in a continuous arc around the patient. Electronic detectors placed opposite the x-ray tube on the other side of the body convert the exiting beam into electrical pulses, the intensity of which depends on the amount of the x-ray beam that was not absorbed by the intervening tissues. This information is then conveyed to a computer, which calculates the x-ray absorption for each voxel and creates the final CT image.

How are modern (third-and fourth-generation) CT scanners different from each other?	Third-generation scanners have one detector array that rotates opposite the tube, while fourth-generation scanners have a fixed array of detectors that extends completely around the gantry.
What is the linear attenuation coefficient (LAC)?	A measure of a tissue's ability to attenuate (i.e., absorb or scatter) an x-ray beam.
What are Hounsfield units (HU)?	A numerical indication of the LAC, and therefore, a measure of the density of a structure on CT
What is the range of HU?	It is most useful to think of the scale as ranging from -1000 (air) to $+1000$ (complete attenuation), although some manufacturers may vary this scale (e.g., -2048 to $+6000$).

What is the approximate value of the HU for:

Water?	0
Muscle and soft tissue?	40
Air?	-1000
Bone?	1000
Fat?	-60
Cerebrospinal fluid (CSF)?	10
Fresh clot?	50
White matter?	30
Gray matter?	40
What does window width refer to?	The range of HU that are displayed on the gray scale of the digital image

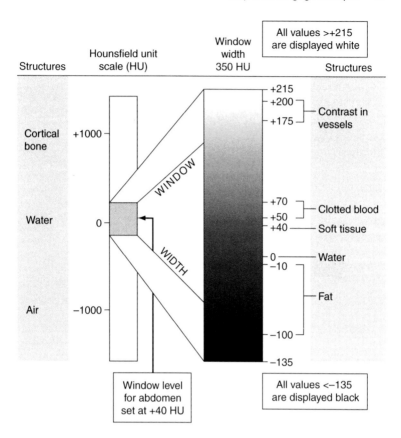

| What is the window level? | The HU value chosen for the middle gray on the gray scale |

If a CT image is viewed with a window width of 100 HU and a level of 75 HU, what are the:

| Lower values of the window (in HU)? | 25 (i.e., 75–100/2) |

| Upper values of the window (in HU)? | 125 (i.e., 75+100/2) |

With this window and level, what will:

| Structures less than 25 HU look like? | Completely black |

Structures more than 125 HU look like?	Completely white
What 2 things determine the beam width in the field of view in CT?	The collimator and the focal spot size

Describe the following artifacts:

Partial volume artifact	Occurs when adjacent structures of different attenuation are "averaged" together to appear as one density; more apparent with thick slices
Streak artifact	Lines of density that extend from the interface of highly contrasted structures (e.g., bone and air)
Motion artifact	"Ghosting" or blurring of a structure that results when a slice is sampled while the structure is in more than one position
Beam hardening	An area of decreased attenuation (i.e., a dark area) immediately adjacent to an object of high attenuation (e.g., metal, bone); caused when a dense object attenuates a greater number of low-energy x-rays than high-energy x-rays
Ring artifact	A ring or series of rings that appear around the center of a CT image; caused by a weak or strong signal from a bad detector; mostly seen with third-generation scanners
Star artifact	High-attenuation materials (e.g., metal) cause streaks to emanate from the object in a star pattern

Spiral (helical) CT

What is the key modification in the CT scanner that allows spiral CT?	Slip rings replace the cables that carry the current to the x-ray tube and from the detectors, allowing the tube to

continuously rotate. In helical CT, the table and the x-ray tubes are moving, while in axial CT, the table is stopped, the image is taken, and the table is moved again.

What is pitch in spiral CT?

The pitch is the longitudinal distance (in millimeters) that the table moves during one revolution of the x-ray tube. The pitch is a variable that is prescribed for a CT protocol (e.g., a pitch of 1.5 or 2).

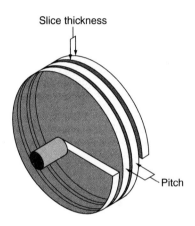

Slice thickness

Pitch

What is the pitch ratio?

The pitch ratio is the pitch divided by the slice thickness. Note that although most people refer to the pitch ratio as "pitch," the two are not technically the same.

What is the advantage of an increased pitch?

Extended coverage and faster scanning of a volume of interest

Name the main advantage of spiral CT over axial CT.

Shorter time necessary to collect data for imaging (i.e., faster acquisition)

What are the other advantages?

Most of the other advantages of spiral CT over axial CT relate to the increased speed of acquisition.
1. Improved lesion detection (leads to faster diagnosis)
2. Decreased radiation dose
3. Minimized motion and partial volume artifacts

4. Capability for retrospective slice reconstruction from the volumetric data
5. Capability for virtual endoscopy
6. Improved 3-dimensional imaging
7. Optimal use of intravenous contrast can be achieved by scanning during the most effective phase
8. Decreased imaging costs

What is multi-ring CT?

In this modification, additional detectors permit the acquisition of multiple datasets during one rotation, providing additional data and enabling faster coverage.

What is CT fluoroscopy (continuous CT)?

The tube continues to rotate and images are generated "on the fly," permitting the radiologist to observe a needle entering a lesion.

MAGNETIC RESONANCE IMAGING (MRI)

What is a tesla?

A measure of magnetic field strength (1 tesla = 10,000 gauss; the earth's field $\cong$ 0.5 gauss)

What is the principle behind MRI?

Hydrogen nuclei have magnetic polarity. When placed in a strong magnetic field, a portion of the nuclei will align with the field. These nuclei precess with a characteristic frequency, called the Larmor frequency. Radio waves, called a "pulse," may be applied selectively in a particular sequence to excite the nuclei by moving them out of alignment with the magnetic field to some degree (e.g., 90°, 180°). As the nuclei return to alignment, they emit the absorbed radio waves, which are then amplified and transmitted to a computer, which generates an image.

What is an MRI sequence?

A sequence of pulses delivered in a repetitive pattern to produce an echo (i.e., a signal); sequences may be repeated numerous times

How are different tissues distinguished by MRI?	Each tissue relaxes (returns to a non-excited state) at a different rate. MRI parameters can be altered to allow us to listen for a particular signal (an echo) at a particular time.
What are T_1 and T_2?	T_1 and T_2 are relaxation times—T_1 is the longitudinal relaxation time, and T_2 is the transverse relaxation time.
What are T_1- and T_2-weighting?	MRI sequences that emphasize, or "weight," these characteristics
What is proton density-weighting?	An MRI sequence that de-emphasizes both T_1 and T_2 characteristics so that the density of the nuclei themselves is imaged.
In MRI, T_1 has units of millimeters, gray-scale value, milliseconds, tesla, or rotations per second?	Milliseconds
What is the repetition time (TR)?	The repetition time for the sequence (i.e., the time between the beginning of two successive pulse sequences)
What is the echo time (TE)?	The time to echo
What characteristics of the MRI pulse sequence help to identify certain sequences as:	
T_1-weighted?	Short TR, short TE (500/20)
T_2-weighted?	Long TR, long TE (> 1000/100)
Proton density-weighted?	Long TR, short TE (~ 1000/20)
What term is used to describe the pixel values on MRI?	Signal intensity (not x-ray attenuation, as in CT)
What characterizes a good image?	A high signal-to-background noise (S:N) ratio

What happens to the signal intensity when the TR is increased?	It increases at a rate that depends on the T_1 of the tissue. Structures with a short T_1 (e.g., fat) increase more rapidly than those with a long T_1 (e.g., fluid). (Note that after a certain point, the signal intensities tend to come together.)

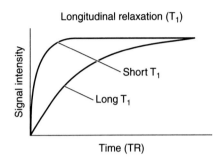

Longitudinal relaxation (T_1)

What happens to the signal intensity when the TE is increased?	It decreases at a rate that depends on the T_2 of the tissue. Structures with a long T_2 (e.g., fluid) decrease more slowly than those with a short T_2.

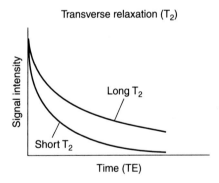

Transverse relaxation (T_2)

What is a spin-echo sequence?	The most common MRI sequence type, a spin-echo sequence uses a 90° pulse followed by a 180° pulse to create an echo.
In a spin-echo sequence, is the 180° pulse applied in the transverse or longitudinal plane?	The transverse plane, so that the transverse plane components of the nuclear dipoles are inverted. This corrects for magnetic field inhomogeneities.

How is signal intensity related to TR and TE in a spin-echo sequence?

The signal is generated as a result of the relaxation related to the closer TR, TE, and the type of tissue.

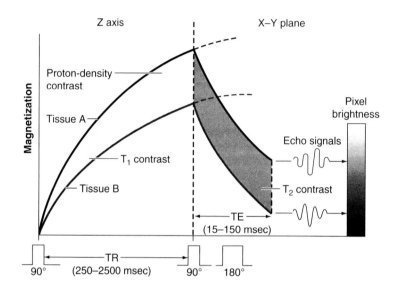

What is a gradient-echo sequence?

A fast MRI sequence that uses a low-angle pulse (i.e., one less than 90°) to create a signal. These sequences generally take less time to image than spin-echo sequences.

What are fluid attenuated inversion recovery (FLAIR) and short-tau inversion recovery (STIR) sequences?

Sequences using inversion recovery (IR), a special technique that allows certain tissue signals to be nulled.

What are averages?

The number of times the sequence is repeated throughout the image. In general, as the number of averages increases, the S:N ratio increases and the image quality improves (to a point).

Coils are used to produce different magnetic field strengths at different locations. The rate at which the field strength changes with changing position is called what?

The gradient

How are these gradients used?	To choose a slice thickness and location ("slice selection")
How can one calculate how long a sequence will take to perform?	The total time for image collection is TR $\times$ N $\times$ n, where N is the number of gradient steps in the phase-encoding direction and n is the number of averages. For a sequence with a TR of 2.5 seconds, a matrix size of 128 $\times$ 256 (phase $\times$ frequency), and 2 averages, the total time for image collection is 640 seconds, or 10 minutes, 40 seconds: 2.5 $\times$ 128 $\times$ 2 = 640. Changing the TR to 0.5 seconds, the total time for image collection changes to 2 minutes, 8 seconds.

On T$_1$-weighted imaging, which tissues are:

High-signal (i.e., bright)?	Fat Bone marrow in the peripheral skeleton Subacute hemorrhage Slow-flowing blood Proteinaceous fluid Melanin
Low-signal (i.e., dark)?	Fluid (CSF, bile, flowing blood, possibly bowel contents) Bone Air

On T$_2$-weighted imaging, which tissues are:

Low-signal (i.e., dark)?	Bone Flowing blood Acute or subacute hematoma Bone Air
High-signal (bright)?	Fluid (CSF, bile)
How are magnetic resonance angiograms (MRA) and magnetic resonance venograms (MRV) created?	Several methods may be used, including time-of-flight (TOF), phase-contrast, and gadolinium techniques. In the most commonly used technique, TOF, blood flows into the selected slice between the time that the radio wave pulse is applied (i.e., when the slice is excited) and when

the echo is returned. The blood flowing in has all of its magnetization and gives a high signal (the "entry slice" phenomenon), producing a clear image of the vessel.

Describe the following artifacts:

Pulsation artifact

A blurred band across the image in one direction; caused by motion from pulsating blood

Wrap-around artifact

The appearance of one portion of the imaged part on the image side opposite its true location; caused by a FOV that is too small

Chemical shift artifact

A white band adjacent to a black band at a water-fat interface; fat and water protons have slightly different frequencies and the software misplaces the location of the fat

Magnetic susceptibility artifact

"Blooming" (expansion) of a low (dark) signal on T_2-weighted images or gradient-echo sequences; caused by metal or hemosiderin in the imaged area

ULTRASOUND

What is ultrasound?

Ultrasound consists of sound waves with frequencies that exceed the audible range [more than 20,000 cycles per second or hertz (Hz)].

What is the primary difference between ultrasound imaging and other imaging?

Unlike radiography, CT, and MRI, ultrasound does not use EM radiation to create an image. In addition, it does not cause ionization because of the relatively low energy of the sound wave.

Describe a sound wave.

Sound waves are a series of compressions and rarefactions that can be represented by a sine wave, and can be characterized by a velocity, a wavelength, and a frequency.

What is a velocity?

The speed with which a sound moves through a medium

What is a wavelength?

The distance between two compressions or two rarefactions (i.e., one cycle)

What is the frequency?

The number of cycles per unit time

How are wavelength (λ), velocity (v), and frequency (f) related?

$v = f \cdot \lambda$

Describe how an ultrasound signal is generated.

A sound wave is produced by electricity within the ultrasound transducer and is directed toward the area of interest. The wave is propagated through the tissue and is attenuated, reflected, or transmitted to different degrees by different tissues. The reflected sound wave is received by the transducer and converted into an electronic signal.

How is an ultrasound image created?

A particular sector of the body is imaged (swept) by delivering multiple sound waves to the sector and receiving echoes back. The image is created by combining signals from the scanned sector. The transducer is either mechanically steered to sweep a sector over time (mechanical sector scanner) or electronically steered with the transducer signal delivered in parts over time (phased array scanner).

What are A-, B-, and M-modes?

Different methods of displaying an ultrasound signal:
A-mode (amplitude mode): Shows amplitude of the signal at various depths; rarely used except in ophthalmology
B-mode (brightness mode): Shows brightness of the echo at each depth or position; the common, familiar display mode
M-mode (motion mode): Shows position of the signal over time; used primarily in echocardiography

What is a spatial resolution?

Spatial resolution is the ability to separate two adjacent structures. This can be two structures deep to one another (axial resolution) or next to one another (lateral resolution). Diminished lateral resolution accounts for most ultrasound "blur." Lateral resolution is improved (less blur) with a high frequency transducer.

What is the effect of motion on spatial resolution?

For a stationary object, spatial resolution is improved by a slow scanner sweep. This is because the transducer sees the object for a longer time, receiving more signals from it to pinpoint its characteristics. If the object moves over time, the result is blurring (because signals at multiple locations are received from the same object). If the object is scanned more rapidly, motion blur is reduced and the object's motion can be accurately seen over time. This is the technique used in echocardiography. However, as nothing is free in physics, rapid scanning reduces spatial resolution.

In ultrasound, does increasing the transducer frequency increase or decrease:

The depth of penetration of the pulses?

Decreases

The resolution?

Increases

What is the range of frequencies employed in transthoracic ultrasound?

2–7 million cycles per second [2–7 megahertz (MHz)]

What is impedance?

Impedance is a property of matter that is determined by the density of the matter and the velocity of sound in that matter. The amount of sound reflected at an interface between two tissues depends on the difference in their impedance. With large differences, there is greater reflection (brighter signal).

Is the acoustic impedance of air greater than or less than that of water?

Less than that of water (by a factor of nearly 4000)

Is the speed of ultrasound in air greater than or less than its speed in tissue?

Less (~330 m/s in air, as compared with ~1540 m/s in tissue)

What is attenuation?

Attenuation is the reduction in beam energy owing to interaction with matter. The primary reduction in energy is caused by absorption, which increases with transducer frequency and tissue thickness (or depth).

In ultrasound, what is the function of time-controlled gain ("gain")?

Gain corrects for the attenuation caused by the depth of a structure.

Define the following terms:

Anechoic

Lacking internal echoes (A)

Acoustic enhancement

Acoustic enhancement occurs deep to a lesion with little attenuation or reflection—the echoes are not attenuated by the lesion as in the adjacent tissue, so there seem to be more echoes deep to the lesion. (B)

Shadowing

Shadowing is loss of the ultrasound echoes deep to an echoreflective surface (e.g., a gallstone). (C)

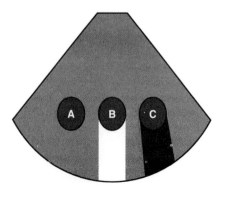

What limits our ability to image vessels with ultrasound?	Overlying gas, excess soft tissue (fat), edema, calcification

DOPPLER ULTRASOUND

What is the Doppler effect?	The Doppler effect is a change in frequency of received sound reflected from a moving object compared with the transmitted sound. If an object moves away from the ultrasound transducer, the wavelength increases (sound waves spread apart) and frequency decreases because the speed of the sound (v) is constant ($v = f \cdot \lambda$). If the object moves toward the transducer, wavelength decreases and frequency increases. For example, recall how the pitch of a whistle on an oncoming train is higher than that of a departing train. The Doppler effect is used in vascular studies. This principle is known as "Doppler shift."
What is the Doppler angle (θ)?	The angle between the moving object and the transducer. An object moving directly toward the transducer has an angle of $0°$, which maximizes the Doppler effect.
What is the optimal Doppler angle?	$60°$ or less; at $90°$, there is no Doppler shift

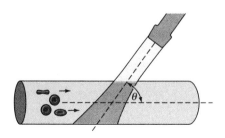

Describe 2 methods of Doppler imaging.

1. **Continuous wave Doppler** uses a continuous signal and is capable of measuring very small velocities. It samples all depths in the beam and thus is poor at determining the position of an individual signal. Continuous wave Doppler is used for peripheral vascular studies in patients with suspected atherosclerosis.
2. **Pulsed wave Doppler** uses pulses of finite length. Received signals are "time gated" to sample only a given depth. Pulsed wave Doppler is less sensitive to low velocity than continuous wave Doppler.

How is Doppler information displayed?

The velocity may be displayed in a graph of velocity versus time (spectral Doppler), or it may be displayed as colors on a scale (color flow Doppler). By convention, blood flow toward the transducer is red, and blood flow away from the transducer is blue. Spectral Doppler generally samples one given area, while color flow Doppler may simultaneously depict flow over the entire imaged area.

What is duplex Doppler ultrasound?

A combination of grayscale B-mode imaging and Doppler ultrasound

What is laminar flow?

Laminar flow is the normal flow within a cylinder or vessel. This occurs if there are no branches or narrow areas that may cause turbulence and all of the particles [e.g., red blood cells (RBCs)] move at the same velocity.

What happens to the flow at a stenosis?

Flow becomes turbulent (non-laminar). The flow velocity is increased (to > 5–6 m/s) within the stenosis and slow eddy flow occurs adjacent to the stenosis.

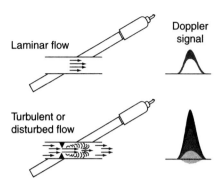

**How is flow at a stenosis
depicted by Doppler?**

Multiple velocities of differing amplitudes
and directions are seen. This is termed
spectral broadening. Similarly, color
Doppler shows multiple colors on both
the blue and red spectrum.

What is aliasing?

Aliasing is the result of flow velocity
exceeding the measuring ability of pulsed
wave Doppler. To measure a velocity,
pulsed Doppler must sample the moving
blood rapidly. In stenosed areas, blood
velocity may exceed sampling ability. The
high-velocity blood is assigned an
incorrect velocity by the system. On
spectral Doppler, this is seen as "wrap-
around," (arrows) with high velocity seen
on the bottom of the scale, rather than on
the top. On color Doppler, it is seen as an
inversion of color (blue within an area of
red or vice versa).

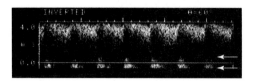

**How do peak velocity
parameters relate to the
severity of a stenosis?**

Doubling of the peak velocity usually
means that the arterial lumen diameter is
narrowed by 50% or more. Tripling of the
peak velocity usually means that the
artery is more than 75% occluded.

What is the resistive index?

A way to indicate the relative resistance to flow

How does one determine a resistive index using Doppler ultrasound?

Measure the peak velocity at systole (PVs) and the peak velocity at diastole (PVd). The resistive index is:

$$\frac{PVs - PVd}{PVs}$$

How is flow to an organ different from systemic arterial flow?

Because organs have a low-resistance capillary bed, blood flow to organs demonstrates a continuous forward flow during diastole. The arteries of the systemic circulation, on the other hand, are characterized by high resistance, usually showing reversal of flow momentarily during diastole. (b) (a = systole)

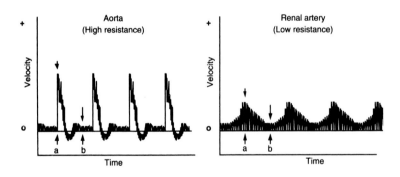

NUCLEAR MEDICINE

What is nuclear medicine?

Nuclear medicine uses radioactive substances to define physiologic processes. Radiopharmaceuticals (tracers) are molecules or cells with physiologic properties that are labeled with radioactive substances called radionuclides. Radionuclides generally emit gamma radiation, which can be detected by a gamma camera system. The amount of radioactivity in an anatomic location or bodily fluid is used to create an image.

How are nuclear medicine images obtained?

The patient is administered the radiopharmaceutical. After a specific amount of time has passed, the patient is placed under a gamma camera system, which is used to generate images on a computer monitor, film, or both.

The gamma camera system consists of a collimator, a sodium iodide crystal, photomultiplier tubes, and a computer. What is the function of each of these components in the system?

The collimator reduces scattered radiation, which can degrade the image. Special collimators can magnify or minimize images. The sodium iodide crystal produces bursts of light when struck by gamma radiation. The photomultiplier tubes turn the light into electric pulses, which are turned into images by the computer.

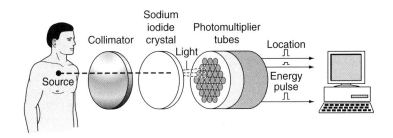

What are planar images?

Images from a single gamma camera held in fixed relation to the patient

Like a plain radiograph, nuclear medicine produces a 2-dimensional image. How can information on depth be obtained?

By obtaining a second planar image at 90° from the first

What is single photon emission computed tomography (SPECT)?

SPECT is a technique that uses one, two, or three gamma cameras to record activity emitted from multiple projections around the patient. The data obtained is used to generate a volumetric dataset, which can be displayed in any plane (typically, however, only sagittal, coronal, and axial planes are employed). SPECT is roughly analogous to CT or MRI in that information on depth is provided.

What is the advantage of SPECT?	Contrast resolution is higher than with planar images
What is the disadvantage?	Spatial resolution is lower
What is activity?	The number of nuclei that decay (i.e., become non-radioactive) per unit time
What are the units of activity?	Becquerels (Bq) or curies (Ci) [1 Bq = 3.7×10^{10} Ci]

BONE SCANS

What is the underlying principle of bone scanning?	Radiolabeled diphosphonate compounds [e.g., methyldiphosphonate (MDP)] are used to demonstrate osseous pathology. It is thought that MDP becomes incorporated into the mineral phase of bone.
How is the standard bone scan performed?	The patient is injected with 15–25 millicuries (mCi) of technetium 99m (Tc-99m)-labeled MDP (Tc-99m MDP). After 2–4 hours, the soft-tissue activity clears and the tracer localizes to bone, enabling planar images, SPECT images, or both to be obtained.
What factors affect the uptake of the tracer?	Osteoblastic activity and blood flow
Tracer uptake is normally seen in what locations?	Bone (should be uniform and symmetric) Kidneys and bladder (tracer is cleared by the kidneys) Soft tissues throughout the body (low levels) Epiphyses (in skeletally immature patients) Breasts (particularly in young women, uptake should be symmetric)
What is a "superscan?"	Diffusely increased osseous uptake Relatively decreased bilateral renal

uptake (be suspicious of a normal-appearing bone scan with faint or no renal activity)

Comparatively low activity in the soft tissues

Higher uptake in the axial skeleton than in the appendicular skeleton

Subtle heterogeneity in the uptake pattern, particularly in the proximal femurs

What are the causes of a "superscan?"

Widespread metastatic disease (e.g., breast cancer, prostate cancer)

Metabolic processes (e.g., renal osteodystrophy, osteomalacia, hyperparathyroidism)

Myelofibrosis

Paget's disease

How is a three-phase bone scan different from a standard bone scan?

A three-phase bone scan includes blood flow and blood pool images, in addition to the delayed images that are normally a part of standard bone scans. In addition, the three-phase bone scan is usually focused on a region of interest, with the FOV generally restricted to the FOV of the gamma camera being employed.

Describe the phases of a three-phase bone scan.

Blood flow phase:

Images are obtained immediately after the injection of the tracer and document arterial flow.

Blood pool phase:

Images are obtained immediately after the blood flow phase. This phase shows the tracer at equilibrium in the extracellular space.

Delayed (late) phase:

Images are obtained 2–4 hours after injecting the tracer, as with a standard bone scan.

What are the indications for a three-phase bone scan?

Infection, reflex sympathetic dystrophy (RSD, Sudeck's atrophy), bone graft (to assess viability)

VENTILATION-PERFUSION (V̇/Q̇) SCANS

How is a V/Q scan performed?

To evaluate ventilation: The patient inhales a radioactive gas (xenon) or Tc-99m-labeled diethylenetriamine penta-acetic acid (DPTA) until equilibrium is reached and a gamma camera is used to evaluate the distribution of the isotope in the airways.

To evaluate perfusion: Tc-99m-labeled macroaggregated albumin (Tc-99m MAA) particles, which are roughly the same size as the capillary diameter, are infused intravenously. A gamma camera is then used to take films showing the distribution of the isotopes trapped in the pulmonary vasculature.

List 3 common indications for a V/Q scan.

1. Suspected pulmonary embolus (PE)
2. Evaluation of relative lung function prior to surgery
3. Suspected right-to-left shunt

What is the main advantage of a V/Q scan?

Noninvasive method of screening for PE

List 3 disadvantages of a V/Q scan.

1. Results may be equivocal in patients with preexisting lung disease, particularly if aerosols are used for ventilation.
2. Equivocal results or results discordant with clinical suspicions require additional testing.
3. Interpretation may be difficult and requires considerable experience.

When should a quantitative V/Q scan be performed?

When it is necessary to determine relative lung function (e.g., prior to performing a pneumonectomy or segmentectomy in a cancer patient or before performing a lung transplant)

How is a quantitative scan performed?

Ventilation and perfusion images are obtained in the posterior projection (perfusion images are typically obtained in all standard projections as well). The relative lung function, expressed as a percentage of total function, is computed for both ventilation and perfusion images.

What are the perfusion scan findings with a right-to-left cardiac shunt?

Activity in the brain and kidneys—activity in the brain with Tc-99m MAA is always a right-to-left shunt; renal activity may be from a poor Tc-99m tag

How should a perfusion scan be altered if there is a suspected right-to-left shunt?

The number of MAA particles should be reduced to approximately 100,000 (from a typical dose of 200,000 to 500,000) to reduce the (largely theoretical) risk of embolism to critical organs.

HEPATOBILIARY SCANS

What is a hepatobiliary scan?

A hepatobiliary scan uses Tc-99m-labeled iminodiacetic acid derivatives (Tc-99m IDA) to detect biliary tract pathology. Tc-99m IDA has uptake, transport, and excretion pathways that are identical to those of bilirubin: it is cleared from the blood stream by the liver, excreted into the biliary ducts, and excreted into the bowel. It also fills the gallbladder under the same physiologic conditions that cause bilirubin to fill the gallbladder (e.g., no recent meals).

What are the common indications for a hepatobiliary scan?

Acute cholecystitis, biliary atresia, biliary leak following cholecystectomy

What are the:

Advantages of a hepatobiliary scan?

It has high specificity for excluding acute cholecystitis and is not operator-dependent.

Disadvantages of a hepatobiliary scan?

It requires at least 1 hour of actual imaging time and patient preparation, and false-positive results may occur.

How is a hepatobiliary scan performed?

1. If acute cholecystitis is suspected, the patient must not have anything orally for 4 hours prior to the study. If the patient has not had anything to eat for more than 24 hours, cholecystokinin

(CCK) should be administered prior to the examination.

2. 5–10 mCi of Tc-99m IDA are administered intravenously. Some institutions increase the dose with increasing bilirubin levels.

3. Images are obtained every 5 minutes for 1 hour. If no filling is seen after 1 hour, late images may be obtained for as long as 4 hours post-injection, or morphine administration can be considered (to contract the sphincter of Oddi and help to fill the gallbladder, if the cystic duct is patent).

What are the findings in a normal scan?

The radiopharmaceutical should be cleared from the blood pool after 5 minutes. Liver activity should decrease over time, with the onset of noticeable liver clearing after 20–30 minutes. The gallbladder and bowel activity should be visualized after 60 minutes (i.e., the biliary-to-bowel transit time).

RENAL SCANS

What are the 2 types of renal scans?

Dynamic (functional) renal scans and cortical scans

Dynamic (functional) renal scans

How is the standard study performed?

Approximately 10–20 mCi of Tc-99m-labeled DTPA, Tc-99m-labeled mercaptylacetyltriglycine (Tc-99m MAG3), or Tc-99m-labeled glucoheptonate (Tc-99m GH) are administered intravenously, and images are obtained posteriorly. Blood flow phase images are obtained with 1-second frames for 60–90 seconds, and static images are obtained every 5 minutes for approximately 25–30 minutes.

What is the difference between the 3 imaging agents?

Tc-99m DTPA is cleared via glomerular filtration. It is a relatively inexpensive agent that is used for patients with native kidneys and normal renal function.

Tc-99m MAG3 is cleared predominately via tubular excretion (80%), with a small amount of clearance occurring by glomerular filtration (20%). It is concentrated more effectively by the kidneys than Tc-99m DTPA, particularly where there is poor renal function.

Tc-99m GH is predominantly cleared via glomerular filtration (80%), although a fraction of the radiopharmaceutical (20%) is tightly bound to sulfhydryl groups on the cortical surface. This allows GH to be used as both a dynamic (functional) imaging agent and a cortical imaging agent.

What are the phases of a normal dynamic (functional) study?

Blood flow phase: The first 30–60 seconds after the injection of the radio-pharmaceutical, this is the phase when the agent arrives at the kidneys.

Cortical phase: Occurring 1–3 minutes after injection of the tracer, this is the phase when the agent is most intensely concentrated in the renal cortex.

Clearance phase: Beginning after the cortical phase, this is the phase where the tracer is cleared from the cortex and excreted into the collecting system (i.e., the renal pelvis and ureters) and, eventually, the bladder.

What is the appearance of a normal blood flow phase?

Renal activity should be seen when there is activity in the adjacent abdominal aorta.

What is normal differential renal function?

Generally, a kidney's function should be within 10% of that of the contralateral side (i.e., a differential function of 55%–45% would be normal).

What are the indications for a dynamic (functional) renal scan in the setting of renal transplantation?

Poor function or a clinically suspected urine leak in the immediate post-operative period

Declining renal function post-transplantation

How is the renal scan performed in this setting?

10–20 mCi of Tc-99m MAG3 are injected intravenously. Images are obtained anteriorly over the pelvis in a manner identical to standard renal dynamic (functional) imaging. Delayed images are obtained approximately 2 hours post-injection if a urine leak is a clinical consideration.

What is the appearance of a normal renal transplant?

Images obtained during the blood flow phase should demonstrate activity within the transplant at the same time activity is seen in the iliac arteries. Images obtained during the cortical and clearance phases should be identical to those seen in standard dynamic (functional) studies. The cortex should demonstrate uniform uptake during the cortical phase.

Furosemide renogram

List 3 uses for a furosemide renogram.

1. To confirm a diagnosis of renal obstruction, often suggested by hydronephrosis on cross-sectional imaging (e.g., ultrasound or CT)
2. To quantitate renal obstruction
3. To follow patients with known obstruction, with or without previous intervention

How is the furosemide renogram performed?

The standard procedure for dynamic (functional) imaging is followed. Static images are inspected after approximately 30 minutes, and if there is still significant activity within the collecting system, furosemide is administered intravenously and static images are obtained for approx-imately 30 minutes following the injection.

What is the theory behind the furosemide renogram?

The furosemide bolus will cause diuresis of non-radioactive urine into the collecting system in patients who respond to the drug. The non-radioactive urine will flush the radioactive urine out of dilated, nonobstructed collecting systems, while activity will remain if there is obstruction.

What factors limit the effectiveness of this study?

Poor renal function makes interpretation difficult (i.e., is there obstruction or is the kidney just unable to respond to the furosemide?)

How are the results interpreted?

"Wash-out" of half of the radioactivity in the collecting system within 10 minutes of injecting the furosemide is normal and consistent with a dilated, nonobstructed system. Wash-out occurring 10–20 minutes after the injection is indeterminant, and washout occurring more than 20 minutes after injection indicates obstruction.

When are late images necessary?

Late images are required occasionally to document the degree of severe obstruction. They may also be used if renal function itself is an issue (i.e., does a hydronephrotic kidney have any function?)

Captopril renogram

When is a captopril renogram indicated?

In the setting of clinically suspected renal artery stenosis (i.e., renovascular hypertension)

What is the physiology behind a captopril renogram?

With untreated renal artery stenosis, the renin-angiotensin mechanism responds to a decreased glomerular filtration rate (GFR) by producing renin, which in turn converts angiotensinogen to angiotensin I. Angiotensin I is then converted to angiotensin II, which constricts the efferent arterioles of the renal glomeruli in order to maintain the GFR. Angiotensin-converting enzyme (ACE) inhibitors, such as captopril, disrupt this compensatory mechanism by dilating the efferent arterioles and decreasing the GFR.

How is a captopril renogram performed?

Tc-99m MAG3 is often the preferred agent. The study may include only a dynamic (functional) scan following ACE inhibitor administration, or it may include a baseline study (i.e., a half-dose of tracer followed by administration of the ACE inhibitor and a study with a full dose of tracer). The patient should be hydrated prior to administering the ACE-inhibitor, and the blood pressure should be monitored throughout.

What constitutes a normal study?

A dynamic (functional) renogram with an ACE inhibitor demonstrates normal renal function and time-activity curves. If a baseline study was performed, there should be no difference between the baseline time-activity curve and the post-ACE inhibitor time-activity curve.

What are potential pitfalls?

Poor renal function from any cause makes interpretation difficult or impossible. A drop in the systemic blood pressure (as a result of ACE inhibitor administration) decreases renal function and makes interpretation difficult or impossible.

Renal cortical scans

What are the indications for a renal cortical scan?

Suspected pyelonephritis or renal scarring

How is a renal cortical scan performed?

5 mCi of Tc-99m-labeled dimercaptosuccinic acid (Tc-99m DMSA) or 15–20 mCi of Tc-99m GH are injected intravenously, and planar or SPECT images are obtained 2 hours post-injection.

How do Tc-99m DMSA and Tc-99m GH agents work to produce an image?

They bind to the sulfhydryl groups in the renal cortex.

What is the benefit of renal cortical imaging?

This study is considered more sensitive than cross-sectional imaging (e.g., ultrasound or CT) for small defects.

THYROID SCANS

How is the thyroid gland imaged with nuclear medicine?

Iodine 123 (I^{123}) is administered orally, or an intravenous dose of Tc-99m pertechnetate may be used. Imaging is performed with a pinhole collimator after about 6 hours (with I^{123}) or 20 minutes (with Tc-99m pertechnetate).

Which radiopharmaceutical is used in cancer patients?

Iodine 131 (I^{131}), to look for metastatic disease

What are the advantages of the pinhole collimator?

Higher resolution images

What should be done to a palpable thyroid abnormality after a scan is performed?

The location of a nodule is confirmed by outlining the palpable nodule with a radioactive marker placed on the patient. The marked image confirms whether the nodule is functioning or nonfunctioning.

What is a thyroid uptake study, and when is it indicated?

A thyroid uptake study is a nuclear medicine study that measures the percentage of a dose of radioactive iodine taken up by the thyroid gland in a given period of time, usually 24 hours. It evaluates the physiologic process whereby the thyroid takes up iodine to manufacture thyroid hormone. The test is indicated when there is thyroid dysfunction, particularly hyperthyroidism.

What constitutes a normal study?

A thyroid scan is normal when the activity is uniform and a normal-sized gland is seen in its usual location. The 24-hour iodine uptake at most institutions is normally in the range of 10%-25% of the administered dose.

PARATHYROID SCANS

What are the clinical indications for parathyroid imaging?

Parathyroid imaging is indicated when it is necessary to localize the source of parathyroid hormone (PTH) production (e.g., in a patient with elevated serum calcium levels and potential hyperparathyroidism).

How is a scan performed?

Parathyroid tissue is capable of concentrating thallium 201 (Tl^{201}) chloride and Tc-99m sestamibi. Because thyroid tissue also concentrates these drugs, it is necessary to image the thyroid tissue by itself (using oral I^{123} or intravenous Tc-99m pertechnate) and then "subtract" (either digitally or visually) the image of the thyroid tissue.

Alternatively, delayed Tc-99m sestamibi images may show retained tracer in parathyroid tissue (for 4–6 hours), allowing direct imaging.

What are the diagnostic possibilities if the parathyroid glands cannot be visualized using either technique?

A hyperactive parathyroid can be ruled out (it is difficult to see normal parathyroid glands using either technique, much less hyperactive ones). However, the patient may have parathyroid hyperplasia and none of the glands is active enough or big enough to be detected. An ectopic location must also be looked for in the chest or other locations in the neck.

What is the primary diagnostic consideration for multiple areas of increased uptake in the expected location of the parathyroid glands?

Parathyroid hyperplasia. Hyperplastic glands are often asymmetric in activity and size.

What are the primary diagnostic considerations for a focal area of increased uptake with either subtraction or wash-out studies?

Parathyroid adenoma (80% of cases), thyroid cancer, focal thyroiditis and parathyroid carcinoma

Why are anterior views of the thorax obtained?

These views are obtained to look for ectopic parathyroid tissue. At times, SPECT is needed to more accurately localize the lesion. Often it is helpful to compare the SPECT images with CT scans of the chest.

3

Pulmonary Imaging

Elizabeth K. Dee

ANATOMY

Identify the structures comprising the mediastinal margins:

A = Right innominate vein
B = Superior vena cava (SVC)
C = Ascending aorta
D = Right atrium
E = Left innominate vein
F = Aortic knob
G = Aortopulmonary window
H = Left pulmonary artery
I = Left ventricle
J = Descending aorta
K = Diaphragm

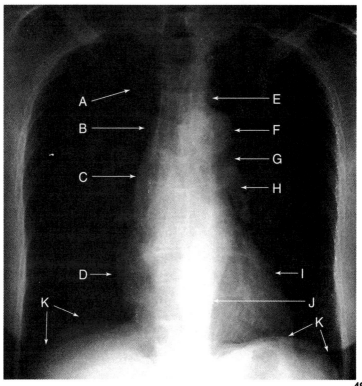

Identify the parts of the lung (*black areas*) adjacent to the mediastinum and diaphragm (*gray areas*):

A = Right upper lobe (RUL)
B = Right middle lobe (RML)
C = Right lower lobe (RLL)
D = Left upper lobe (LUL)
E = Lingula
F = Left lower lobe (LLL)

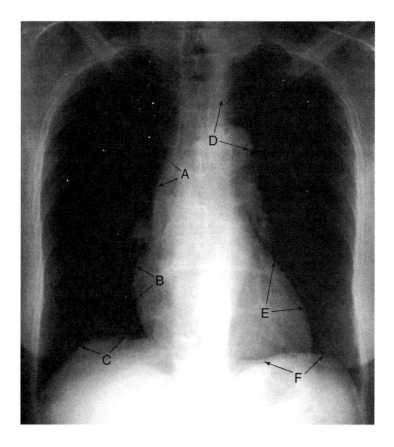

Identify the location of the lobes of the lung on:

Posterior-anterior (PA) view

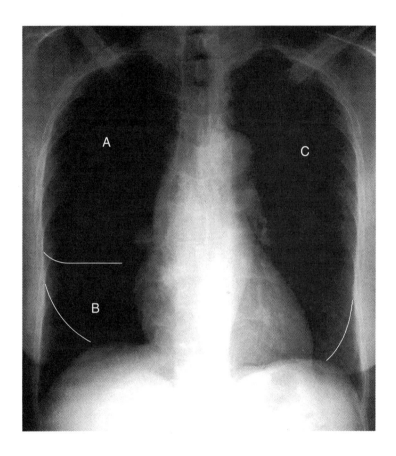

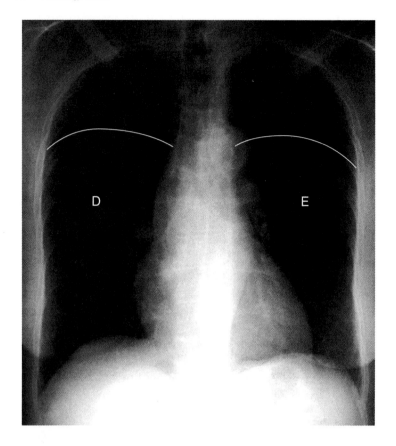

Lateral view

Upper lobes lie anteriorly; lower lobes lie posteriorly.

A = RUL
B = RML
C = LUL
D = RLL
E = LLL

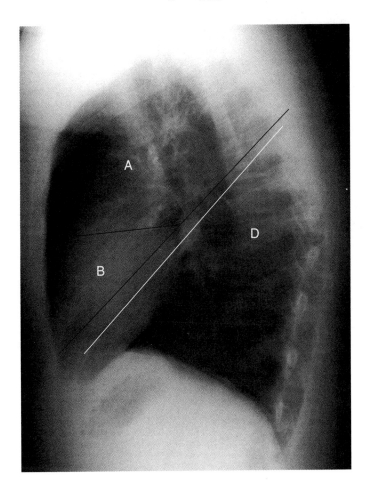

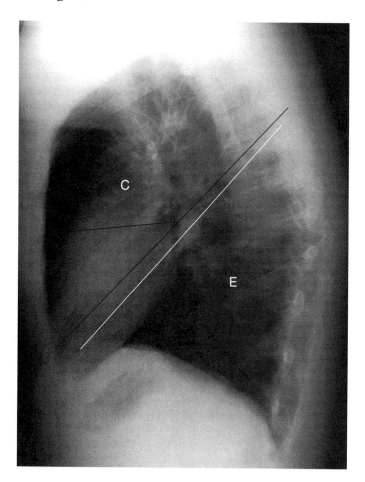

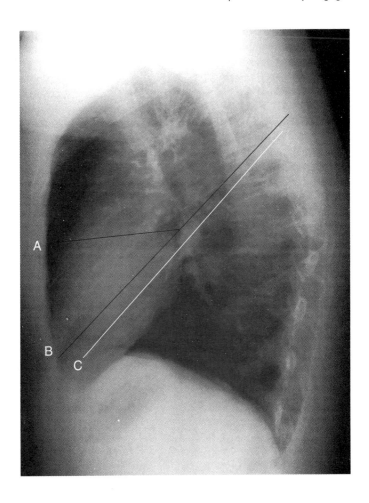

Identify the fissures of the lung:

A = Minor fissure (horizontal)
B = Right major fissure (oblique)
C = Left major fissure (oblique)

Identify the bronchi of the lungs:

A = Right main stem bronchus
B = Right upper lobe bronchus
  B_1 = Apical segmental bronchus
  B_2 = Anterior segmental bronchus
  B_3 = Posterior segmental bronchus
C = Bronchus intermedius
D = Right middle lobe bronchus
  D_4 = Lateral segmental bronchus
  D_5 = Medial segmental bronchus

E = Right lower lobe bronchus
Suppose My Aunt Loves Peaches **_m_**

E_6 = **S**uperior segmental bronchus
E_7 = **M**edial basal segmental bronchus
E_8 = **A**nterior basal segmental bronchus
E_9 = **L**ateral basal segmental bronchus
E_{10} = **P**osterior basal segmental bronchus

F = Left main stem bronchus

G = Left upper lobe bronchus
G_1, G_2 = Apicoposterior segmental bronchus
G_3 = Anterior segmental bronchus

H = Lingular bronchus
H_4 = Superior lingular segmental bronchus
H_5 = Inferior lingular segmental bronchus

I = Left lower lobe bronchus
I_6 = **S**uperior segmental bronchus
I_7 = **M**edial basal segmental bronchus
I_8 = **A**nterior basal segmental bronchus
I_9 = **L**ateral basal segmental bronchus
I_{10} = **P**osterior basal segmental bronchus

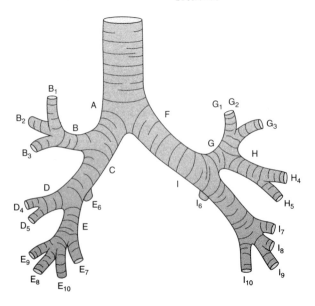

Identify the airways and pulmonary vessels on the lateral view:

A = Right pulmonary artery
B = Trachea
C = Left pulmonary artery
D = Right upper lobe bronchus orifice
E = Left upper lobe bronchus orifice
F = Posterior wall of bronchus intermedius
G = Bronchus intermedius
H = Left lower lobe bronchus

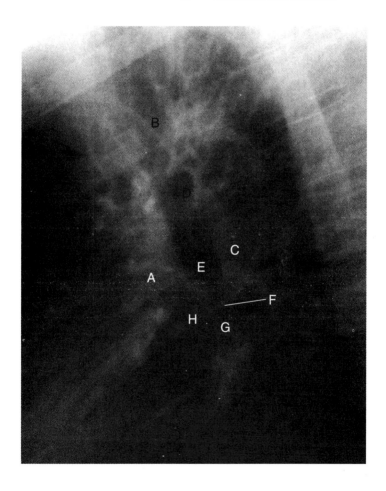

Identify the following hilar structures:

A = Apical segmental bronchus
B = Posterior segmental bronchus
C = Anterior segmental bronchus
D = Bronchus intermedius
E = Truncus anterior
F = Carina
G = Right main pulmonary artery
H = Left main pulmonary artery
I = Right inferior pulmonary artery
J = Right superior pulmonary vein
K = Right middle lobe bronchus
L = Right lower lobe bronchus
M = Right inferior pulmonary vein
N = Left atrium
O = Left superior pulmonary vein
P = Apicoposterior segmental bronchus
Q = Left upper lobe bronchus
R = Lingular bronchus
S = Left inferior pulmonary artery
T = Left inferior pulmonary vein

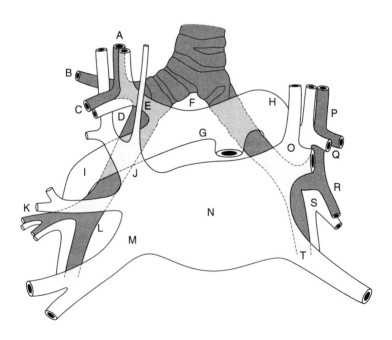

Identify the following mediastinal structures:

A = SVC
B = Left brachiocephalic vein
C = Right subclavian vein
D = Right subclavian artery
E = Right internal jugular vein
F = Right common carotid artery
G = Right brachiocephalic artery
H = Left common carotid artery
I = Left internal jugular vein
J = Left subclavian artery
K = Left subclavian vein
L = Left brachiocephalic vein

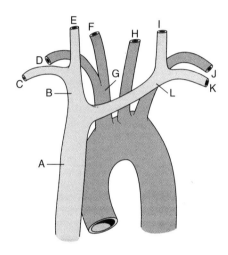

Identify the structures on this series of computed tomography (CT) sections:

A = Aorta
B = Ascending aorta
C = Descending aorta
D = SVC
E = Right brachiocephalic artery
F = Left common carotid artery
G = Left subclavian artery
H = Right brachiocephalic vein
I = Left brachiocephalic vein
J = Esophagus
K = Azygos arch
L = Azygos vein
M = Hemiazygos vein
N = Truncus anterior
O = Right pulmonary artery
P = Left pulmonary artery
Q = Pericardium
R = Coronary sinus
S = Root of aorta
T = Pulmonary outflow tract
U = Left atrium
V = Right atrium
W = Right ventricle
X = Interventricular septum
Y = Left ventricle
Z = Inferior vena cava (IVC)
1 = Right superior pulmonary vein
2 = Left superior pulmonary vein
3 = Azygoesophageal recess
4 = Sternum
5 = Trachea
6 = Right upper lobe bronchus
7 = Left upper lobe bronchus
8 = Anterior segment right upper lobe bronchus
9 = Posterior segment right upper lobe bronchus
10 = Bronchus intermedius
11 = Left upper lobe bronchus
12 = Left upper lobe spur
13 = Left lower lobe bronchus
14 = Left lower lobe, superior segment
15 = Right lower lobe bronchus
16 = Right lower lobe, superior segment
17 = Right middle lobe bronchus
18 = Right middle lobe, medial segment
19 = Right middle lobe, lateral segment

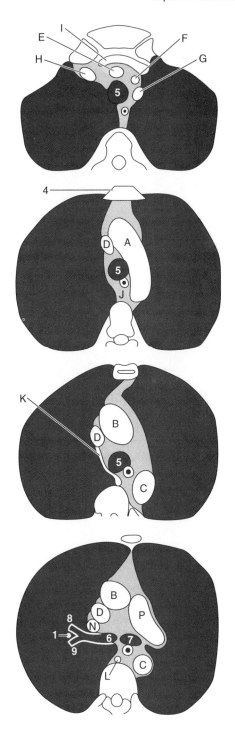

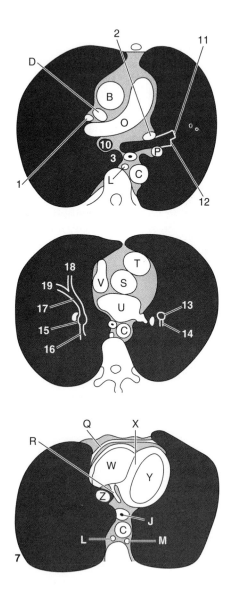

Where is the azygos vein seen on a frontal CXR?

The azygos vein is seen end-on as an ovoid mass in the right tracheobronchial angle.

DEFINITIONS

Define the following terms:

Alveolar (airspace) disease	Disease that results in filling of the alveoli with material other than air
Anterior and posterior junction lines	The interface of the two lungs anteriorly and posteriorly
Atelectasis	A decrease in the amount of air in part or all of a lung with resultant loss of volume; often termed "collapse"
Aortopulmonary window	A region under the aortic arch and above the left pulmonary artery that contains the recurrent laryngeal nerve and the ligamentum arteriosum; masses in this region can cause vocal cord paralysis and hoarseness
Azygoesophageal line	The interface between the lung tissue and the esophagus that is seen on frontal radiographs
Azygoesophageal recess	The space occupied by lung tissue behind the right bronchus intermedius, adjacent to the right wall of the esophagus
Azygos lobe fissure	An accessory fissure in the RUL that appears as a curvilinear density terminating in a small round or ovoid density (i.e., the azygos vein); seen in 1% of the normal population
Bronchiectasis	Dilatation of a bronchus, seen on chest radiographs (CXRs) or computed tomography (CT) scans as a loss of the normal tapering, often with thickening of the bronchial wall
Bulla	A thin-walled round or oval air space; most often seen in patients with emphysema
Cardiophrenic angles	The normally acute angles formed by the intersection of the diaphragm contour with the right and left heart borders (i.e., the right atrium and left ventricle, respectively)

Cephalization

Prominence of the upper zone pulmonary vessels (normally, in the upright position, the lower zone vessels are larger); most often seen in patients with congestive heart failure (CHF)

Costophrenic angles

The sulci where the diaphragm meets the chest wall

Eventration of the diaphragm

Idiopathic incomplete muscularization of all or part of a hemidiaphragm that permits the abdominal contents, usually the liver, to bulge into the chest

Granuloma

A nodular aggregation of chronic inflammatory cells in response to certain infectious (e.g., histoplasmosis) and non-infectious (e.g., sarcoidosis) processes; often calcified

Interstitial disease

Disease involving mainly the extra-alveolar tissue (i.e., the interstitium) of the lungs; tends to spare the alveolar spaces

Lung markings

Normal structures visible within the lungs, such as pulmonary vessels, bronchial walls, fissures, and interstitial lines. Over 90% of markings are vascular structures. In the outer third of normal lungs, markings are few.

Right paratracheal stripe

The interface between the trachea and the right lung; seen in the frontal view as a 2- to 4-mm line

Superior pericardial recess

The superior pericardial recess communicates with the pericardium and extends cephalad posterior to the aorta. It can be confused with mediastinal adenopathy, but the recess is crescentic and adenopathy is round or oval in shape.

IMAGING STUDIES

CHEST RADIOGRAPH (CXR)

Technical considerations

How do you read a CXR?

Patient data: Name, history number, age, sex, old films?

Technique: AP or PA, exposure, rotation, supine or erect position, portable?

Trachea: Midline or deviated, caliber?

Lungs: Abnormal shadowing?

Pulmonary vessels: Artery or vein enlargement?

Hila: Masses, lymphadenopathy?

Heart: Ratio of the thoracic width to the cardiac width (normal is $> 2:1$), valve calcifications, cardiac configuration?

Mediastinal contour: Widening mass?

Pleura: Effusion, thickening, calcification?

Bones: Lesions, fractures?

Soft tissues: Check every part of the CXR for abnormalities, including below the diaphragm. Don't miss a mastectomy!

Tubes and lines: Proper positioning?

How does this pattern change when evaluating films from a patient in the intensive care unit (ICU)?

Identify tubes first and always look for pneumothoraces.

What defines a technically adequate CXR:

On a PA film?

Good inspiration: Diaphragm is at or below ribs 8–10 posteriorly and ribs 5–6 anteriorly

Penetration: Disk spaces are visible but there is no bony detail of the spine; bronchovascular structures are seen through the heart

Rotation: Clavicular heads are equidistant from the thoracic spinous processes

On a lateral film?

Spine should darken caudally owing to more air in the lower lobes and less chest wall mass

Sternum should be edge-on

The ribs closer to the x-ray source should be projected more posteriorly owing to beam divergence

Why is a frontal CXR routinely taken with the x-ray beam traversing from posterior to anterior?

To reduce heart shadow magnification and provide a more accurate estimation of heart size (objects closer to the x-ray source are more magnified than those closer to the film owing to the divergence of the x-ray beam)

Why does it matter whether the patient is upright or supine when the CXR is taken?

The appearance of air or fluid in the pleural space, the heart size, and the appearance of the pulmonary vessels are significantly affected by position.

List the potential blind spots on a:

Frontal CXR (List 4)

1. In the lung apices behind the clavicles and first ribs
2. Below and behind the diaphragm
3. Behind or in front of the hilar shadows
4. Behind the heart

Lateral CXR (List 3)

1. In the apices
2. In the anterior mediastinum
3. Over the vertebral bodies

How can the right ribs be differentiated from the left ribs on a left lateral CXR?

The right ribs appear larger and more posterior than the left ribs because lateral CXRs are routinely taken with the patient's left side against the film cassette to minimize heart magnification; therefore, the right ribs are more magnified owing to divergence of the beam.

When are oblique views of the chest helpful?

Oblique views are useful for showing lesions hidden by bony or soft tissue structures in the more conventional views and for demonstrating the chest wall. CT is better for all of this, but is more expensive.

List 5 disadvantages of portable CXRs.

1. Heart overmagnification (because the film is taken anteroposteriorly)
2. Poor positioning
3. Poor respiratory effort of bedridden patients
4. Radiation exposure to other patients and staff
5. Poor results in obese patients (longer exposure times are needed because the x-ray output of a portable apparatus is lower than that of standard equipment)

Common radiographic signs

What is a "bat wing" or "butterfly" pattern?

Bilateral perihilar airspace shadowing

List 5 causes of a "bat wing" pattern.

1. Pulmonary edema, especially cardiogenic edema
2. Pneumonia, especially aspiration or *Pneumocystis carinii* pneumonia (PCP)
3. Noxious gas or liquid inhalation
4. Alveolar proteinosis
5. Pulmonary hemorrhage

What are Kerley (septal) lines?

The interstitium made visible by thickening of the connective tissue septae

Kerley A lines (**A** = **A**pex): Nonbranching deep septal lines 4–6 cm long, extending radially from the hilum into the upper lobes

Kerley B lines (**B** = **B**ase): Horizontal lines less than 2 cm long, commonly found in the lower zone periphery, although they may be seen as high as the clavicles

List 6 causes of Kerley lines.

1. Pulmonary edema (virtually diagnostic if lines are transient or rapid in development)
2. Lymphangitis carcinomatosa and malignant lymphoma
3. Viral and mycoplasmal pneumonia
4. Interstitial pulmonary fibrosis
5. Pneumoconiosis
6. Sarcoidosis

What is the "phantom" or "vanishing" tumor sign (pseudotumor)?

An interlobar effusion, seen in patients with CHF, that mimics a parenchymal tumor but disappears as cardiac status improves; most often seen in the minor fissure and can recur in the same area with subsequent episodes of heart failure

How can a phantom tumor be confirmed?

On a lateral film, an interlobar fluid collection will have an elliptical shape and is bisected by the fissural line on the long axis

What is an air bronchogram?

The tubular outline of an airway (arrows on CT) made visible by filling of the surrounding alveoli by fluid or inflammatory exudates

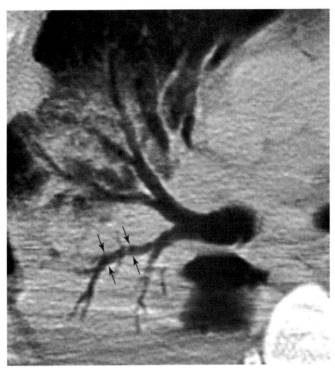

List 6 causes of an air bronchogram.

1. Lung consolidation
2. Pulmonary edema
3. Nonobstructive pulmonary atelectasis
4. Severe interstitial disease
5. Neoplasm (e.g., bronchoalveolar carcinoma, lymphoma)
6. Normal expiration

Describe the following signs and when they are most likely to be seen:

Golden S sign

Upper lobe collapse caused by a central mass results in an "S"-shaped (or reverse "S"-shaped) contour

Silhouette sign

Loss of the normal border (silhouette) of a soft-tissue structure; contrast between the aerated lung and the nonaerated soft tissue forms the border

Hilum overlay sign

If the pulmonary artery is seen clearly through a lesion, the lesion is either in front of or behind the hilum (i.e., not a hilar mass).

Extrapleural sign

A mass within the extrapleural space appears as a smoothly contoured mass with tapered edges that bulges into the parenchyma from the periphery. A parenchymal mass abutting the pleural surface has acute angles at the pleural interface.

Incomplete border sign

An extrapleural or pleural mass has an obscured lateral border where it merges with the pleura or the extrapleural space. This sign helps to distinguish protruding extrapleural or pleural masses from peripheral parenchymal masses.

Cervicothoracic sign

Clearly demarcated lesions above the clavicles on a frontal view are within the posterior mediastinum or lung apices. A lesion extending down from the neck will have an obscured upper border.

Double lesion sign

If two or more segments are collapsed and not contiguous, a central cancer is not the cause.

Open bronchus sign

If the bronchi within the opacified lung are open, an obstructing lesion completely occluding a more central bronchus is unlikely.

Air crescent (meniscus) sign	A crescent-shaped shadow at the edge of a lung lesion formed by gas separating the outer wall of the lesion from the inner mass; most commonly seen with an intracavitary fungus ball (*Aspergillus fumigatus*)
Anterior sulcus (double diaphragm) sign	A sign of a pneumothorax seen on a frontal radiograph taken when the patient is supine; gas localizes anteriorly, resulting in a sharply delineated hyper-lucency of the upper diaphragm
Apical cap sign	Blood in the extrapleural space forms a crescent-shaped cap over the left lung apex; classically seen with a ruptured aorta
Bulging fissure sign	Bulging fissures occur when consolidated lobes become large; may be seen with *Klebsiella pneumoniae* pneumonia
Continuous diaphragm sign	Mediastinal gas between the heart and the diaphragm permits visualization of the normally obscured central diaphragm (i.e., the entire diaphragm contour is seen); indicative of pneumomediastinum
Double contour sign	Two right heart borders; seen with increased left atrial size
Hampton's hump	A rounded opacity with its base at the pleural surface; represents an area of pulmonary infarction
Melting sign	A wedge of opacity decreases in size like a melting snowman; seen with a resolving infarct
Westermark's sign	A local reduction of pulmonary blood volume (i.e., oligemia) distal to a large-vessel pulmonary embolus (PE) causes hyperlucency of the involved portion of lung
Fleischner's sign	Enlargement of a main pulmonary artery when a pulmonary thromboembolism causes either pulmonary hypertension or distention of the artery

Gloved finger sign	Mucus-filled bronchiectatic airways extending from the hilum form homogenous band-like densities akin to gloved fingers
Signet ring sign	The "ring" (i.e., a dilated bronchus) is accompanied by a "signet") (i.e., a pulmonary artery); seen in bronchiectasis
What is mediastinal widening?	A superior mediastinum that is wider than 8 centimeters or that occupies more than 25% of the transverse thoracic diameter at the level of the aortic arch
List 4 differential diagnoses for acute mediastinal widening.	Postsurgical bleeding Aorta or great vessel rupture Esophageal rupture Mediastinal abscess
What are the pitfalls in the diagnosis of mediastinal widening?	Typical trauma film (taken AP and supine) magnifies the anterior mediastinum Excessive mediastinal fat may cause widening Rotated film
What is mediastinal shift?	Significant deviation of the mediastinum to one side (most easily seen as tracheal shift away from the midline)
List 3 causes of mediastinal shift and the direction of the shift associated with each.	1. Decreased lung volume, such as occurs in patients with atelectasis, following pneumonectomy, and in patients with a hypoplastic or agenetic lung (mediastinum shifts toward the lesion) 2. Increased lung volume, such as occurs in patients with a massive tumor or severe expansile pneumonia, such as that caused by *K. pneumoniae* or anaerobic organisms (mediastinum shifts away from the lesion) 3. Pleural disease, such as tension pneumothorax, large pleural effusion, or large diaphragmatic hernia (mediastinum shifts away from the lesion)

Which way will the mediastinum shift if there is both atelectasis and pleural effusion?	There may be no shift in this case.

List 8 common causes of hemidiaphragm elevation.	1. Atelectasis or lobar collapse 2. Eventration 3. Phrenic nerve injury (neoplastic, traumatic, or iatrogenic) 4. Subpulmonic effusion 5. Subphrenic abscess 6. Hepatomegaly 7. Diaphragmatic hernia 8. Bowel distention

List 6 common causes of bilateral diaphragmatic elevation.	1. Poor inspiration 2. Bilateral lower lobe atelectasis 3. Restrictive pulmonary disease 4. Abdominal disorders (e.g., ascites, abdominal mass) 5. Obesity 6. Neuromuscular disease [e.g., amyotrophic lateral sclerosis (ALS), myasthenia gravis]

CXRs in the intensive care unit (ICU)

When should CXRs be done on ICU patients?	Daily in intubated patients and those with a Swan-Ganz catheter or chest tubes After any invasive procedure (e.g., central line placement, intubation, thoracentesis) After any significant change in the patient's status

What is the most common CXR abnormality in the ICU patient?	Atelectasis

What other abnormalities are often found on an ICU CXR?	Pulmonary edema, pleural effusion, lung consolidation, barotrauma (e.g., pneumothorax, pneumomediastinum), adult respiratory distress syndrome (ARDS), malpositioned lines

List 6 common causes of pneumothorax in the ICU patient.	1. Barotrauma secondary to positive-pressure ventilation 2. Central line insertion

3. Thoracentesis
4. Surgery
5. Perforation of the pleural space by a feeding tube
6. Tracheostomy

What is a tension pneumothorax and what does it look like?

A pneumothorax with mass effect; characterized by mediastinal shift away from the affected side and a small heart

Why is it important to recognize tension pneumothorax?

It may cause cardiac tamponade and death.

Use of CXRs to verify tube, line, catheter, and pacemaker placement

On a CXR, what is the ideal position for a:

Swan-Ganz catheter?

Tip in the right or left main pulmonary artery, usually no more than 1 centimeter lateral to the mediastinal margin

Central venous catheter?

Tip in the SVC, below the brachiocephalic veins and above the right atrium

Endotracheal tube?

Tip at or below the clavicles and at least 2 centimeters above the carina

Transvenous ventricular pacemaker?

At the apex of the right ventricle, lodged within the trabeculae

What are the complications of:

Central line placement? (List 7)

1. Pneumothorax
2. Adjacent artery puncture
3. Erosion of line tip through the SVC
4. Arrhythmias
5. Damage to the tricuspid valve
6. Line infection
7. Venous thrombosis

Endotracheal tube positioning? (List 2)

1. Esophageal intubation, leading to gastrointestinal overdistention and failure to ventilate the patient

2. Main stem bronchus intubation (usually the right bronchus), leading to ipsilateral lung distention, contralateral lung collapse, and hypoxia

Nasogastric tube placement? (List 3)

1. Coiling or looping in the pharynx or esophagus
2. Intubation of the lung, potentially causing pneumothorax
3. Sinusitis

Transvenous ventricular pacemaker placement? (List 3)

1. Malposition (e.g., in the coronary sinus, right atrium, or pulmonary artery)
2. Cardiac perforation
3. Wire breakage

What is the best indicator that the pacer is in the coronary sinus?

The tip travels posteriorly as seen on the lateral view

COMPUTED TOMOGRAPHY (CT)

List 3 of the best uses for CT in patients with chest disease.

1. Localizing masses prior to biopsy
2. Revealing fine detail of pulmonary processes [with high resolution CT (HRCT)]
3. Diagnosing mediastinal masses

VENTILATION-PERFUSION (V/Q) SCAN

Describe the appearance of a normal V/Q scan.

Perfusion and ventilation should be uniform throughout both lungs.

Defects may be seen at the location of normal structures, such as the hila, aorta, or fissures. If xenon gas is used, the agent should "wash out" of the lungs 2–3 minutes after the patient ceases breathing the agent.

What conditions can cause:

Bilateral perfusion defects? (List 4)

1. PE
2. Extrinsic compression of the pulmonary artery (e.g., by neoplasm,

fibrosing mediastinitis, surgical
ligation)
3. Physiologic response from decreased
or absent ventilation
4. Pleural effusions

**Unilateral perfusion
defects? (List 6)**

1. Mucus plug
2. Compression of pulmonary artery by
tumor
3. Fibrosing mediastinitis
4. PE
5. Massive effusion
6. Pneumonectomy

**Ventilation abnormalities?
(List 3)**

1. Chronic lung disease
2. Mucus plugging
3. Alveolar (airspace) disease (e.g.,
pneumonia, pulmonary edema,
tumors)

**What is the difference
between segmental and
nonsegmental defects?**

Segmental defects correspond to
anatomic lung segments and may
represent a PE. Nonsegmental defects do
not follow segmental anatomy, do not
extend to the pleural base, and are
unlikely to represent a PE.

**What is the "stripe sign"
and what is its significance?**

An area of normal perfusion peripheral to
a perfusion defect; decreases likelihood of
a diagnosis of PE

**What is the terminology
used in describing V/Q
scan findings?**

Matched defect: Not ventilated and not
perfused
Mismatched defect (V/Q mismatch):
Ventilated but not perfused
Reverse mismatched defect: Perfused
but not ventilated

What conditions can cause:

A matched defect? (List 6)

1. Chronic obstructive pulmonary disease
(COPD)
2. Airspace disease
3. Tumors and other mass lesions
4. Asthma
5. Pleural effusion
6. Lung infarction

A mismatched defect? (List 4)	1. PE 2. Pulmonary artery compression (e.g., tumor, fibrosing mediastinitis) 3. Radiation therapy 4. Vasculitis
A reverse mismatched defect? (List 3)	1. Pneumonia 2. Alveolar pulmonary edema 3. Mucus plugging
What is the physiologic significance of a reverse mismatch?	It represents a functional right-to-left shunt, which may lead to clinically significant hypoxia.
List 3 causes of V/Q mismatch that involve the entire lung.	Tumor causing compression of pulmonary artery, fibrosing mediastinitis, PE
What is the generally accepted terminology for describing V/Q mismatches?	Small defect: Less than 25% of a segment Moderate defect: 25%–75% of a segment Large defect: More than 75% of a segment

PATHOLOGY

How can one approach interpreting diffuse (interstitial, alveolar, or mixed) lung shadows?	Determine the answers to the following questions: Is the process acute or chronic? Is the patient immunocompromised? What type of pattern is noted (nodular, reticular, or reticulonodular)? Is there miliary or diffuse airspace disease? What is the zonal predominance? Is there a known primary tumor? Is there adenopathy? Are there effusions? Are there septal lines or bronchial wall thickening?
What are the differential diagnoses for acute pulmonary infiltrates?	**I HEAD** toward the diagnosis. **m** Infection (viral pneumonia, PCP, tuberculosis) Hemorrhage (anticoagulant therapy, trauma, Goodpasture's syndrome, leukemia, bone marrow transplant) Edema (cardiogenic or noncardiogenic)

Adult respiratory distress syndrome (ARDS) or aspiration
Drug reaction (nitrofurantoin)

What does airspace disease look like on a CXR?

Amorphous inhomogeneous areas of opacity without evidence of volume loss; air bronchograms are diagnostic

List 5 substances that can fill the alveolar spaces in disease and give examples of situations where this may occur.

Water: CHF, neurogenic edema, ARDS
Blood: Contusion, Goodpasture's syndrome
Pus: Bacterial pneumonia, tuberculosis
Proteinaceous fluid: alveolar proteinosis
Cells: bronchoalveolar cell carcinoma, lymphoma

What are the differential diagnoses for:

Diffuse shadows with Kerley B lines? (List 5)

Pulmonary edema, lymphangitis carcinomatosa, pneumoconiosis, sarcoidosis, idiopathic pulmonary fibrosis (IPF)

Diffuse shadows with adenopathy? (List 6)

1. Sarcoidosis
2. Silicosis
3. Lymphangitis carcinomatosa
4. Infection (tuberculosis or histoplasmosis)
5. Metastases
6. Lymphoma

Localized airspace disease? (List 11)

1. Pneumonia
2. Atelectasis
3. Infarction or hemorrhage associated with PE
4. Pulmonary contusion
5. Collagen vascular disease or vasculitis
6. Drug and allergic reactions
7. Neoplasm
8. Radiation pneumonitis
9. Eosinophilic pneumonia, usually multifocal
10. Amyloidosis
11. Bronchiolitis obliterans, organizing pneumonia (BOOP)

Unilateral white out? (List 8)

1. Massive pleural effusion with underlying lung collapse

2. Pneumonia with total consolidation
   (look for air bronchograms)
3. Massive tumor
4. Total lung collapse
5. Pneumonectomy
6. Unilateral pulmonary edema
7. Massive aspiration
8. Agenesis of the lung

What does interstitial disease generally look like radiographically?

An architectural pattern of lines and nodules that is more structured than that seen in alveolar disease

What are the radiologic types of interstitial lung disease?

Miliary: Tiny nodular densities, 2–3 mm in diameter
Reticular: A net-like pattern of intersecting lines
Nodular: Nodular densities, 3–10 mm in diameter
Reticulonodular: A combination of reticular and nodular shadowing

What are the differential diagnoses for:

An upper zone-predominant reticulonodular pattern? (List 5)

PAGES
Pneumoconioses
Allergic alveolitis or **A**nkylosing spondylitis
Granulomatous disease (most common cause)
Eosinophilic granuloma
Sarcoidosis

m

A lower zone-predominant reticulonodular pattern? (List 3)

CIA
Connective tissue disease, especially scleroderma
Idiopathic (most common)
Asbestosis

m

What characterizes "end-stage lung"?

A honeycomb pattern of dense interstitial fibrosis and multiple cysts seen in many diffuse diseases (e.g., sarcoidosis, silicosis, IPF)

List 7 causes of linear and band-like shadows.

1. Skin fold
2. Clothing or tubes
3. Bleb or pneumatocele wall

4. Pleuroparenchymal scar
5. Discoid, linear, or plate-like atelectasis
6. Anomalous blood vessels
7. Thickened fissures

List 8 factors that can cause hyperlucency of a lung.

1. Rotation of the patient
2. Pneumothorax
3. Emphysema
4. Mastectomy
5. Contralateral effusion on a supine film
6. Ipsilateral lobar collapse
7. PE
8. Congenitally absent pectoralis muscle

List 5 causes of localized increases in radiolucency.

Compensatory emphysema secondary to lobar excision or collapse, pneumothorax, less soft tissue (e.g., mastectomy), COPD, PE

ATELECTASIS

What causes atelectasis?

Bronchial obstruction (e.g., by tumor, mucus, or a foreign body) with resorption of air behind the obstruction; pressure from masses or pleural fluid

What are the radiologic signs of atelectasis?

Rapidly appearing (and disappearing) opacification of part or all of a lung with evidence of volume loss (e.g., displacement of fissures, the diaphragm, or the mediastinum). Diaphragm elevation and mediastinal shift only occur with severe atelectasis.

What is linear, discoid, or plate-like atelectasis?

Horizontal or oblique opacified bands of volume loss in the lungs, often visible in two projections and often transient

How can atelectasis be distinguished from pneumonia?

Atelectasis is frequently linear and may change rapidly, and is most often seen in the lower lobes. Pneumonia is patchy with an irregular shape; segmental or lobar consolidation may be seen, and air bronchograms are common.

Why is it sometimes impossible to differentiate atelectasis from pneumonia?

An atelectatic lung can have the same radiographic density as a consolidated lung. Atelectasis and pneumonia may also coexist, particularly at the lung bases.

What are the radiographic signs of lobar collapse?

HE DROVE ME to lobar collapse.
Hilar displacement
Elevated hemidiaphragm
Displaced fissure
Rib crowding
Opacity of lung tissue
Vascular and bronchial stretching in noncollapsed lobes
Emphysema (compensation in noncollapsed lobes)
MEdiastinal shift

For each set of views, identify which lobe is collapsed:

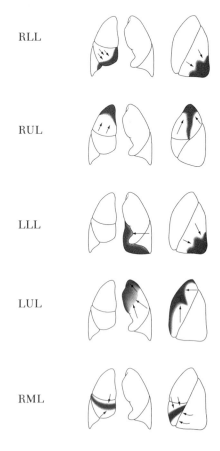

RLL

RUL

LLL

LUL

RML

How can one confirm the diagnosis of lobar collapse using CT?	Carefully follow the bronchus into the collapsed lobe; "cut off" suggests lobar collapse. Fluid-filled, distended bronchi beyond an obstruction may be noted.
Do air bronchograms in an opacity completely rule out atelectasis?	Not entirely. The mucus plugging may be peripheral or the atelectasis may be compressive due to a pleural effusion.

PULMONARY EDEMA

What are the two basic types of pulmonary edema?	Cardiogenic edema, caused by increased hydrostatic pulmonary capillary pressure
	Noncardiogenic edema, caused by either altered capillary membrane permeability or decreased plasma oncotic pressure
What are the causes of noncardiogenic pulmonary edema?	**NOT CARDIAC** **m** **N**ear-drowning **O**xygen therapy **T**ransfusion or **T**rauma (fat embolism) **C**entral nervous system (CNS) disorder **A**RDS, **A**spiration, or **A**ltitude sickness **R**enal disorder or **R**esuscitation **D**rugs (e.g., narcotics, salicylates, tricyclic antidepressants) **I**nhaled toxins (e.g., smoke, toxic gas) **A**llergic alveolitis **C**ontrast (intravenous) or **C**ontusion
What does cardiogenic pulmonary edema look like on CXR?	Cephalization of pulmonary vessels, Kerley B lines or septal lines, peribronchial cuffing, "bat wing" pattern, patchy shadowing with air bronchograms, increased cardiac size
What are some atypical patterns of cardiac pulmonary edema, and when are they most often seen?	Unilateral edema, miliary edema, and lobar or lower zone edema are atypical patterns of cardiac pulmonary edema. A unilateral pattern may be caused by lying preferentially on the right side. Miliary edema is probably a transitory phase in the development of full-scale edema. Lobar or lower zone edema may be found in patients with COPD who have predominant upper lobe emphysema.

PULMONARY NODULES

What findings indicate a benign pulmonary nodule on CXR?	Slow growth (if no growth in 2 years, the nodule is almost always benign) and calcification (central, laminated, or diffuse calcification is typical for a granuloma)

What are the differential diagnoses for a:

Solitary pulmonary nodule? (List 10)

1. Granuloma caused by fungal infection (e.g., histoplasmosis) or tuberculosis
2. Primary carcinoma
3. Abscess
4. Hamartoma (popcorn calcification is virtually diagnostic)
5. Solitary metastasis (colon, breast, kidney, ovary, or testis most common)
6. Sequestration
7. Arteriovenous malformation (AVM); usually single (if multiple, consider Osler-Weber-Rendu disease)
8. Fluid in an interlobar fissure
9. Pleural plaques
10. Skin lesion (e.g., nipple shadow, mole, lipoma)

Solitary pulmonary mass larger than 4 cm in diameter? (List 12)

1. Bronchial carcinoma
2. Metastasis
3. Lung abscess
4. Lymphoma
5. Round pneumonia
6. Round atelectasis
7. Sequestration
8. Blastomycosis or actinomycosis
9. Wegener's granulomatosis
10. Hydatid cyst
11. Amyloid
12. Sarcoid

Large nodular shadows ("cannonballs") in the lungs? (List 7)

1. Metastases
2. Abscesses or septic emboli
3. Wegener's granulomatosis
4. Granulomas (e.g., histoplasmosis or tuberculosis)
5. Necrobiotic nodules (in patients with rheumatoid arthritis)
6. Multiple hydatid cysts
7. Amyloid

Cavitary masses? (List 6)

CAVITY

Cancer (i.e., bronchial carcinoma, especially squamous cell carcinoma, metastasis, and lymphoma)

Autoimmune disease (e.g., rheumatoid arthritis, Wegener's granulomatosis)

Vascular disorders (e.g., pulmonary infarct)

Infection (e.g., staphylococcal or Gram-negative pneumonia, lung abscess, septic emboli, tuberculosis)

Trauma

Youth (i.e., congenital disorders, such as sequestration or cyst)

Miliary nodules? (List 7)

1. Tuberculosis, usually uniform distribution
2. Fungal infection (e.g., blastomycosis, histoplasmosis, cryptococcus, coccidioidomycosis)
3. BOOP
4. Silicosis or coal miner's pneumoconiosis
5. Sarcoidosis
6. Metastases (e.g., thyroid tumors, melanoma, gastrointestinal tumors)
7. Eosinophilic granuloma of the lung

ADULT RESPIRATORY DISTRESS SYNDROME (ARDS)

List 13 factors that put a patient at risk for developing ARDS.

1. Inhalation of toxins (e.g., smoke) and oxygen therapy
2. Sepsis (bacterial and viral pneumonia, Gram-negative septicemia)
3. Aspiration of gastric contents or hydrocarbons
4. Major surgery, especially cardiopulmonary bypass surgery
5. Metabolic disorders (e.g., acute pancreatitis, diabetic ketoacidosis, uremia)
6. Disseminated intravascular coagulation (DIC)
7. Trauma
8. Burns
9. Bowel infarction

10. Drugs (e.g., heroin, salicylates, ethchlorvynol, chemotherapy)
11. Blood transfusion
12. Hemodynamic shock
13. Fat embolism

How does ARDS develop radiographically?

Radiographic changes become apparent approximately 12 hours after the onset of symptoms and include bilateral, wide-spread, ill-defined densities that become confluent and occur in all lung zones.

What is the pulmonary wedge pressure in a patient with ARDS?

The pulmonary wedge pressure is normal or only mildly elevated.

List 5 complications of ARDS.

Multiple organ failure, septicemia, pneumonia, barotrauma, pulmonary fibrosis

How is cardiac pulmonary edema or fluid overload differentiated from ARDS on CXR?

In general, ARDS is not associated with cardiomegaly, cephalization, or pleural effusion, all of which are seen in patients with pulmonary edema.

HILAR ADENOPATHY

What distinguishes hilar adenopathy from pulmonary artery enlargement?

Lymphadenopathy has a "lumpy-bumpy" appearance. An enlarged pulmonary artery has a smooth appearance and appears larger than the bronchus intermedius in the RLL.

List 3 common causes of hilar lymphadenopathy.

1. Inflammation (e.g., sarcoidosis, silicosis)
2. Neoplasm (e.g., lymphoma, metastases, leukemia, bronchogenic carcinoma)
3. Infection (e.g., tuberculosis, infectious mononucleosis, histoplasmosis)

List 5 causes of eggshell calcification of the hilar and mediastinal lymph nodes.

Pneumoconioses (e.g., silicosis), sarcoidosis, granulomatous disease (e.g., histoplasmosis, tuberculosis), treated lymphoma, amyloidosis

List 4 causes of unilateral enlargement of the hilar lymph nodes.

Bronchogenic carcinoma, metastases, lymphoma, infection (especially tuberculosis and histoplasmosis)

What can cause markedly enhancing hilar lymph- adenopathy on CT?	Diseases that are very vascular (e.g., metastatic thyroid, renal cell, or small cell carcinoma; Castleman's disease)

DISORDERS OF THE PLEURA

PLEURAL EFFUSION

List 7 common causes of pleural effusion.	1. CHF (usually bilateral) 2. Tumor 3. Infection (parapneumonic or tubercular) 4. Autoimmune disease [e.g., rheumatoid arthritis, systemic lupus erythematosus (SLE)] 5. Renal failure 6. Trauma 7. PE
What are the signs of a pleural effusion on a CXR taken while the patient is:	
Upright?	Blunting of the lateral and posterior costophrenic sulci; large effusions cause mediastinal shift away from the effusion and can completely opacify the hemithorax
Supine?	A graded haze, more dense at the base, that veils the lung tissue; a fluid cap over the apex; fissural thickening
What is the minimum amount of fluid needed to detect a pleural effusion on a lateral film and a frontal film, respectively?	75 ml and 200 ml
What are the radiologic signs of a loculated pleural effusion along the chest wall?	The fluid fails to move with a change in position and appears as a dome-shaped projection into the lung.

How can a pleural effusion in a bedridden patient be confirmed?

By obtaining a lateral decubitus film with the patient lying on the side of the suspected effusion. Fluid will "layer out" along the chest wall, unless the fluid is loculated. (arrows)

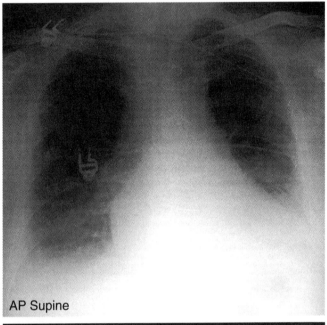

AP Supine

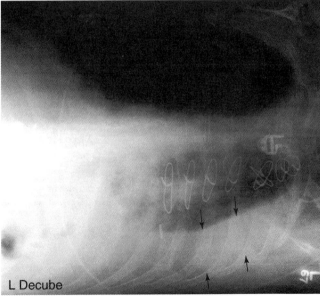

L Decube

List 4 ways ultrasound is helpful in the evaluation and management of pleural fluid.

1. Distinguishes fluid from solid pleural processes
2. Identifies fluid in unusual sites (e.g., a subpulmonic location)
3. Localizes fluid and masses for aspiration or biopsy
4. Identifies septations better than CT

EMPYEMA

What is an empyema?

Suppurative inflammation of the pleural space

Which one of the following CT scans shows an abscess, and which shows an empyema?

A is the empyema. It has a lenticular shape and smooth, uniform walls formed by the thickened pleura, which seems to split around the empyema (i.e., the "split pleura" sign). The adjacent lung tissue is compressed.

B is the lung abscess. It has a spherical shape and thick, irregular walls, often containing air bubbles. The adjacent lung tissue is less compressed; the abscess may be surrounded by airspace disease.

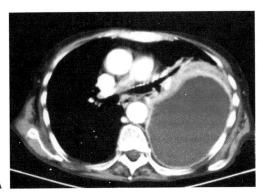

A

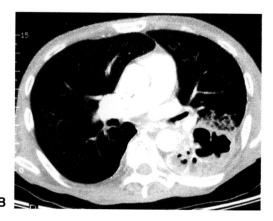

B

Why is it important to distinguish an empyema from a lung abscess?	Treatment for the two conditions differs. Empyemas are drained by a catheter or surgical decortication, whereas abscesses may resolve with antibiotic treatment.

PNEUMOTHORAX

What is a spontaneous pneumothorax?	A pneumothorax occurring without any obvious inciting cause
List 8 causes of spontaneous pneumothorax.	1. Idiopathic (often associated with a long, slender build) 2. COPD or asthma 3. Pulmonary infection (e.g., bacterial pneumonia, tuberculosis, PCP) 4. Neoplasms, particularly primary lung cancer and metastatic osteosarcoma 5. Diseases causing "honeycomb lung" (e.g., sarcoidosis, eosinophilic granuloma of the lung) 6. Marfan's syndrome 7. Catamenial pneumothorax (i.e., a recurrent pneumothorax related to menses caused by endometriosis of the pleura; right lung affected more often than the left) 8. Smoking cocaine (i.e., "crack")
What is the radiographic appearance of a pneumothorax?	Air without lung markings is seen outside the white pleural line (i.e., a distinct pencil-like line seen when the lung is normally aerated)
Where is a pneumothorax best seen on an upright CXR?	In the apices of the thorax

How can a pneumothorax be made more visible on CXR?

A film taken in full expiration can make a subtle pneumothorax more obvious.

Pneumothoraces can be difficult to appreciate on supine CXRs. What subtle signs do you look for?

Hyperlucency in the lung bases, especially at the heart border (*horizontal arrows*)

The "double diaphragm" sign (*vertical arrows*)

The "deep sulcus" sign (i.e., deepening of the costophrenic angle caused by air collecting in a subpulmonic location), indicated by the *D*

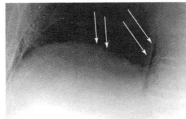

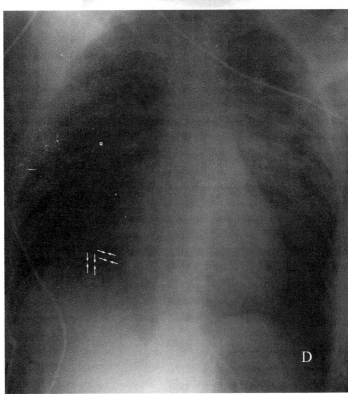

Which type of pneumo-thorax is most likely to be missed on a supine CXR?	An anterior pneumothorax can be invisible.
What should you do if you suspect an anterior pneumothorax?	Obtain a lateral decubitus film with the affected side up. CT is also extremely reliable.
What finding is often confused with a pneumo-thorax?	Overlying skin folds. A skin fold has white shading on its inner margin and is not a distinct line. A pneumothorax has a white pleural line.
What is a hydropneumo-thorax?	Air and fluid in the pleural space; characterized by an air-fluid level on upright or decubitus CXR in a patient with a pneumothorax
List 5 causes of a hydro-pneumothorax.	Trauma, thoracentesis, surgery, ruptured esophagus, empyema

PLEURAL MASS

List 5 differential diagnoses for multiple pleural densities.	1. Metastases, especially adenocarcinoma and malignant thymoma (can spread along pleural surfaces) 2. Loculated pleural effusions (pseudotumor) 3. Malignant mesothelioma (unilateral densities) 4. Pleural plaques from asbestosis (bilateral densities) 5. Lymphoma
List 4 differential diagnoses for an extrapleural mass.	1. Rib tumor (e.g., metastases, myeloma, Ewing's sarcoma, fibrous dysplasia, osteosarcoma) 2. Rib infection, including chest wall fungal infection 3. Neurofibroma or schwannoma (may erode a rib, but does not destroy it) 4. Lipoma
How can a pleural process be differentiated from an extrapleural process?	Differentiation can be difficult. If the center of the lesion is inside the chest wall, a pleural process is likely. Rib destruction indicates extrapleural extension and possibly the origin of the mass.

List 4 causes of pleural calcification.

I **HATE** pleural calcification.
Hemothorax (previous)
Asbestos exposure
Tuberculosis (previous)
Empyema (previous)

m

DISORDERS OF THE MEDIASTINUM

PNEUMOMEDIASTINUM

List 7 causes of pneumo-mediastinum.

1. Asthma
2. Surgery (postoperative complication)
3. Traumatic tracheobronchial rupture
4. Abrupt changes in intrathoracic pressure, such as those caused by vomiting, coughing, strenuous exercise, or parturition
5. Ruptured esophagus
6. Barotrauma
7. Smoking cocaine (i.e., "crack")

Describe 3 radiographic findings in a patient with pneumomediastinum.

1. Streaky lucencies over the mediastinum that extend into the neck
2. "Continuous diaphragm" sign
3. Elevation of the parietal pleura along the mediastinal borders

ACUTE MEDIASTINITIS

List 3 causes of acute mediastinitis.

1. Surgery (postoperative complication)
2. Infection from the cervical region
3. Spontaneous esophageal rupture (Boerhaave's syndrome)

What are the radiologic manifestations of acute mediastinitis?

CXRs and CT scans show mediastinal widening, pneumomediastinum, diffuse tissue infiltration and abscess formation, and pleural effusions

What are the clinical and radiographic features of Boerhaave's syndrome?

Clinical signs include the sudden onset of severe chest pain following forceful vomiting. Radiographs may show pneumomediastinum and a pleural effusion, with the left lung affected more often than the right.

MEDIASTINAL MASS

List the "4 Ts" that can cause an anterior mediastinal mass.	**4 Ts** Terrible lymphadenopathy, notably Hodgkin's lymphoma Thymic tumors Teratoma (germ cell tumors) Thyroid mass
List 3 more differential diagnoses for an anterior mediastinal mass.	Aortic aneurysm, pericardial cyst, epicardial fat pad
What is the best method for diagnosing an anterior mediastinal mass?	CT is usually required to diagnose an anterior mass. In many patients, fine needle aspiration is necessary for definitive diagnosis.
List the 7 thymic tumors.	1. Thymoma 2. Thymic carcinoma 3. Thymolipoma 4. Thymic cyst 5. Thymic lymphoma 6. Thymic carcinoid 7. Thymic hyperplasia
Which thymic tumor is most common?	Thymoma
What percentage of thymomas are malignant?	15%–40%
What percentage of patients with myasthenia gravis have thymomas?	10%–23%
What percentage of patients with thymoma have myasthenia gravis?	35%–40%
What is a teratoma?	A neoplasm derived from a multipotent primitive germ cell
What is the radiographic appearance of a teratoma?	A rounded mass that grows slowly and contains fat and calcified areas

List 6 causes of a middle mediastinal mass.

1. Lymphadenopathy caused by sarcoidosis, lymphoma, infection, or neoplasm
2. Primary neoplasm
3. Hiatal hernia, usually near the gastroesophageal junction
4. Aortic aneurysm
5. Thyroid mass extending down from the neck
6. Bronchogenic cyst, usually near the carina

List 8 differential diagnoses for a cardiophrenic angle mass.

1. Epicardial fat pad
2. Pericardial cyst
3. Lymph node
4. Anterior mediastinal mass
5. Left ventricular aneurysm (left) or aortic aneurysm (right)
6. Adjacent lung or pleural tumor
7. Dilated right atrium
8. Diaphragmatic (Morgagni's) hernia

List 6 differential diagnoses for a posterior mediastinal mass.

1. Neoplasms (e.g., neurogenic tumors, spinal tumors, lymphoma)
2. Lymphadenopathy
3. Aortic aneurysm
4. Adjacent pleural or lung mass
5. Neurenteric cyst or lateral meningocele
6. Extramedullary hematopoiesis

List 7 neurogenic tumors that are found in the chest.

1. Ganglioneuroma
2. Neuroblastoma
3. Ganglioneuroblastoma
4. Neurofibroma
5. Schwannoma
6. Paraganglioma
7. Pheochromocytoma

DISORDERS OF THE LUNG

LUNG CANCER

According to the TNM staging criteria for lung cancer, which tumors are unresectable?

T_4, N_3, and M_1 tumors

Describe the criteria for each of these stages.

T_4: Invasion of the mediastinum or involvement of the heart, great vessels, trachea, esophagus, vertebral body, or carina; or neoplasia associated with a malignant pleural or pericardial effusion, or satellite nodules in the same lobe

N_3: Metastasis to contralateral mediastinal and hilar nodes, ipsilateral or contralateral scalene or supraclavicular nodes

M_1: Distant metastasis present

On a CT scan, how large must a lymph node measure to be considered lymphadenopathy (pathologic)?

A lymph node that measures 1 cm across the short axis is at the lower limit of abnormal (sensitivity 95%, specificity 70%).

Identify the nodal stations as classified by the American Thoracic Society.

A = Right upper paratracheal
B = Left upper paratracheal
C = Right lower paratracheal
D = Right intrapulmonary
E = Right tracheobronchial
F = Left lower paratracheal
G = Aortopulmonary
H = Paraesophageal
I = Subcarinal
J = Left tracheobronchial
K = Left intrapulmonary
L = Diaphragmatic

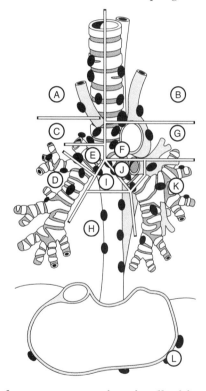

What divides the upper paratracheal nodes from the lower ones?

The "take-off" of the great vessels

Name the 6 types of primary lung carcinomas and the prevalence of each.

1. Adenocarcinoma: 35%–50%
2. Squamous cell carcinoma: 30%
3. Small cell: 15%–20%
4. Large cell: 10%–15%
5. Bronchoalveolar: 3%
6. Carcinoid: Less than 1%

What is a carcinoid tumor?	A tumor derived from a neuroendocrine precursor cell

Describe the radiographic appearance of each of the following lung cancers:

Adenocarcinoma	Peripheral, sometimes associated with scars, high incidence of early metastases
Squamous cell carcinoma	Central with hilar involvement, cavitation common, slow growing
Small cell carcinoma	Central, cavitation rare, hilar and mediastinal masses often the dominant feature, rapid growth and early metastases
Large cell carcinoma	Peripheral, large, cavitation present
Bronchoalveolar carcinoma	Peripheral, rounded appearance, pneumonia-like infiltrate (air bronchograms), occasionally multifocal
Carcinoid	Typically a well-defined endobronchial lesion; nodal, liver and brain metastases may enhance densely (i.e., they may be hypervascular)
What is a Pancoast (superior sulcus) tumor?	Apical bronchogenic carcinoma most often associated with squamous cell carcinoma that causes Horner's syndrome and ipsilateral hand atrophy or pain owing to brachial plexus invasion
What is SVC syndrome?	Brawny edema of the upper extremity, face, and neck caused by obstruction of the SVC; the classic clinical finding is venous distention that is not relieved by elevation
List 2 causes of SVC syndrome.	Tumor (especially small cell bronchogenic carcinoma) and fibrosing mediastinitis
What is fibrosing mediastinitis?	A progressive fibrotic reaction that results in adherence of mediastinal structures to each other, fibrosis, and narrowing of the great vessels; most often associated with histoplasmosis

List 11 of the paraneoplastic syndromes seen with bronchogenic carcinoma.

1. Cushing's syndrome
2. Syndrome of inappropriate antidiuretic hormone (SIADH)
3. Carcinoid syndrome
4. Hypercalcemia
5. Hypoglycemia
6. Neuromyopathies
7. Clubbing
8. Pulmonary hypertrophic osteoarthropathy
9. Anemia
10. Acanthosis nigricans
11. Thrombophlebitis

With what type of lung cancer are paraneoplastic syndromes most often associated?

Small cell carcinoma

What cell type is associated with hypercalcemia?

Squamous cell carcinoma

List 8 types of tumors that can metastasize to the lung.

1. Female reproductive (e.g., breast, uterine, choriocarcinoma)
2. Male reproductive (e.g., prostate, testicular)
3. Gastrointestinal
4. Renal
5. Lung
6. Skin (i.e., melanoma)
7. Bone (e.g., osteosarcoma, Ewing's sarcoma)
8. Head and neck (e.g., thyroid)

List 4 extrathoracic primary tumors that commonly metastasize to the ribs.

Breast, prostate, kidney, thyroid

What is lymphangitis carcinomatosa?

Neoplastic spread into the pulmonary lymphatics

List 6 types of tumors that commonly spread in this manner.

Bronchial, breast, pancreatic, gastric, colon, prostatic

What are some of the intrathoracic manifestations of lymphoma?	Adenopathy, diffuse pulmonary infiltration, pulmonary masses, pleural involvement with nodules and effusions

INFECTION

Pneumonia and pneumonitis

What are the radiographic features of a broncho-pneumonia?	Patchy airspace disease in a lobar or greater distribution, may be associated with volume loss
What are the radiographic features of a lobar pneu-monia?	Patchy airspace opacity that is often progressive, with coalescence leading to sublobar or lobar consolidation; air bronchograms and cavitation; parapneumonic pleural effusion
What type of pneumonia commonly causes consol-idation of an entire lobe?	Bacterial pneumonia, especially that caused by *Streptococcus pneumoniae*
What is "round pneumonia"?	An infiltrate that looks remarkably like a lung mass
Name the 2 atypical pneumonias.	Viral and mycoplasmal
Can viral pneumonias be differentiated from other pneumonias on the basis of the CXR findings?	No.
In an upright patient with aspiration pneumonia, which lobes are most commonly affected?	The posterior segments of the upper and lower lobes, usually bilateral or right-sided
When is pneumonia asso-ciated with volume loss in a lobe?	A minor degree of volume loss is not infrequent in a lobar consolidation.
When does radiographic clearing take place follow-ing treatment for pneumo-nia in:	
Otherwise healthy patients?	6–8 weeks

Older, debilitated patients or patients with COPD?	2–3 months
When is hilar adenopathy usually seen on plain films in adults with pneumonia?	In patients with tuberculosis, a fungal infection, or a neglected lung abscess (rare)
List 4 of the most common causes of pneumonia characterized by consolidation and cavitation.	*Staphylococcus aureus*, gram-negative bacteria (*Klebsiella*, *Pseudomonas*), anaerobic bacteria, *Mycobacterium tuberculosis*
List 3 causes of a lung abscess.	Aspiration, infection beyond an obstructing lesion, septic emboli (particularly in drug addicts)
List 4 of the most common causes of septic emboli.	Infected venous catheters, endocarditis or septic thrombophlebitis (especially in intravenous drug abusers), indwelling prosthetic devices
What are the radiographic and CT findings in a patient with septic emboli?	Multiple pulmonary nodules (of any size) that frequently cavitate Feeding vessel to the nodule (commonly found on CT) Pleural effusions and empyemas are also common

Tuberculosis and mycobacterial infection

How does one acquire pulmonary tuberculosis?	Inhalation of droplets containing *M. tuberculosis*
What is primary tuberculosis?	Pulmonary infection without prior exposure
What is post-primary tuberculosis?	Reactivation of a focus of primary tuberculosis, or continuation of initial infection
What percentage of patients with primary tuberculosis develop the post-primary form without any latent interval?	10%
What is this form of the disease called?	Progressive primary tuberculosis
What are the radiographic features of primary tuberculosis?	Infiltrate, consolidation, adenopathy (less common in adults), pleural effusion

What is a Ghon focus?

An area of consolidation in a patient with primary tuberculosis

Does a Ghon focus have a preferred lobe or zone?

Any portion of the lung may be involved because tuberculosis is caused by inhaling infectious material; however, statistically, Ghon foci are more common in the mid- and lower lung zones.

What is a Ghon (Ranke) complex?

A Ghon focus plus hilar adenopathy

List 5 radiographic features of post-primary tuberculosis.

1. Focal patchy infiltrates or "cotton wool" shadows
2. Cavitation (single or multiple), fluid levels in cavities are unusual
3. Fibrosis
4. Nodal calcification
5. Calcific flecks of caseous material

Post-primary tuberculosis has a predilection for which areas of the lung?

Favored sites are the apical and posterior segments of the upper lobes and the superior segments of the lower lobes.

List 3 radiographic findings that suggest active disease.

Cavitation, fresh "cotton wool" shadows, pleural effusions

Can tuberculosis cause lobar pneumonia?

Yes

How does pulmonary tuberculosis disseminate and what is the result?

Hematogenously, leading to miliary tuberculosis or involvement of other organ systems
Via the airways, leading to tuberculous bronchopulmonary pneumonia
Via extension into the pleura, leading to tuberculous pleurisy

Can tuberculous pleural effusions exist as an isolated entity?

Yes, but they are usually associated with evidence of upper zone tuberculosis.

How does reactivation tuberculosis in HIV-positive patients differ from the classic description?

It resembles primary tuberculosis

What is endobronchial tuberculosis?

Tuberculosis involving the wall of a major bronchus

What complications are associated with endobronchial tuberculosis?	Cicatricial stenosis and obstruction
What is a broncholith?	A calcified nodal mass associated with histoplasmosis or tuberculosis that erodes into a major bronchus; may be coughed out
What complications are associated with a broncholith?	Obstruction and hemoptysis

Does the CXR show tuberculous involvement when tuberculosis affects the:

Kidneys?	Possibly (CXR may be normal, but in 10%–15% of patients shows evidence of old pulmonary tuberculosis, and in fewer than 5% shows evidence of active pulmonary tuberculosis)
Bones?	Possibly (CXR normal in 50% of patients with active pulmonary tuberculosis)
Gastrointestinal tract?	Possibly, but in most patients with tubercular involvement of the gastrointestinal tract, there is no evidence of active pulmonary tuberculosis on CXR
Brain and meninges?	Usually abnormal (CXR shows signs of active or old pulmonary tuberculosis in 60% of patients)
What are the radiographic features of atypical mycobacterial infections of the lung?	Often indistinguishable from classic tuberculosis; disease may be slowly progressive and resistant to standard therapy
Name 5 of the most common atypical mycobacteria associated with lung disease.	*Mycobacterium avium-intracellulare, Mycobacterium kansasii, Mycobacterium fortuitum, Mycobacterium xenopi, Mycobacterium simiae*

Mycoses (fungal infections)

What causes histoplasmosis and how is it transmitted?	Histoplasmosis is caused by inhalation of aerosolized bird or bat droppings that contain the fungus *Histoplasma capsulatum*.

What symptoms are associated with histoplasmosis?

Most cases are asymptomatic.

What radiologic findings are initially seen in typical histoplasmosis?

A single or several isolated peripheral areas of consolidation, lymphadenopathy (rare)

What are the results of infection seen on later CXR?

Granulomas (i.e., single or multiple calcified foci), lymphadenopathy (often calcified), histoplasmomas (i.e., well-defined spherical nodules), nodules with concentric laminated calcification (specific for histoplasmosis)

List 3 types of pulmonary aspergillosis.

Acute bronchopulmonary aspergillosis (ABPA), semi-invasive aspergillosis (mycetoma), invasive aspergillosis

What is ABPA and what are the associated CXR findings?

In patients with atopic asthma, the central bronchi may become plugged with mucus and *Aspergillus.* Secondary bronchiectasis may result. Dilated, plugged bronchi are seen as opacities extending from a hilum into a portion of the lung ("gloved finger" sign).

What are the clinical and radiologic features of blastomycosis?

Patients are often asymptomatic but may have cough, fever, dyspnea, chest pain, or papular to raised verrucous skin lesions. Radiographic signs include destructive and proliferative lesions (particularly of the vertebrae and ribs) and unifocal or multifocal consolidation in the lungs, possibly with cavitation and hilar adenopathy.

Where is a patient most likely to contract coccidioidomycosis?

In the southwestern United States and northern Mexico

What are the radiologic features of coccidioidomycosis?

Unifocal or multifocal segmental consolidation; hilar and mediastinal lymphadenopathy and pleural effusions are seen in 25% of patients

What are the radiographic features of nocardiosis?

CXR findings are variable, but unifocal or multifocal large pulmonary consolidations that can cavitate are often seen.

What disease predisposes a patient to nocardiosis?

Alveolar proteinosis

What radiographic features suggest pulmonary actino-mycosis?

The lung lesion is usually a consolidation or cavitary mass, which may cross the pleura to involve adjacent lobes or the chest wall.

Pulmonary infections in immunocompromised patients

List 4 common causes of pneumonia in HIV-infected patients.

PCP, bacterial pathogens, *M. tuberculosis*, fungi

What are the radiographic findings of PCP on CXR?

The CXR may be normal, or bilateral, symmetric, diffuse infiltrates in the parenchyma with a "ground glass" appearance and no zonal predominance may be seen. In the very early stages, the infiltrates look interstitial. A slight perihilar distribution may be detected.

What is the most common fungal pneumonia in patients with AIDS?

Cryptococcosis

What is the most common viral pneumonia in immuno-compromised hosts?

Cytomegalovirus

What are the 2 most common intrathoracic malignancies in patients with AIDS?

Kaposi's sarcoma and non-Hodgkin's lymphoma

Should biopsy be performed to confirm intrapulmonary Kaposi's sarcoma?

No. There is a high risk of bleeding and patients with intrapulmonary Kaposi's sarcoma usually have skin manifestations.

IDIOPATHIC DISEASE

What is alveolar proteinosis?

An idiopathic disease in which proteinaceous material fills the alveoli, causing bilateral, diffuse pulmonary shadowing

What is the classic radiographic appearance of sarcoidosis?

Right paratracheal and bilateral hilar adenopathy

List 5 parenchymal changes seen in patients with sarcoidosis.

1. Reticulonodular infiltrates extending from the hilar regions
2. Alveolar sarcoidosis (i.e., multifocal, ill-defined foci of airspace disease, often associated with obvious hilar adenopathy)
3. Large nodular sarcoidosis
4. Miliary sarcoidosis
5. Severe, coarse fibrosis radiating from the hila, bulla formation, mycetoma formation, and bronchiectasis; suggestive of progression to more severe disease (seen in only 5%–10% of patients)

How is sarcoidosis staged?

Stage 0: Clear chest radiograph
Stage I: Hilar node enlargement only
Stage II: Hilar node enlargement and parenchymal shadowing
Stage III: Parenchymal shadowing alone

What other organs may be affected by sarcoidosis?

Skin, eyes, CNS, salivary glands, liver, spleen, bones

What is BOOP?

Also known as cryptogenic organizing pneumonia (COP), BOOP is a form of pneumonia without a defined cause that is responsive to steroid therapy.

List 4 clinical features of BOOP.

Cough, malaise, mild fever, and elevated erythrocyte sedimentation rate (ESR)

What are the radiographic features of BOOP?

Multifocal, bilateral, patchy peripheral opacities; alternatively, a diffuse pattern of parenchymal infiltration may be seen

List 4 CXR findings in patients with rheumatoid arthritis.

1. Pleural effusions and thickening (common and usually unilateral)
2. Interstitial fibrosis in the bases
3. Necrobiotic nodules (single or multiple nodules up to 5 cm in diameter that may cavitate and are associated with subcutaneous nodules; rare)
4. BOOP

What is Caplan's syndrome?	A syndrome that affects coal miners and is characterized by necrobiotic nodules and rheumatoid arthritis, or detection of rheumatoid factors on laboratory analysis.
What are the findings on CXR in a patient with SLE?	The CXR is usually normal, but pleural effusion and cardiac enlargement (owing to pericardial effusion) may be seen. Rarely, lupoid pneumonia or diffuse interstitial lung disease and fibrosis are noted.
What are the clinical features of Goodpasture's syndrome?	Pulmonary hemorrhage and renal failure or hematuria
What are the radiographic features of Goodpasture's syndrome?	Patchy, ill-defined shadows that are bilateral and symmetric, caused by hemorrhage
What is Wegener's granulomatosis?	Necrotizing granulomatous vasculitis of the entire respiratory tract and kidneys
What radiographic findings are associated with Wegener's granulomatosis?	CXRs reveal single or multiple discrete focal opacities that often show evidence of cavitation.

Sinus CT scans show evidence of diffuse disease, often with bone destruction |
| **What is the prognosis for patients with treated and untreated Wegener's granulomatosis?** | If untreated, the patient usually dies within 5 months of renal failure. If the patient receives treatment with cyclophosphamide and steroids, the 5-year survival rate is 90%–95%. |

PULMONARY VASCULAR DISEASE

Pulmonary embolus (PE) [see also Chapter 5]

Is PE rare?	No. PE occurs commonly, especially in the inpatient setting.
What is the usual source of to the pulmonary arteries?	Thrombus from the deep venous system of the legs

What percentage of pulmonary emboli result in infarction?

10%

What modalities are used to investigate possible PE?

Venous ultrasound [evaluation for deep venous thrombosis (DVT)], V/Q scan, pulmonary arteriogram, CT angiogram (CTA)

What is the purpose of getting a plain chest film when PE is suspected?

To exclude other diagnoses (e.g., pneumothorax, pneumonia, CHF, rib fracture] as the cause of dyspnea or hypoxia

List 6 radiologic signs of PE on CXR.

Although the CXR is often normal, the following may be seen:
1. Westermark's sign (oligemia in area of involvement)
2. Increased size of a hilum (caused by thrombus impaction)
3. Atelectasis with elevation of hemidiaphragm and linear or disk-shaped densities
4. Pleural effusion (usually unilateral, often bloody)
5. Consolidation (multifocal, lower lobe predominance), seen with infarction
6. Hampton's hump

What is the main radiologic feature of pulmonary infarction?

Multifocal consolidation, pleural based, usually in the lower lung fields

What is the risk of a PE in a patient with a normal perfusion scan?

Less than 5% (essentially nil)

What is the finding on V/Q scan most suggestive of PE?

A normal ventilation scan with at least two localized perfusion defects

Does a normal perfusion scan exclude PE?

Yes, a ventilation scan need not be performed in these patients.

How are the results of a V/Q scan reported in patients with suspected PE?

Normal, low (10%) probability, intermediate (40%) probability, or high (90%) probability

What are the modified Prospective Investigation of Pulmonary Embolism Diagnosis (PIOPED) criteria for:

A high probability scan?

Two or more large mismatched segmental defects or any combination of mismatched defects equivalent to two large segmental defects (all moderate and large defects may be added; therefore, two moderate defects equal one large)

Perfusion defect unaccompanied by a radiographic abnormality; if one is present, the perfusion defect must be substantially larger

An intermediate probability scan?

Any combination of large and moderate-sized defects not equal to two large segmental defects

Difficulty categorizing as high or low probability

Failure to meet the stated criteria for high or low probability

A low probability scan?

Nonsegmental perfusion defects

Any perfusion defect accompanied by a substantially larger radiographic abnormality

Matched defects with a normal CXR

Small subsegmental defects

Roughly what percentage of V/Q scans are interpreted as being in the low or intermediate probability range?

Over 50%

Pulmonary arterial hypertension

What are the radiographic signs of pulmonary arterial hypertension?

Enlargement of the central pulmonary arteries (pulmonary artery larger than the accompanying bronchus)

Peripheral pruning of vascularity (i.e., diminished vascularity)

Right ventricular enlargement

List 7 causes of pulmonary arterial hypertension.	1. Left-sided heart failure 2. Left-sided valvular disease 3. Shunt lesions [e.g., atrial septal defect (ASD), ventricular septal defect (VSD)] 4. Chronic lung disease or ventilatory disorders (e.g., sleep apnea) 5. Chronic pulmonary embolic disease 6. Primary or idiopathic disease 7. Obesity

AIRWAY DISEASE

There are three major types of airway obstruction: luminal, mural, and extramural.

List 5 luminal causes of airway obstruction	Mucus plug, primary neoplasm, metastases, foreign body, broncholith
List 5 mural causes of airway obstruction.	Lung cancer, inflammatory stricture secondary to tuberculosis, bronchial rupture, stricture following surgery for airway rupture, tracheomalacia
List 5 extramural causes of airway obstruction.	Adenopathy, mediastinal mass, aortic aneurysm, cardiomegaly, large pleural effusion

Asthma

What are the pathologic changes in asthma?	Lungs are overinflated secondary to mucus plugging, submucosal edema, vascular congestion, and bronchospasm.
What radiographic changes are seen in an acute exacerbation of uncomplicated asthma?	Hyperinflation, bronchial wall thickening, hilar prominence
List 5 complications of asthma that can be detected on a CXR.	Atelectasis, mucoid impaction, pneumothorax, pneumomediastinum, ABPA

Chronic obstructive pulmonary disease (COPD)

What are the two classic clinical descriptions of COPD patients and the radiographic features of each?

"Pink puffer" (oxygen saturation is maintained with no carbon dioxide retention): marked emphysema, small heart, mild pulmonary arterial hypertensive changes

"Blue bloater" (oxygen saturation is not maintained and the patient has marked carbon dioxide retention): enlarged heart, absence of obviously hyperexpanded lungs, pulmonary plethora (pulmonary hypertension and effects of polycythemia)

List 4 signs of emphysema on a CXR.

Hyperinflation (flattened diaphragms, increased AP diameter, and increased retrosternal airspace on the lateral CXR)

Bullae (lucent, air-containing spaces that have no vessels and are not perfused)

Pruning of pulmonary vessels

Pulmonary hypertension

What are the best radiographic predictors of emphysema?

Hyperinflation and bullae

Describe a typical patient with COPD attributed to α_1-antitrypsin deficiency.

Young, nonsmoking patient with a family history of emphysema

What radiographic signs may be seen in this patient?

Lower lung zones involved more often than the upper lung zones (the reverse of the usual situation with smokers)

In patients with emphysema, is there good correlation between the radiographic findings and the pulmonary function tests?

No. Correlation is poor, particularly in patients with mild to moderate disease.

What is the radiographic change associated with chronic bronchitis?

Bronchial wall thickening

Bronchiectasis

What are the clinical symptoms of bronchiectasis?

Persistent cough, copious purulent sputum, recurrent pulmonary infections, fever

List 6 signs of bronchiectasis on the CXR.

There are frequently no changes, particularly in patients with mild cases. Dilated tubular bronchi (which appear as "ring shadows" or "tram lines," depending on the angle), cystic structures, peribronchial thickening, mucus plugging of dilated bronchi, and fibrosis and lung contraction may be seen.

How is bronchiectasis investigated further?

By bronchoscopy, HRCT, or both

List 8 radiographic features of cystic fibrosis

1. Upper lobe predominance
2. Enlarged hilar shadows (owing to reactive nodal hyperplasia and large pulmonary arteries)
3. Cystic cavities with air-fluid levels
4. Fibrosis
5. Bronchiectasis with ring shadows, mucus plugging, and cysts
6. Emphysematous changes
7. Atelectasis and focal infiltration with peribronchial cuffing
8. Pneumothorax

INTERSTITIAL LUNG DISEASE

List 6 of the most common causes of diffuse interstitial pulmonary fibrosis.

1. IPF (more than 50% of cases)
2. Collagen vascular disease
3. Cytotoxic agents and nitrofurantoin
4. Pneumoconioses
5. Radiation
6. Sarcoidosis

What are the clinical findings associated with IPF?

Progressive exertional dyspnea and a nonproductive cough

What are the radiographic findings associated with IPF?

Early disease: Hazy, "ground glass" opacification

Late disease: Volume loss with linear opacities bilaterally, honeycomb lung

What is the prognosis associated with IPF?	Poor. Death usually occurs 3–6 years after diagnosis.
How is IPF treated?	With steroids; occasionally, penicillamine or cytotoxic agents are used as well

INHALATIONAL LUNG DISEASES

Silicosis

Name 4 types of people who are at risk for silicosis by virtue of their professions.	Quarry workers, boiler cleaners, quartz miners, sandblasters

On a CXR, what is the pattern of:

Acute silicosis (silicoproteinosis)?	Patchy scattered opacity
Chronic silicosis?	Bilaterally symmetric nodular infiltrates (5 mm or less in diameter), often with a slight reticular component Maximal involvement of the upper zones, fading to the bases Hilar lymphadenopathy with eggshell calcification
Complicated silicosis?	Progressive massive fibrosis—fibrotic nodules coalesce into areas of dense fibrosis in the upper zones that migrate inward to form hilar masses
Does progressive massive fibrosis occur only on one side or in the lower lung zones?	Not usually.
Does adenopathy occur in silicosis?	Yes, the nodes may also calcify, producing eggshell calcification.

Coal workers' pneumoconiosis

How does coal workers' pneumoconiosis appear on CXR?	Similar to silicosis
Is there a complicated form of coal workers' pneumoconioses?	Yes. Coal workers may develop progressive massive fibrosis.

Asbestosis

What is asbestosis?

Interstitial lung disease that develops in the setting of exposure to asbestos

List 7 radiographic abnormalities related to asbestos exposure.

1. Benign asbestos pleural effusion (most common within 10 years of exposure)
2. Pleural plaque formation (localized areas of pleural thickening, ± calcification)
3. Pleural thickening (may be a sequela of a pleural effusion)
4. Rounded atelectasis (associated with pleural thickening)
5. Pulmonary fibrosis (usually not apparent until at least 20 years after exposure)
6. Malignant mesothelioma
7. Bronchial carcinoma

Which is more common in asbestos-exposed individuals: bronchogenic carcinoma or mesothelioma?

Bronchogenic carcinoma

How many times more likely are smokers than nonsmokers to develop bronchogenic carcinoma following exposure to asbestos?

60–70 times more likely than nonsmoking individuals exposed to asbestos

What are the radiographic features of malignant mesothelioma on CXR?

Circumferential, lobulated pleural masses are usually seen.

How is malignant mesothelioma best assessed?

Using CT

Is the development of a localized fibrous tumor of the pleura (i.e., a benign mesothelioma) associated with asbestos exposure?

No.

Extrinsic allergic alveolitis

What causes extrinsic allergic alveolitis?	Exposure to organic dusts
What are the clinical manifestations of extrinsic allergic alveolitis?	Dry cough, fever, wheezing, and dyspnea shortly after exposure
What are the radiographic manifestations of extrinsic allergic alveolitis?	Radiographic findings may include lower lung-predominant mixed interstitial and alveolar infiltrates; chronic lung damage and fibrosis may be seen following recurrent exposure
Name 5 forms of dust exposure that can cause extrinsic allergic alveolitis.	1. Cotton dust (byssinosis,"Monday morning fever") 2. Moldy hay (farmer's lung) 3. Molds in air conditioners (Pandora's lung) 4. Moldy sugar cane (bagassosis) 5. Protein in pigeon droppings or feathers (bird fancier's lung)

TRAUMA

What are the common forms of traumatic lung injury?	The most common form of lung trauma is simple contusion. More severe injury causes lung shearing and the development of spaces filled with air (i.e., pneumatoceles) or blood (i.e., hematomas).
How is a pneumatocele treated?	No treatment necessary (it usually resolves with time)
What are the findings of pulmonary contusion on CXR?	A diffuse, ill-defined patchy alveolar pattern that often resolves within 48 hours (may be at site of impact or can be contrecoup)
What are the clinical manifestations of fat embolism syndrome?	Hypoxia, petechial rash, altered mental status
What pattern does fat embolism syndrome have on CXR?	ARDS pattern

In a trauma patient, what is the possible significance of fractures of the:

Upper three ribs?

Increased risk of aortic injury (because severe trauma is required to fracture these ribs)

Lower three ribs?

Can be associated with liver or spleen injury

What chest finding is associated with child abuse?

Multiple bilateral rib fractures in various stages of healing

List 5 findings of traumatic aortic rupture on CXR.

1. Widening of the mediastinum (> 8 cm) on an upright PA film
2. Downward displacement of the left main bronchus
3. Displacement of the trachea and esophagus to the right
4. Apical capping
5. Left pleural effusion

What percentage of patients with traumatic rupture have normal CXRs initially?

7%

What is the best method for working up a suspected case of traumatic aortic rupture?

The gold standard is aortography, although CT and CTA are increasingly used as screening tools or even as substitutes for aortography.

What are the CXR signs of diaphragmatic rupture:

On the left side?

Air-containing viscera in the chest, or angling of the nasogastric tube upward into the chest at the gastroesophageal junction

On the right side?

A high diaphragm may be the only indication

Which hemidiaphragm most commonly ruptures?

The left (the liver probably has a protective effect on the right side)

What methods (other than surgical inspection) can be used to diagnose diaphragmatic rupture?

CT, ultrasound, or magnetic resonance imaging (MRI) may show disruption of the diaphragm and can demonstrate viscus or solid organ herniation

List 4 immediate radiographic findings in a burn victim with inhalational injury.

Subglottic edema, diffuse peribronchial infiltration, pulmonary edema, atelectasis

List 5 delayed radiographic findings in the same patient.

Pneumonia, ARDS, barotrauma, atelectasis, fluid overload

What radiographic abnormalities may be seen in foreign body inhalation?

Overinflation (caused by a ball valve effect), atelectasis or pneumonia distal to the obstruction, possibly the foreign object

What percentage of foreign bodies are identifiable on CXR?

5%–15%

What maneuvers can one perform to demonstrate foreign bodies in the airways?

Inspiration-expiration CXRs or bilateral decubitus films may demonstrate air trapping in a lung or lobe. Fluoroscopy of the chest may show a pendulum movement of the heart and mediastinum with breathing (also the result of air trapping in a lung or lobe).

What is the time course for radiographic clearing of massive aspiration of gastric contents?

Aspiration worsens over the first 36 hours and gradually clears over 4–5 days.

What are the radiographic manifestations of near-drowning?

The CXR may be normal, especially in children, if laryngospasm, (i.e., the "diving reflex,") occurs. Otherwise, a pattern of pulmonary edema with "bat wing" shadows is seen. The clinical situation may be complicated by the development of ARDS.

Which lung looks worse immediately after lung transplant—the native or the graft?

The graft looks worse secondary to alveolar and interstitial edema, which clears in 72 hours. This phenomenon is known as the "reimplantation response."

IATROGENIC INJURY

What is the characteristic radiographic feature of pneumonitis secondary to radiation therapy?	The damaged area is usually a strikingly geometric shape confined to the radiation port.

What are the features of the:

Acute phase of radiation pneumonitis?	After 1–6 months, a diffuse haze appears with obscured vascular outlines. Patchy consolidations appear confined to the area of the radiation port.
Chronic (fibrotic) phase of radiation pneumonitis?	The opacities become more linear and structured as they fibrose and condense.

What are the potential pulmonary complications of:

Oral contraceptive use?	Pulmonary thromboembolism
Amiodarone therapy?	Phospholipidosis (i.e., the abnormal accumulation of phospholipids in the lungs), multiple peripheral areas of consolidation on CXR

CONGENITAL DISORDERS

In a patient with chronic pulmonary infections, what radiographic clues would suggest Kartagener's (immotile cilia) syndrome as the diagnosis?	Situs inversus and bronchiectasis
What is pulmonary sequestration?	An area of the lung without a normal connection to a bronchus or pulmonary artery, fed by the systemic arterial system, generally found posteromedially at one of the lung bases, more common on the left side
What are the two types of pulmonary sequestration and their characteristics?	Intralobar: Located within the normal lung and its pleural covering, most common type, usually presents as

recurrent pneumonias or abscesses in young adults, incidence equal in men and women, drains via the pulmonary vein, not associated with other congenital abnormalities

Extralobar: Separate from lung and has its own pleural covering, often discovered incidentally, associated with other congenital abnormalities, four times more common in men than in women, drains via the systemic venous system

PERCUTANEOUS LUNG BIOPSY

What are the relative contraindications for a lung biopsy?	Severe COPD, coagulopathy, contralateral pneumonectomy, inaccessible lesion
What 3 factors are essential prior to biopsy?	Coagulation studies, patient consent, patient cooperation
List 4 potential complications of biopsy.	1. Pneumothorax. Patients with COPD are more likely to have a pneumothorax as a complication of lung biopsy, although pneumothorax occurs in 30% of patients without underlying lung disease who undergo lung biopsy. 10% require a chest tube.
	2. Hemoptysis (rarely significant)
	3. Pulmonary or pleural hemorrhage
	4. Air embolus

4   Cardiac Imaging

Robert A. Pelberg
Jared L. Antevil

ANATOMY

Where are each of the four cardiac chambers found on posterior-anterior (PA) and lateral chest radiographs (CXRs)?

The **right atrium (*RA*)** forms the right heart border on the PA view.

The **right ventricle (*RV*)** is the most anterior chamber. Its borders are not normally seen on the PA view. On the lateral view, the right ventricle lies just behind the sternum.

The **left atrium (*LA*)** is the most posterior and superior chamber. It is nearly midline. The only border seen on a PA view is that of the left atrial appendage at the top of the left cardiac silhouette.

The **left ventricle (*LV*)** forms all of the left heart border below the left atrial appendage on the PA view. On the lateral view, it forms the lower posterior border of the heart.

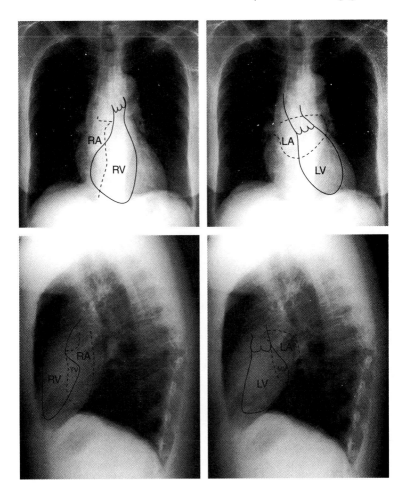

Which cardiac chamber normally forms the right heart border?

The right atrium

Which cardiac chambers contribute to the left heart border?

The left ventricle and the left atrium (i.e., the left atrial appendage)

Which chamber normally forms the anterior heart border?

The right ventricle

Which structures drain into the right atrium?

The superior vena cava (SVC), the inferior vena cava (IVC), and the coronary sinus

How can the structures that drain into the right atrium be identified on a CXR?

SVC: Seen at the right upper mediastinal border, below the right main stem bronchus

IVC: The curvilinear structure at the diaphragm, just behind the heart shadow on a lateral view

Coronary sinus: Cannot be seen on plain film but is visible in the posterior atrioventricular groove on angiography, computed tomography (CT), and magnetic resonance imaging (MRI)

What structures normally drain into the left atrium?

The four pulmonary veins

What is the venous drainage of each lobe of the lungs?

The **right superior pulmonary vein** drains the right upper and middle lobes **(RUL, RML).**

The **right inferior pulmonary vein** drains the right lower lobe **(RLL).**

The **left superior pulmonary vein** drains the left upper lobe **(LUL).**

The **left inferior pulmonary vein** drains the left lower lobe **(LLL).**

How does one identify the pulmonary veins on CXR?

The **superior pulmonary veins** are **diagonally oriented** toward the left atrium.

The **inferior pulmonary veins** are **horizontally oriented** toward the left atrium.

How can the left pulmonary artery be identified on a CXR?

The left pulmonary artery is the second bump after the aortic knob. The left pulmonary artery arches over the left main stem bronchus and then descends posterior to it.

What is the course of the right pulmonary artery?

It passes behind the ascending aorta and bifurcates within the mediastinum. The truncus anterior passes anterior to the RUL bronchus superiorly into the RUL and the right descending pulmonary artery lies lateral to the bronchus intermedius.

What is the upper limit of normal for the transverse diameter of the right descending pulmonary artery?

16 mm

What are the sinuses of Valsalva?

Three small dilatations of the ascending aorta located just above the aortic valve (i.e., the anterior right sinus, the posterior right sinus, and the left sinus)

Which sinuses give rise to the coronary arteries?

The anterior right sinus (R) gives off the right coronary artery (RCA) and the left sinus (L) gives off the left coronary artery (LCA). The posterior right [noncoronary (NC)] sinus does not give off a coronary artery.

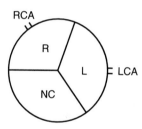

What is the aortic isthmus?

The junction of the aortic arch and the descending aorta, located just distal to the left subclavian artery

What structure runs from the aortic isthmus to the main pulmonary artery?

The ligamentum arteriosum

What embryologic structure gives rise to the ligamentum arteriosum?

The ductus arteriosus

Define the following terms:

Cardiac base

The heart's superior pericardial attachment

Cardiac apex

The tip of the left ventricle

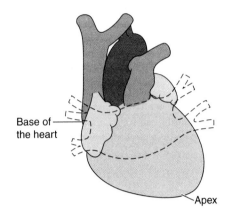

Base of the heart

Apex

What is the name of the groove between the:

Two ventricles?

The interventricular groove

The atria and the ventricles?

The atrioventricular groove

What structures do the interventricular and atrioventricular grooves contain?

The coronary arteries

CORONARY ARTERY ANATOMY

How can the location of the coronary arteries be identified, in all planes of imaging?

Visualize the atrioventricular groove as a circle and the interventricular groove as a loop. You can then use the circle and the loop to place the coronary arteries, regardless of whether the plane of imaging is PA, lateral, left anterior oblique (LAO), or right anterior oblique (RAO).

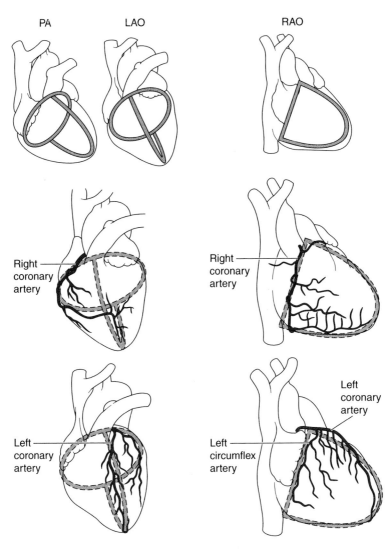

PA   LAO   RAO

Right coronary artery

Right coronary artery

Left coronary artery

Left coronary artery

Left circumflex artery

Left coronary artery

Which artery travels in the right atrioventricular groove?

Right coronary artery

Identify the 7 branches of the right coronary artery on the following LAO and RAO views:

1. Sinoatrial node branch
2. Conus branch
3. Right ventricular (marginal) branches
4. Posterior descending artery
5. Atrioventricular node branch
6. Posterolateral branch
7. Atrial branches

A. LAO view

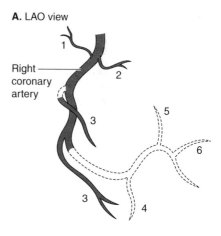

B. RAO view

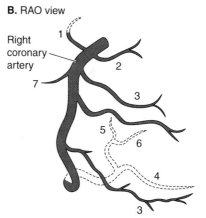

What is meant by "coronary dominance?"

The posterior descending artery supplies the diaphragmatic surface of the left ventricle and the posterior ventricular septum. If the posterior descending artery is a branch of the right coronary artery, as it is in 75% of patients, then the system is "right dominant." If the posterior descending artery is a branch of the left coronary artery, then the system is "left dominant." If the posterior descending artery is supplied by both the right and the left coronary arteries, then the system is "balanced or codominant."

What are the 2 main branches of the left coronary artery?

The left anterior descending artery (anteriorly) and the left circumflex artery (posterolaterally). In some patients, a third branch, the ramus intermedius, arises between the left anterior descending artery and the left circumflex artery.

Identify the segments and branches of the left coronary artery on the following LAO and RAO views:

1. Left anterior descending artery
2. Left circumflex artery
3. Diagonal branches
4. Obtuse marginal branches (to the lateral and posterolateral left ventricle)
5. Septal perforators

A. LAO view

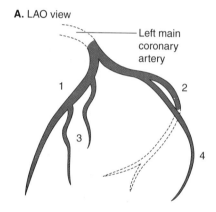

B. RAO view

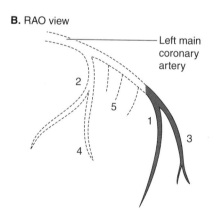

What is the course of the left anterior descending artery?

It courses anteriorly in the anterior interventricular groove.

What is the course of the left circumflex artery?

It runs posteriorly in the atrioventricular groove.

What areas of the myocardium are typically supplied by the:

Right coronary artery?

Inferior wall

Left anterior descending artery?

Anterolateral wall, apex, anterior two thirds of the interventricular septum

Left circumflex artery?

Posterolateral wall

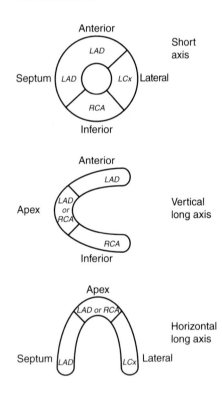

VALVULAR ANATOMY

What approach may be used to understand cardiac valvular anatomy?

Use the same loop and circle approach and place the mitral valve (i.e. the left atrioventricular valve) and the tricuspid valve (i.e., the right atrioventricular valve) in the plane of the circle. Then note that the pulmonic valve is superior and

anterior to the aortic valve and that the
aortic valve is superior and contiguous
with the mitral valve.

A. PA view

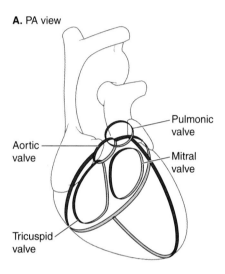

B. Lateral view

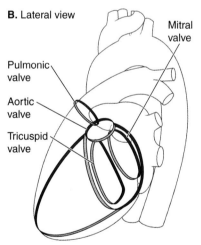

| **How can you distinguish between aortic and mitral valve calcification on a lateral CXR?** | If a line is drawn on the lateral view between the left main bronchus and the sternodiaphragmatic junction, the aortic valve usually lies above the line and the mitral valve below it. |

What is the relationship of the pulmonic valve to the aortic valve?	The pulmonic valve is superior, anterior, and to the left of the aortic valve.
What is the relationship of the mitral and aortic valves?	They are contiguous and the aortic valve is superior.
What is the relationship of the tricuspid and pulmonic valves?	They are not contiguous. The infundibulum of the pulmonary outflow tract is between them.
What structures make up the mitral apparatus?	The annulus, anterior and posterior leaflets, chordae tendineae, and papillary muscles

IMAGING STUDIES

CHEST RADIOGRAPHY

What feature of a plain film reveals proper exposure for evaluating the cardiac structures?

The spine should be just visible behind the heart.

How does one assess cardiac structure and function on a CXR?

1. Assess the cardiac silhouette to evaluate the heart size. Note any calcifications.
2. Note the size of the individual chambers.
3. Note the size and position of the great vessels.
4. Is the pulmonary vascularity increased or decreased?
5. Look at the extracardiac structures (i.e., the ribs and chest wall).

What musculoskeletal findings on CXR may be useful in cardiac diagnosis?

1. Sternal or rib deformities, wires, surgical clips, or the absence of ribs may suggest a prior surgical procedure.
2. Pectus excavatum may be associated with Marfan's syndrome and mitral valve prolapse.
3. Rib notching, caused by dilated subcostal arteries, may be seen in aortic coarctation and other types of congenital heart disease (CHD).

List 5 other causes of rib notching on CXR.

1. Subclavian artery obstruction
2. Pulmonary atresia
3. SVC obstruction
4. Neurofibromatosis
5. Hyperparathyroidism

Cardiac silhouette and chamber size

What is the differential diagnosis of an enlarged cardiac shadow on CXR?

1. Congestion [i.e., congestive heart failure (CHF) or fluid overload]
2. Cardiomyopathy (ischemic, idiopathic, or valvular)
3. Intracardiac shunt
4. Pericardial effusion
5. Valvular disease
6. Massive mediastinal mass

What is the pathophysiology behind cardiac or chamber enlargement?

The heart is a pump with two circulatory systems in series—a high pressure side (i.e., the left) and a low pressure side (i.e., the right):

An abnormal connection (i.e., a shunt) causes increased flow (i.e., volume overload), leading to cardiac enlargement.

An insufficient valve also causes volume overload, leading to chamber enlargement.

A stenotic valve causes pressure overload, leading to hypertrophy (which can be difficult to assess on CXR).

What is the epicardial fat pad?

An accumulation of fat at the apex of the heart, seen primarily in obese patients

How does the epicardial fat pad appear on CXR?

It usually tapers toward the left chest wall and is more lucent than the myocardium. On a lateral view, it typically has a triangular shape and covers the anterior heart at the apex.

What is the cardiothoracic ratio?

$$\frac{\text{Maximum transverse cardiac diameter}}{\text{Maximum thoracic diameter}}$$

Be careful not to include the epicardial fat pad when measuring the transverse cardiac diameter. The maximum thoracic diameter is measured using the inner border of the ribs.

What is the definition of an enlarged cardiac shadow on CXR?

A cardiothoracic ratio greater than 0.5 on a PA view, or 0.6 on an AP view (the AP view makes the heart appear larger)

Atrial enlargement

How does right atrial enlargement appear on CXR?

Right atrial enlargement can be difficult to assess, but lateral bulging of the right heart border, possibly accompanied by enlargement of the SVC or IVC, may be noted.

List 5 causes of right atrial enlargement.

1. Right ventricular failure
2. Tricuspid insufficiency
3. Pulmonic stenosis
4. Intracardiac shunts [i.e., ventricular septal defect (VSD), atrial septal defect (ASD), total anomalous pulmonary venous return (TAPVR)]
5. Other congenital lesions (e.g., pulmonic stenosis or atresia, Ebstein's anomaly)

What are the signs of left atrial enlargement on a:

PA view?

A double contour below the carina (caused by projection of the enlarged left atrium through the right atrium)
A bulge along the upper left cardiac border, resulting from the enlarged left atrial appendage
Elevation of the left main stem bronchus

Lateral view?

Posterior displacement of the left main stem bronchus
Leftward displacement of the descending aorta (Bedford sign)

List 6 causes of left atrial enlargement.

1. Aortic valve stenosis or insufficiency
2. Mitral valve stenosis or insufficiency
3. Intracardiac shunts [e.g., VSD, patent ductus arteriosus (PDA)]
4. Left ventricular failure
5. Cardiac restriction
6. Diastolic dysfunction (e.g., as a result of idiopathic hypertrophic subaortic stenosis, old age, hypertension)

Ventricular enlargement

How does right ventricular enlargement appear on CXR?

Right ventricular enlargement is best appreciated on a lateral CXR as a decrease in the retrosternal space (normally, the heart contacts the sternum for less than 40% of its length).

List 8 causes of right ventricular enlargement.

1. Pulmonary embolus (PE)
2. Pulmonary hypertension of any cause
3. Pulmonic stenosis
4. ASD
5. VSD
6. Tricuspid regurgitation
7. Pulmonic insufficiency
8. Congenital disorders

How does left ventricular enlargement appear on CXR?

The cardiac apex is displaced to the left, downward, and posteriorly, and the cardiothoracic ratio is increased. Note that right ventricular enlargement can cause upward and outward displacement of the left ventricle and cardiac apex, whereas left ventricular enlargement tends to cause downward and outward displacement.

A. Left ventricular enlargement

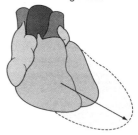

B. Right ventricular enlargement

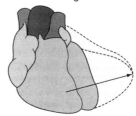

What is the "2 up, 2 back" rule?

On a lateral CXR, measure 2 centimeters up from the junction of the shadow of the IVC with the diaphragm and measure 2 centimeters posteriorly. If the ventricular shadow projects posterior to this point, the left ventricle is likely enlarged.

List 5 causes of left ventricular enlargement.

1. End-stage hypertension
2. Left-sided heart failure
3. Aortic insufficiency
4. End-stage mitral regurgitation
5. Intracardiac shunts

What is a radiographic sign of left ventricular hypertrophy?

Rounding of the left heart border (similar to a flexed biceps muscle)

What can cause a focal bulge involving the left heart border?

A ventricular aneurysm

Pulmonary vascularity

What characterizes the normal pulmonary vascularity?

On an upright film, the pulmonary vessels are smaller in caliber in the upper zones than in the lower zones. The vessel margins are crisp and taper gradually.

What are 3 cardiac causes of increased pulmonary vascularity (pulmonary venous hypertension)?

1. Left-sided heart failure
2. Left-sided valvular pathology (e.g., aortic stenosis or regurgitation, mitral stenosis or regurgitation)
3. Intracardiac shunts

List 5 signs of increased pulmonary vascularity (pulmonary venous hypertension) on CXR.

1. Cephalization (i.e., increased diameter of the upper lobe vessels)
2. Interstitial prominence with Kerley A and B lines
3. Indistinct pulmonary vascular margins
4. Alveolar infiltrates
5. Pleural effusion

What radiographic findings are generally associated with:

Mild pulmonary venous hypertension [central venous pressure (CVP) = 15–20 mm Hg]

The pulmonary vascular diameter is equal in the upper and lower lobes (normally, the upper lobe vessels are smaller than the lower lobe vessels, but they dilate with venous overload).

The vessels in the first interspace should not exceed 3 mm in diameter. (Compare the upper lobe veins with the lower lobe veins equidistant from the hilum.)

Moderate pulmonary venous hypertension (CVP = 20–30 mm Hg)

Increased vascular pressure prevents the lymphatics from effectively transporting fluid out of the interstitium, leading to an interstitial infiltrate and increased density on CXR. Indistinct pulmonary vessel borders, hilar haziness or enlargement, and Kerley A and B lines may also be seen.

Severe pulmonary venous hypertension (CVP = 25–30 mm Hg)

Alveolar edema, evidenced by ill-defined, diffuse areas of increased density with a predilection for the perihilar area and lower lobes, and pleural effusions may be seen.

Note that when the underlying condition is chronic, all of these changes tend not to occur until higher pressures are reached.

How can a CXR be used to detect increased systemic venous pressure resulting from right ventricular failure?

Enlargement of the azygos vein (seen as a discrete "knob" above the right main stem bronchus) suggests increased systemic venous pressure as a result of right ventricular failure.

Cardiac calcifications

List 7 cardiac structures that can be calcified.

1. Myocardium
2. Valve leaflets and annuli (usually on the left side)
3. Coronary arteries
4. Pericardium
5. Aneurysm
6. Thrombus
7. Tumor

How is valvular calcification best assessed by plain film?

A lateral view often allows the best definition of the site.

Which patients are more likely to have calcified valve leaflets or annuli?

Elderly patients and patients with diabetes or renal failure

What is the significance of valve calcification?

Calcification is often predictive of a stenotic or incompetent valve, although this finding is not diagnostic and the calcification may not have hemodynamic consequences.

ECHOCARDIOGRAPHY

Name the 2 primary means of evaluating cardiac structures by ultrasound echocardiography.

Transthoracic echocardiography (TTE) and transesophageal echocardiography (TEE)

What are the limitations of TTE?

The modality depends on an adequate echocardiographic window. Imaging may be poor in patients with obstructive lung disease because ultrasound transmission through air is poor. Calcified or metallic substances (e.g., the rib cage, prosthetic heart valves) may block ultrasound transmission and cause shadowing.

What is TEE?

An ultrasound transducer mounted at the end of a flexible tube is used to image the heart from the esophagus.

Why is the transesophageal approach useful?

1. The heart lies in close proximity to the esophagus. Therefore, higher frequency transducers may be used, resulting in higher resolution ultrasound images.
2. Posterior structures, which are difficult to image transthoracically, are much more clearly seen with TEE.
3. TEE allows imaging of patients with poor transthoracic windows.

List 6 indications for TEE.

1. Evaluation of native and prosthetic cardiac valves
2. Identification of vegetations and complications of endocarditis
3. Identification of intracardiac shunts
4. Evaluation of diseases of the aorta
5. Visualization of atrial thrombi
6. Characterization of intracardiac masses

How safe is TEE?

Although TEE is an invasive procedure, it is quite safe. The complication rate is reported to be 0.2%–0.5%.

List 10 possible complications of TEE.

1. Esophageal trauma (e.g., rupture of the esophagus)
2. Aspiration
3. Damage to the teeth
4. Respiratory depression as a result of conscious sedation
5. Hemorrhage
6. Angina
7. Cardiac dysrhythmias and cardiac arrest
8. Hypotension
9. Pulmonary edema
10. Death (fewer than 0.001% of patients)

What patient preparation is necessary prior to performing TEE?

1. Screen for esophageal disorders (i.e., diverticula, inflammation, varices, and tumors). Check the patient history for dysphagia, odynophagia, liver disease, or irradiation.
2. Evaluate the airway, paying particular attention to the teeth.
3. Assess the likelihood of adequate patient cooperation.
4. Be prepared to intubate if respiratory depression ensues.

Two-dimensional echocardiography (2DE)

What is two-dimensional echocardiography (2DE)?

2DE (a tomographic technique) is a real time, rapidly acquired B-mode ("brightness mode") image. An imaging sector is scanned with multiple lines of ultrasound and the information is electronically recorded. After the entire sector has been scanned, the information is displayed in a two-dimensional, spatially oriented format.

Is 2DE the same as other ultrasound examinations?

Yes, 2DE and ultrasound are the same, except for the mode of archival. In general, 2DE images are stored on videotape and ultrasound images are stored on film.

What types of abnormalities can be discerned using routine 2DE?

1. Abnormal cardiac structures and anatomy (e.g., congenital malformations, pericardial effusions, pleural effusions, vegetations, masses, thrombi)

2. Abnormalities of normal cardiac structures (e.g., the valves, myocardium, and great vessels)
3. Functional abnormalities [e.g., abnormal left or right ventricular function (global or regional), abnormal valve function]

How does one select the appropriate transducer?

In most adult patients, a low frequency (2–2.5 MHZ) transducer is used to increase penetration. In thin patients, a higher frequency (3.5–5 MHZ) transducer may be used to increase resolution. Remember, higher frequency transducers yield increased resolution, but penetration of the ultrasound beam is decreased.

What are the 3 2DE orthogonal imaging planes?

The short-axis plane, the long-axis plane, and the four-chamber plane

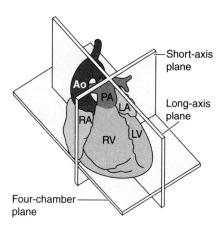

List the 4 most common transducer positions (windows) used in 2DE and the planes they interrogate.

Left parasternal (parasternal): Long-axis and short-axis
Left apical (apical): Four-chamber and long-axis
Subcostal: Four-chamber and short-axis
Suprasternal: Long-axis and short-axis planes of the aorta and pulmonary artery

Name 2 other positions that can be used.

Right parasternal position: Rarely used; may be useful for visualizing the aorta

Right apical position: Useful in dextrocardia

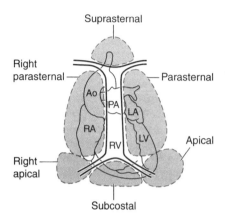

The standard transducer positions must be tailored to suit each individual.

Parasternal position (window)

What structures are visualized in the standard parasternal long-axis plane?

Ao = Aorta
AV = Aortic valve
IVS = Interventricular septum
LA = Left atrium
LV = Left ventricle
MV = Mitral valve
PM = Papillary muscle
RV = Right ventricle

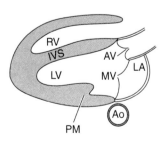

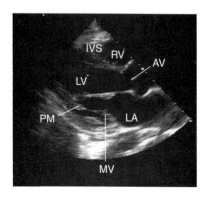

Can the tricuspid valve and right atrium be seen from the parasternal window?

Yes. In fact, it is standard to angle the transducer toward the right ventricle to obtain the right ventricular inflow view [i.e., a view of the right atrium (*RA*), tricuspid valve (*TV*), and right ventricle (*RV*)]. The interventricular septum (*IVS*) and inferior vena cava (*IVC*) are also visible.

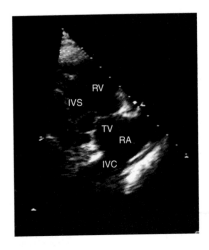

What specific imaging sections are used when obtaining parasternal short-axis views?

Imaging planes through the aortic valve, mitral valve, mid-papillary muscles, and apex

What structures are seen in the standard parasternal short-axis plane at the:

Level of the aorta?

Ao	=	Aorta
IAS	=	Interatrial septum
LA	=	Left atrium
PA	=	Pulmonary artery
PV	=	Pulmonic valve
RA	=	Right atrium
RVOT	=	Right ventricular outflow tract
TV	=	Tricuspid valve

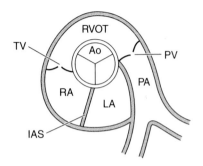 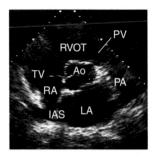

Level of the mitral valve?   *IVS* = Interventricular septum
MV = Mitral valve
LV = Left ventricle wall
RV = Right ventricle

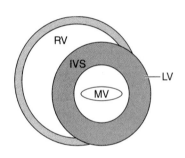 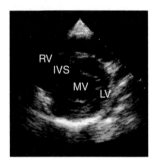

Mid-papillary level?   *IVS* = Interventricular septum
LV = Left ventricular cavity
PM = Papillary muscle
RV = Right ventricle

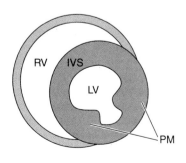 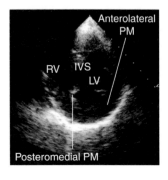

Level of the apex?

The apical cavity

Apical position

**What structures are visible
on the apical four-chamber
plane?**

Ao	=	Aorta
LA	=	Left atrium
LV	=	Left ventricle
MV	=	Mitral valve
RA	=	Right atrium
RV	=	Right ventricle
TV	=	Tricuspid valve

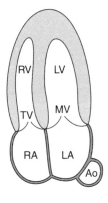 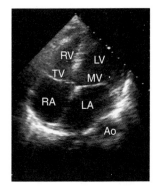

**What structure can be
visualized on the apical
four-chamber plane by
angling the transducer
more posteriorly?**

The coronary sinus

**How is the apical five-
chamber plane obtained?**

By angling the transducer posteriorly

**In addition to the structures
visible on the apical four-
chamber plane, what structures are visible on the
apical five-chamber plane?**

The left ventricular outflow tract (*LVOT*)
and the aortic valve (*AV*)

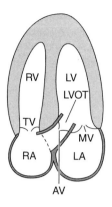

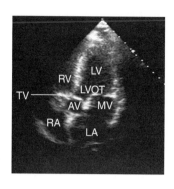

What structures are visible on the apical two-chamber plane?

Ao = Aorta
LA = Left atrium
LV = Left ventricle
MV = Mitral valve
TV = Tricuspid valve

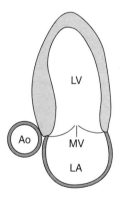

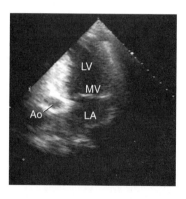

In addition to the structures visible on the apical two-chamber plane, what structures are visible on the apical three-chamber plane?

The left ventricular outflow tract ($LVOT$) and the aorta (Ao)

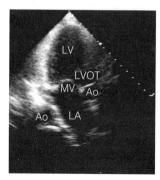

Subcostal position

**What structures are seen
on the subcostal four-
chamber plane?**

The subcostal four-chamber plane is
similar to the apical four- and five-
chamber planes. This image is often
obtained through part of the liver (*L*).
The right ventricle (*RV*), tricuspid valve
(*TV*), right atrium (*RA*), left atrium (*LA*),
mitral valve (*MV*), left ventricle (*LV*), and
aorta (*Ao*) can be visualized on the subcostal four-chamber plane:

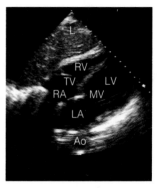

**The subcostal short-axis
plane is similar to what
other plane?**

The parasternal short-axis plane

**At what levels are subcostal
short-axis planes obtained?**

The same levels that are used for the
parasternal short-axis plane (i.e., at the
aortic valve, mitral valve, papillary
muscles, and apex).

**What structures can be
visualized on the IVC inflow
view?**

The inferior vena cava (*IVC*), liver (*L*),
and right atrium (*RA*) are visible on the
IVC inflow view.

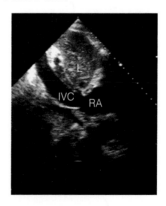

Suprasternal position

What structures are seen in the suprasternal:

Long-axis plane?

AA   = Ascending aorta
ARCH = Aortic arch
DA   = Descending aorta
LA   = Left atrium
LCA = Left carotid artery
LSA = Left subclavian artery
RPA = Right pulmonary artery

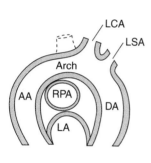 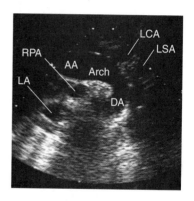

Short-axis plane?

Ao = Aorta
LA = Left atrium
RPA = Right pulmonary artery

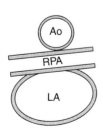 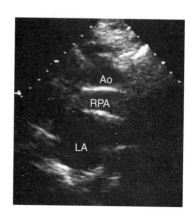

Doppler ultrasound

What is Doppler ultra-sound?

A technique in which shifts in frequency between emitted sound waves and their echoes are used to measure the velocities of moving objects, based on the Doppler principle (see Chapter 2, "Imaging Techniques")

What hemodynamic information may be obtained from Doppler ultrasound?

1. The **pressure gradient across a stenosis** (in a heart valve or blood vessel) may be obtained using the modified Bernoulli equation, $\Delta p = 4 \times v^2$, where Δp is the pressure gradient (in mm Hg) and v is the peak velocity (in m/s), as determined by continuous wave Doppler ultrasound.
2. **Flow through a region** may be measured by the equation $F = a \times v$, where F is flow, a is the area of the orifice defined by 2DE, and v is the velocity through that orifice as determined by Doppler ultrasound.
3. Valve area using the continuity equation $a \times v = a \times v$

What are the 3 primary uses of Doppler ultrasound?

1. Evaluation of stenotic or regurgitant valves
2. Evaluation of shunts
3. Evaluation of abnormal intracardiac or great vessel flow

Contrast echocardiography

What is contrast echocardiography?

A technique that employs tiny bubbles (agitated saline and air or commercially produced microbubbles consisting of high-molecular-weight gases encased within a shell) to enhance the returning ultrasound signal

What are 2 advantages of contrast echocardiography?

1. Better definition of intracardiac shunts
2. Enhancement of Doppler wave forms

What are the advantages of the commercially produced microbubbles over agitated saline and air?

The commercially produced micro-bubbles are the size of red blood cells (RBCs) and have similar rheologic properties. They can be used to opacify the left ventricular cavity, allowing enhanced assessment of global and regional cardiac function. They can also be used to opacify the myocardium to assess myocardial perfusion.

Echocardiographic evaluation of cardiac function

What functional information is obtained when evaluating the chambers of the heart using 2DE?

1. The cardiac chambers are measured.
2. Global and regional right and left ventricular function is assessed.
3. The thickness of the myocardial wall is assessed.
4. Both atria and the great arteries are measured.

For each standard cardiac measurement, state the normal value:

Left and right atria (anterior to posterior)	< 3.8 cm
Left and right atria (lateral dimension)	< 4.5 cm
Left and right atria (apex to base)	< 6.0 cm
Left ventricle at end-systole	< 4.0 cm
Left ventricle at end-diastole	< 5.2 cm
Right ventricle	< 3.8 cm
Interventricular septum and posterior myocardium	< 1.1 cm
Aortic root	< 3.5 cm
IVC	< 2.0 cm

How is regional left ventricular function assessed?

The myocardium is divided into sixteen "segments," and myocardial thickening is assessed in each segment. Note that many segments are seen in more than one window.

How is global left ventricular function assessed?

Qualitatively: The examiner evaluates wall thickening in each myocardial segment and uses this as a basis for describing left ventricular function in general terms (i.e., "normal," "mildly diminished," "moderately diminished," "severely diminished").

Quantitatively: The percent fractional shortening index (diastolic area − systolic area / diastolic area) may be measured in the parasternal short-axis plane at the mid-papillary level. This measurement is the echocardiographic representation of the ejection fraction.

How might Doppler echo-cardiography be used to assess cardiac function?

Cardiac output may be obtained by measuring the area of the left ventricular outflow tract (a) and the velocity (v) at that location. These values can then be plugged into the equation $f = a \times v$ to obtain the flow-per-beat, or stroke volume. Cardiac output is the product of the stroke volume and the heart rate.

Describe 3 ways that dia-stolic function can be assessed using echocardi-ography.

1. Evaluate the thickness of the myo-cardium. A thickened myocardium suggests increased stiffness and decreased diastolic function.
2. Evaluate the size of the atria. Enlarged atria suggest abnormal diastolic function.
3. Obtain a mitral inflow velocity profile using Doppler ultrasound. A reversed E:A ratio of the mitral valve suggests diminished diastolic function.

COMPUTED TOMOGRAPHY (CT)

What type of CT is gener-ally best for imaging cardiac structures?

Ultrafast CT scanning, also known as electron beam CT (EBCT), allows for the best temporal and spatial resolution of cardiac structures. These instruments can acquire an image in 100 msec (1/10 of a second).

How long does it take to obtain an image using a spiral CT scanner?

Recent developments have enabled spiral CT scanners to acquire an image in 500 msec.

Are noncontrast scans use-ful?

Calcification of coronary arteries can be seen readily on EBCT or spiral CT scans without using contrast. The scans are scored electronically to obtain a "calcification score." These scores have been found to correlate reasonably well with the presence of coronary artery disease (CAD), suggesting that EBCT or spiral CT scanning may have a role in screening for CAD.

Why is intravenous contrast used in CT of the heart?

Blood and myocardial tissue are of similar density and therefore difficult to distinguish on a noncontrast scan; using contrast differentiates one from the other.

What is the appearance of infarcted myocardium on CT?

Infarcted myocardium has a lower-than-normal attenuation, thought to be related to edema in the infarcted tissue. Myocardial thinning or myocardial calcification may be seen in patients with chronic myocardial infarction.

What is the CT appearance of a stenotic valve?

The valve is thickened and calcified and relatively immobile on EBCT scanning. However, these findings are anatomic in nature and may not be of physiologic significance.

List 4 pericardial abnormalities that may be diagnosed using CT.

1. Pericardial effusion
2. Constrictive pericarditis
3. Pericardial neoplasm
4. Congenital pericardial absence or deformity

What CT findings help to differentiate constrictive cardiomyopathy from restrictive cardiomyopathy?

The pericardium is thickened (i.e., > 4 mm) in constrictive cardiomyopathy, but not in restrictive cardiomyopathy. Pericardial calcification is more suggestive of constrictive cardiomyopathy.

List 4 intracardiac masses that may be detected using CT.

1. Thrombus (most common in the left atrium)
2. Metastasis (the most common intracardiac neoplasm)
3. Myxoma
4. Lipoma (most common in the right atrium)

MAGNETIC RESONANCE IMAGING (MRI)

**What advantages does
MRI cardiac imaging have:**

    Over CT?

No exposure to ionizing radiation or
iodinated contrast
Images can be generated in any planar
orientation

    Over echocardiography?

Not limited by an acoustic window
Images can be generated in any planar
orientation
Less operator-dependent

**What disadvantages are
associated with MRI
cardiac imaging?**

Expensive, not always available, patient
compatibility is sometimes an issue (e.g.,
not appropriate for patients with pacemakers, aneurysm clips, or claustrophobia)

**How can MRI be acquired
so that each slice of the
heart is obtained at the
same point in the cardiac
cycle?**

Each MRI acquisition is triggered by the
R wave of the ECG.
This may not be possible in patients who
lack a consistent R wave (e.g., those with
atrial fibrillation or very irregular cardiac
rhythms).

**What 3 cardiac parameters
are assessed effectively with
MRI?**

1. Cardiac dimensions
2. Ventricular function (i.e., stroke
   volume and ejection fraction)
3. Normal anatomy of the great vessels
   and myocardium

**What types of disorders can
be assessed using MRI?**

1. Myocardial disease
2. Intracardiac masses and thrombus
   extension into adjacent structures
3. Pericardial disease
4. Tissue dysfunction and infarction
5. Valvular dysfunction
6. CHD

**What MRI technique pro-
vides maximum contrast
between the heart and the
blood?**

On spin-echo sequences, blood appears
black, providing maximum contrast
between the heart and the vessels.

Why does the blood appear black?

The blood that is imaged did not receive an excitation pulse because it was outside the area of scanning.

What MRI technique can be used to determine the velocity of blood flow?

Gradient-echo sequences

How can MRI be used to calculate the ventricular stroke volume and ejection fraction?

By determining the end-systolic and end-diastolic ventricular volumes in a short-axis view, one can calculate the stroke volume and ejection fraction.

How can cardiac function be estimated using MRI?

Cine sequences are obtained during the cardiac cycle. On each slice, systolic wall thickening is identified and measured.

In addition to the axial, sagittal, and coronal planes, what 2 special oblique sections are used for MRI of the heart?

The **long-axis view** is nearly an axial plane, oriented to show the heart from base to apex. The plane of section is defined between the apex of the left ventricle and the mitral valve. The **short-axis view** shows the left ventricle in true cross-section (perpendicular to the long axis). These sections are analogous to the views obtained during 2DE.

Why is standard MRI currently of minimal value in assessing the patency of the coronary arteries?

Sectioning at oblique angles often leads to artifact formation, and it is impossible to include any of the coronary arteries completely in a single section.

What diagnosis is suggested by localized thinning of the ventricular wall on MRI?

Previous myocardial infarction

How might one detect an ischemic segment of myocardium on MRI?

By noting a localized decrease or absence of the normal systolic myocardial thickening

How might an acute infarct appear on a spin-echo sequence?

An area of increased signal density may be seen on T_2-weighted imaging; however, this finding is not entirely sensitive or specific for myocardial infarction.

How can the sensitivity for an acute infarct be increased?

Using a contrast agent [e.g., gadolinium-diethylenetriamine penta-acetic acid (Gd-DTPA)] and T_1-weighted imaging increases the sensitivity for an acute infarct. The infarct shows increased signal intensity at the margin (i.e., enhancment).

How can myocardial perfusion be evaluated using MRI?

Myocardial perfusion can be evaluated by administering an intravenous contrast agent (e.g., Gd-DTPA)—the ischemic myocardium exhibits less uptake and therefore appears less bright than normal. Concomitant infusion of a pharmacologic stress agent, such as dipyridamole, is necessary.

What finding on gradient-echo sequencing indicates valvular incompetence or regurgitation?

A transient decrease in signal intensity at the tips of the valve leaflets suggests valvular incompetence. The size of the void is roughly proportional to the degree of valve dysfunction.

How may MRI demonstrate valvular stenosis?

Gradient-echo sequences reveal a region of signal loss distal to the stenotic valve's leaflets.

How is the pericardium best viewed using MRI?

Spin-echo sequences in the transverse or coronal planes

What pericardial thickness is considered abnormal?

> 4 mm

Is MRI useful in determining whether an effusion is hemorrhagic?

Yes. High-signal intensity on T_1-weighted images suggests a hemorrhagic effusion.

List 4 signs of constrictive pericarditis on MRI.

1. Thickened pericardium (> 4 mm)
2. Dilated IVC and hepatic veins
3. Enlarged right atrium
4. Small or normal right ventricle

How are these findings different from those of restrictive cardiomyopathy?

In restrictive cardiomyopathy, the pericardium is a normal thickness.

What MRI finding characterizes hypertrophic cardiomyopathy?

Thickening of the interventricular septum

NUCLEAR MEDICINE

Perfusion imaging

What is the basic principle of perfusion imaging?

Images of the myocardium are obtained in two phases, stress and rest, following administration of a radionuclide tracer.

How does the appearance of ischemic areas differ from that of infarcted areas on perfusion imaging?

Ischemic areas show poor uptake of the radiotracer on the stress images as compared with the rest images (a reversible defect); infarcted areas show poor uptake on both images (a nonreversible defect).

What 5 areas are examined on perfusion imaging?

1. Myocardial perfusion
2. Global and regional function
3. Lung uptake of tracer (on stress thallium imaging)
4. Left ventricular cavity dilatation (on stress imaging)
5. Myocardial viability

List 4 applications of perfusion studies.

1. Diagnosis of CAD
2. Assessment of myocardial viability
3. Risk stratification (post-myocardial infarction, angina)
4. Risk stratification (preoperatively)

What is the approximate sensitivity and specificity of radionucleotide testing for CAD?

80%–90%

Describe how a perfusion imaging study is performed.

The patient exercises to a maximum point, and then a radionuclide tracer is administered intravenously and stress images are obtained. For thallium, the patient returns hours later so that rest images can be obtained. For sestamibi, low dose rest images are obtained, followed 3 hrs later by a stress exam and reinjection.

According to the most commonly used protocol, the "Bruce protocol," when is the exercise test terminated?

When the patient reaches 85% of his maximal heart rate

When ST segment depression exceeds more than 3 mm

When symptoms of ischemia become intolerable

When hypotension develops
When a greater-than-10-beats ventricular
    arrhythmia develops

What agents are used to produce pharmacologic stress in a patient who cannot exercise?

Dipyridamole, dobutamine, or adenosine

What medication can be administered to reverse the effects of dipyridamole should severe ischemia or other adverse effects occur after its administration?

Aminophylline

Which radionuclide tracers are most often used for the clinical evaluation of myocardial perfusion?

Technetium 99m (Tc-99m) sestamibi and thallium 201 (Tl^{201})

What is the difference between Tc-99m sestamibi and Tl^{201}?

Tl^{201} redistributes; therefore, only one injection is necessary.
Tc-99m sestamibi does not redistribute; therefore, a second injection is required for rest images. Its longer half-life allows images to be obtained much later. Tc-99m sestamibi has less attenuation than Tl^{201} owing to the higher energy of technetium.

What 2 major factors influence the initial myocardial distribution (first pass) of tracer following intravenous injection?

Regional blood flow and extraction of the tracer from the blood (i.e., the extraction fraction)

How are Tc-99m sestamibi and Tl^{201} taken up by the myocardium?

Tc-99m sestamibi binds to mitochondria. Tl^{201} behaves like potassium; therefore, an intact cellular membrane is required for uptake.

Which determinant of uptake predominates at normal blood flow—regional blood flow or the extraction fraction?

Regional blood flow. The extraction fraction is constant (around 90%) with all but very low or very high flow rates. Therefore, tracer uptake is used to represent regional blood flow.

What is "wash-out?"

"Wash-out" occurs only when Tl^{201} is used. Activity decreases in normal myocardium owing to "wash-out" of the tracer from the myocardium.

What is "redistribution?"

"Redistribution" also only occurs with Tl^{201} and is actually a misnomer. Tl^{201} exits the myocardium more slowly from ischemic segments. Therefore, on delayed imaging, the more rapid exit of Tl^{201} from the normal segments results in equilibration among the normal and abnormal segments, giving the appearance of "redistribution."

What is suggested by a:

Reversible defect?

Ischemic myocardium

Partially reversible defect?

Mixture of ischemic and infarcted myocardium

Nonreversible defect?

Infarct (scar)

How do perfusion studies assess for myocardial viability?

On **rest imaging,** a tracer uptake of more than 50% and "redistribution" (when Tl^{201} is used) are fairly sensitive for viable myocardium.

On **stress imaging,** an ischemic response (i.e., a reversible defect) is tantamount to viability.

What 2 imaging techniques may be used in radionuclide scanning?

Planar imaging (single plane imaging) and single photon emission computed tomography (SPECT) imaging, which uses multiple planes

What are the 3 standard planar views?

Anterior, LAO (45°), LAO (70°)

What are the 3 standard SPECT views?

Short-axis, horizontal long-axis, vertical long-axis

How are SPECT images displayed?

The format may vary among institutions, but generally, the stress and rest tomographic slices are displayed side by side and an overall quantification scheme is presented in a "bull's eye" format (i.e., all short-axis images are summed by a computer and displayed).

How can ischemic areas of myocardium be overlooked?

Because tracer counts are relative (all areas are compared to the most normal segment and displayed as a percent of normal), all areas in a diffusely ischemic heart display diminished uptake. Therefore, global ischemia may be interpreted as a normal study because there are no areas of relative under-perfusion. This phenomenon is known as "balanced ischemia."

Name 2 ways the misinter-pretation of "balanced ischemia" can be avoided.

1. Use the exercise portion of the stress test. ECG abnormalities or an abnor-mal blood pressure response suggest "balanced ischemia."
2. Use gated SPECT imaging to assess concomitant wall thickening. Abnormal wall thickening is unusual in nonischemic myocardium.

What artifact may cause reduced uptake:

Anteriorly?

Attenuation of counts by the breast

Inferiorly?

Attenuation of counts by the liver or bowel

What is "hibernating" myocardium?

"Hibernating" myocardium is persistently dysfunctional myocardium with dimin-ished resting perfusion in which function improves after revascularization. Prior to revascularization, perfusion imaging reveals diminished tracer uptake and diminished function (matched).

What is "stunned" myo-cardium?

"Stunned" myocardium is myocardium with normal resting blood flow but abnormal function (mismatch).

What is the significance of lung uptake of Tl^{201} during stress imaging?

This finding suggests the presence of extensive CAD.

Multiple-gated equilibrium radionucleotide cineangiography (MUGA scanning)

What is a MUGA scan?

A cineangiographic technique that uses Tc-99m-labeled RBCs (gated technique) or Tc-99m sestamibi to assess wall motion and cardiac function during rest and exercise

What information does MUGA scanning yield?

Assessment of regional and global myo-cardial function and quantification of the ejection fraction

Describe 2 applications for MUGA scanning.

1. Evaluation of the ejection fraction in patients with a poor echocardiographic window or in those who have contra-indications to angiography
2. Assessment of the ejection fraction prior to adriamycin therapy

How are the ventricular end-systolic and end diastolic volumes determined using MUGA scanning?

By using "area counts" (of tracer)

What equation is used to calculate the ejection fraction?

$$EF = \frac{EDV - ESV}{EDV}$$

In other words,

$$EF = \frac{\text{End-diastolic tracer count} - \text{End-systolic tracer count}}{\text{End-diastolic tracer count}}$$

What is a normal EF?

60%

How are wall motion ab-normalities diagnosed in MUGA scanning?

Viewing the scan results in a dynamic movie format allows qualitative or semi-quantitative evaluation of wall motion.

CARDIAC CATHETERIZATION

What is cardiac catheter-ization?

A technique that involves passing a small catheter from a peripheral vessel into either the left or right side of the heart, enabling the examiner to obtain blood samples, assess intracardiac pressures, and detect cardiac or valvular abnormalities by ventriculography

What is the normal:

Mixed venous oxygen saturation?

70%

Arterial oxygen saturation?

> 95%

What is suggested by a mixed venous oxygen saturation of:

More than 70%?

Intracardiac shunting or a high-output state (e.g., sepsis)

Less than 70%?

Low cardiac output

What does each wave represent on this normal pressure tracing from the right atrium? (Remember that this tracing is transmitted into the vena cava.)

a: Atrial contraction
c: Ventricular contraction and bulging of the tricuspid valve into the atrium
x: Ventricular relaxation
v: Venous inflow into the atrium
y: Early ventricular filling (atrial emptying)

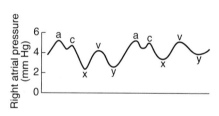

What finding would be expected on a pressure tracing from the right atrium in a patient with tricuspid regurgitation?

Large v waves

How is the left atrial pressure estimated?

Using the pulmonary capillary wedge pressure

What 5 standard views are used for selective cardiac angiography and ventriculography?

1. LAO with cranial angulation
2. LAO with caudal angulation
3. RAO with cranial angulation
4. RAO with caudal angulation
5. Lateral

The function of the left ventricle is evaluated by segment during ventriculography. What are these segments?

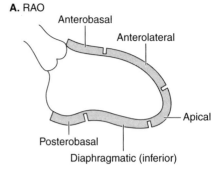

A. RAO

Anterobasal

Anterolateral

Apical

Posterobasal

Diaphragmatic (inferior)

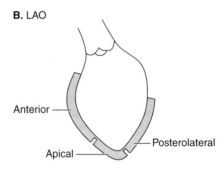

B. LAO

Anterior

Posterolateral

Apical

Can angiography accurately diagnose valvular pathology?

An ascending aortogram can assess aortic regurgitation, and a left ventriculogram can assess mitral regurgitation. Although restrictive leaflet motion may be seen by fluoroscopy, stenotic lesions are assessed by hemodynamic evaluation.

CORONARY ANGIOGRAPHY

What is coronary angiography?

Following selective catheterization of each of the coronary arteries, images of the lumen can be obtained via the injection of contrast.

What are the 4 major types of complications associated with coronary angiography?

1. **Cardiovascular complications** (e.g., CHF, myocardial infarction, stroke, peripheral embolization, thrombosis, arrhythmia, cholesterol emboli syndrome)
2. **Groin complications** (e.g., hematoma, thrombosis, dissection, arteriovenous fistula, pseudoaneurysm)

3. **Renal complications** (e.g., renal failure or anaphylaxis) as a result of intravenous contrast administration
4. **Anesthesia-associated complications**

What percentage of patients undergoing coronary angiography experience complications?

Fewer than 1%

How can one differentiate between an atherosclerotic plaque and coronary artery vasospasm on an angiogram?

A plaque is an eccentric or concentric lesion with sharp edges, while a spasm is a fusiform lesion with smooth edges and a tapered transition. Nitroglycerin administration may help differentiate these two entities, which can be difficult to distinguish from one another.

What is the appearance of an intraluminal thrombus on an angiogram?

A filling defect surrounded by contrast media

How does a collateral cardiac vessel appear on an angiogram?

Collaterals tend to be atypically located and have a serpiginous appearance (i.e., they are "corkscrew"-shaped).

Coronary occlusion is generally deemed to be of hemodynamic significance when what percentage of the vessel diameter is occluded?

An occlusion of more than 75% is considered hemodynamically significant; however, stenosis of more than 95% is required to impair resting myocardial perfusion.

How is angiographic coronary stenosis quantified?

Generally, coronary stenosis is quantified by estimating the percent stenosis as compared with a normal reference segment. Some centers use computerized calculations that compare the diameter of the diseased vessel with that of a normal referenced segment.

What is the major limitation of applying an angiographically determined percent stenosis to clinical practice?

The angiographic percent stenosis does not always correlate with the physiology and the hemodynamic consequences of a lesion.

DISORDERS OF THE HEART AND CORONARY VESSELS

VALVULAR DISEASE

Mitral stenosis

What is the most common cause of mitral stenosis?	Rheumatic fever
List 3 other causes of mitral stenosis.	1. Mitral annular calcification 2. Congenital defect 3. Supravalvular ring
Name 3 of the potential complications of mitral stenosis.	Atrial fibrillation, left atrial thrombus, and pulmonary hypertension
What are 4 signs of mitral stenosis on CXR?	1. Left atrial enlargement 2. Calcification of the mitral valve (best seen on fluoroscopy) 3. Interstitial edema as a result of pulmonary venous hypertension 4. Right-sided heart enlargement secondary to pulmonary hypertension (possibly)
Describe the normal appearance of the mitral apparatus on 2DE.	The **annulus** is free of calcium. The **leaflets** are delicate (i.e., less than 0.5 cm thick) and move in an unrestricted fashion. The anterior leaflet is normally longer than the posterior leaflet and is contiguous with the non-coronary leaflet of the aortic valve. The **chordae tendineae** are delicate and free of calcium.
After systole, does the mitral valve open before or after the aortic valve?	The following figure demonstrates the motion of the aortic and mitral valve leaflets, correlated with the ECG. The mitral valve opens (like the University of Virginia "wah-hoo-wah" cheer) after the aortic valve in diastole:

The **E wave** represents early diastolic filling of the left ventricle (the y descent on a left atrial pressure tracing). The **A wave** reflects atrial contraction. The **F point** is the nadir between the E and A waves.

What is the E-F slope?

The slope of the line connecting the peak of the E wave to the F point

How might atrial fibrillation affect the mitral inflow pattern?

Loss of the A wave

What is the typical 2DE appearance of rheumatic mitral stenosis?

The mitral leaflets and chordae tendineae are thickened and calcified. The leaflets are tethered at the tips, so that the most severely restricted motion is found at the point of coaptation. Tethering results in the classic **"hockey stick"** appearance of the anterior mitral leaflet in diastole and is responsible for doming of the valve. The posterior leaflet is often totally immobile. Although the "hockey stick" appearance of the anterior leaflet and the fixed posterior leaflet are specific for rheumatic mitral stenosis, restricted leaflet motion and doming of the valve are found in all forms of mitral stenosis.

What conditions other than mitral stenosis result in diminished mobility of the mitral leaflets?

Any condition that decreases mitral inflow, such as left ventricular dysfunction.
Significant aortic regurgitation (i.e., the

regurgitant jet hinders movement of
the mitral leaflets)

**Name 3 conditions that
clinically mimic mitral
stenosis.**

1. Left atrial thrombus
2. Left atrial myxoma
3. Cor triatriatum

**What are the classic Doppler findings of mitral
stenosis?**

Increased transmitral velocities owing to a
    pressure gradient
Decreased mitral valve area
Prolonged E-F slope, representing
    restricted early mitral filling
Turbulent mitral inflow

A. Normal   **B.** Mitral stenosis

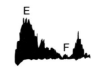

**What is the normal mitral
valve pressure gradient?**

Near zero

**How can the pressure
gradient be calculated?**

From the peak E wave velocity, using the
modified Bernoulli equation

**What is the pressure half-
time ($P_{1/2}$)?**

The time required for the peak pressure
gradient to be reduced by one half

What is the normal $P_{1/2}$?

Less than 60 milliseconds

**Is the $P_{1/2}$ increased or
decreased in mitral stenosis?**

Increased

**What is the equation for
calculating the valve area?**

Valve area $= 220/P_{1/2}$

**What is the normal valve
area of the mitral annulus?**

Approximately 4.5 cm^2

**How is mitral stenosis
graded using echocardiography?**

According to the mean pressure gradient,
the valve area, and the $P_{1/2}$

Grade	Mean gradient	Valve area(cm²)	$P_{1/2}$ (msec)
Mild	0	> 1.5	< 150
Moderate	5–10	1–1.5	150–220
Severe	> 10	< 1	> 220

Mitral regurgitation

List the 5 primary causes of mitral regurgitation.

1. Mitral annular calcification
2. Rheumatic fever
3. Myxomatous degeneration
4. Mitral valve prolapse, with or without flail leaflet
5. Cleft mitral valve (associated with endocardial cushion defects)

List the 3 secondary causes of mitral regurgitation.

1. CAD
2. Idiopathic dilated cardiomyopathy
3. Endocarditis

List 4 ways CAD can lead to secondary mitral regurgitation.

1. Dilatation of the left ventricle can lead to annular dilation.
2. Posterior wall akinesis or dyskinesis may restrict motion of the posterior leaflet.
3. Papillary muscle dysfunction or rupture can occur secondary to myocardial infarction, leading to mitral regurgitation.
4. Poor left ventricular systolic performance can lead to incomplete mitral leaflet closure.

What are the signs of mitral regurgitation on CXR?

Enlargement of the left ventricle and atrium
Pulmonary venous hypertension (evidenced by interstitial edema, alveolar edema, or both)

How might acute mitral regurgitation (e.g., that caused by papillary muscle rupture following a myocardial infarction) appear radiographically?

Pulmonary edema may be present without chamber enlargement

How can echocardiography be used to estimate the severity of mitral regurgitation?

There are various ways to estimate the severity of mitral regurgitation using echocardiography.

1. Identify the cause of the regurgitation (this is the most reliable method). For example, flail leaflet invariably suggests severe regurgitation, while mitral annular calcification suggests mild to moderate regurgitation.
2. Estimate the size of the jet at the level of the valve orifice using 2DE. This estimation correlates with the area of the regurgitant orifice and is a highly qualitative assessment.
3. Measure the jet size at the regurgitant orifice using color flow Doppler. This technique is not reliable because it depends on many variables other than the regurgitant volume, including the left atrial size and pressure, the left ventricular function, and the Doppler gain settings.
4. Identify the direction of the jet using color flow Doppler. This exercise helps determine the cause of the regurgitation. For example, an eccentric jet is almost always seen when there is a flail or prolapsing leaflet, while a central jet is seen predominantly with mitral annular calcification.
5. Evaluate the associated findings. Associated findings, such as left atrial enlargement and pulmonary hypertension, signify long-standing, more severe mitral regurgitation.
6. Identify reversal of pulmonary venous flow during systole. This finding suggests significant mitral regurgitation.

What are 5 echocardiographic criteria for diagnosing mitral valve prolapse?

1. Thickened mitral leaflets (> 0.5 cm) with myxomatous degeneration
2. Redundancy of the leaflets
3. Posterior displacement of any leaflet more than 3 mm beyond the mitral annular plane in the parasternal long axis (the apical window is far less sensitive for this finding owing to the "saddle" shape of the mitral annulus)
4. Posterior displacement of the

posterior leaflet on M-mode echocardiography
5. Late systolic regurgitation

Which patients with mitral valve prolapse should be followed closely?

Patients with severely degenerative, redundant leaflets and significant regurgitation

List 4 complications that may be associated with mitral valve prolapse.

1. Endocarditis
2. Thromboembolism from thrombi on the valve
3. Flail mitral leaflet
4. Pulmonary hypertension

In an asymptomatic patient with mitral regurgitation, how can echocardiography be used to determine the optimal time for mitral valve replacement?

The goal is to replace the valve before irreversible left ventricular dysfunction develops. Patients with mitral regurgitation should exhibit hyperdynamic left ventricular function owing to unloading of the ventricle into the low-pressure left atrium. Normal fractional shortening actually represents suboptimal ventricular performance. Therefore, if the ejection fraction falls below 60% or the end-systolic dimension is more than 45 mm, valve replacement should be considered.

Aortic stenosis

List 3 causes of aortic stenosis.

1. Calcification (adult calcific aortic stenosis, seen in the elderly population)
2. Bicuspid aortic valve (congenital anomaly, usually presents in middle adulthood)
3. Rheumatic fever

List 5 signs of aortic stenosis on CXR.

1. Valvular calcification on a lateral CXR or fluoroscopy (indicates severe disease)
2. Convex right upper cardiac border with a normal aortic knob (caused by poststenotic dilatation of the ascending aorta)
3. Left atrial enlargement
4. Left ventricular enlargement (seen in advanced disease)

5. Increased pulmonary vascularity or pulmonary edema (seen in advanced disease)

How is critical aortic stenosis defined?

By a valve area of less than 0.5 cm^2-0.6 cm^2

What are the clinical signs of critical aortic stenosis?

Angina, syncope, heart failure

What are the classic 2DE findings associated with:

    Adult calcific aortic stenosis? (List 3)

1. A calcified, thickened aortic valve with diminished excursion
2. Doming of the aortic leaflets
3. Associated mitral annular calcification

    Bicuspid aortic valve? (List 4)

1. Only two leaflets in the parasternal short axis
2. Systolic doming of both leaflets in the parasternal long axis
3. Eccentric aortic orifice, secondary to the asymmetry of the two leaflets
4. Absence of calcium early in the disease process

    Rheumatic aortic stenosis? (List 2)

1. Thickened leaflets with commissural fusion
2. Concomitant rheumatic involvement of the mitral valve

What are the classic findings of aortic stenosis on:

    Color flow Doppler?

Turbulent flow

    Spectral Doppler?

A high-velocity profile through the aortic valve

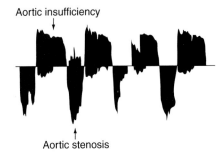

Aortic insufficiency

Aortic stenosis

Which form of spectral Doppler is best for assessing aortic stenosis and why?

Continuous wave Doppler, because it allows mapping of high-velocity jets

What other diagnoses must one consider for an increased gradient on continuous wave Doppler across the aortic valve?

1. Idiopathic hypertrophic subaortic stenosis
2. Subaortic membrane
3. Supra-aortic membrane

How might one differentiate among valvular aortic stenosis, idiopathic hypertrophic subaortic stenosis, subaortic membrane, and supra-aortic membrane?

Pulsed wave Doppler can be used to **precisely** locate the high-velocity jet. **2DE** can be used to search for asymmetric septal hypertrophy or a sub- or supra-aortic membrane. Normal-appearing aortic leaflets argue against valvular aortic stenosis. Associated aortic regurgitation may be seen with a subaortic membrane, although this finding is not specific because mixed aortic valve disease is quite common. **TEE** may be necessary to further evaluate the aortic valve.

How can aortic stenosis be quantified using Doppler echocardiography?

The pressure gradient across the valve can be calculated using the modified Bernoulli equation. The severity of the aortic stenosis is directly related to the gradient. The valve area is calculated using the continuity equation.

What are some pitfalls of using Doppler echocardiography for assessing the severity of aortic stenosis?

When the cardiac output is low, the gradient across the valve may be underestimated, owing to the small stroke volume. In addition, the jet of aortic stenosis may be confused with the jet of mitral regurgitation, leading to errors in estimating the stenosis severity.

What are some of the echocardiographic findings associated with long-standing aortic stenosis?

Left ventricular hypertrophy as a result of pressure overload of the left ventricle

Left ventricular failure and pulmonary hypertension

Aortic insufficiency

List 4 causes of acquired aortic insufficiency.

1. Calcific degenerative aortic insufficiency (may result in aortic valve prolapse)

2. Rheumatic fever
3. Endocarditis
4. Diseases of the aorta (e.g., aneurysm, dissection, Marfan's syndrome, atherosclerosis, syphilis)

List 2 congenital disorders that can be associated with aortic insufficiency.

1. Bicuspid aorta
2. Aortic valve prolapse

List 3 signs of aortic insufficiency on CXR.

1. Left ventricular enlargement
2. Enlargement of the ascending aorta and a prominent aortic knob, with or without enlargement of the descending aorta
3. Increased pulmonary vascularity or pulmonary edema (only seen late in the disease process)

How can aortic insufficiency be differentiated from aortic stenosis on CXR?

Left ventricular enlargement is more likely with aortic insufficiency.
Localized enlargement of the ascending aorta in the thoracic area is more suggestive of aortic stenosis.

What are the classic findings of aortic insufficiency on:

Color flow Doppler?

High velocity, turbulent flow from the aorta into the left ventricle during diastole

Spectral Doppler?

High-velocity diastolic flow across the aorta into the left ventricle

How can echocardiography be used to estimate the severity of aortic insufficiency?

As in mitral regurgitation, there are various ways to estimate the severity of aortic insufficiency using echocardiography.
1. Estimate the jet size at the regurgitant orifice using color flow Doppler. This method is even less reliable in aortic insufficiency than in mitral regurgitation because the size of the jet in aortic insufficiency also depends on the left ventricular end-diastolic pressure and the systemic vascular resistance.

2. Measure the width of the regurgitant jet at the level of the valve orifice using 2DE (best seen in the parasternal short axis).
3. Calculate the $P_{1/2}$. Contrary to the situation with mitral stenosis, the shorter the $P_{1/2}$, the more severe the regurgitation. A short $P_{1/2}$ reflects a rapid equilibration of pressures between the left ventricle and aorta.

What 3 findings suggest severe aortic insufficiency?

1. Presystolic closure of the mitral valve (best seen in M-mode)
2. Presystolic mitral regurgitation
3. Presystolic opening of the aortic valve

In an asymptomatic patient with aortic insufficiency, how can echocardiography be used to judge the timing of valve replacement?

Left ventricular function and the severity of the regurgitation can be followed echocardiographically. It is commonly felt that valve replacement should be considered when left ventricular function is diminished or the ventricle has an end-systolic dimension of more than 55 mm.

Tricuspid stenosis

List 4 causes of acquired tricuspid stenosis.

1. Rheumatic fever (most common)
2. Carcinoid (paraneoplastic effect)
3. Endocardial fibroelastosis
4. Eosinophilic endomyocardial fibrosis (Löffler's endocarditis)

List 2 congenital disorders that can be associated with tricuspid stenosis.

1. Tricuspid atresia
2. Right ventricular hypoplasia

What are the CXR signs of tricuspid atresia?

1. Right atrial enlargement (large right heart border)
2. Enlargement of the azygos vein

What are the echocardiographic characteristics of tricuspid stenosis?

Leaflet thickening, diminished leaflet excursion, and doming are seen on 2DE. Doppler examination reveals turbulent right ventricular inflow and an increased tricuspid inflow velocity.

How is the severity of tricuspid stenosis assessed?

Tricuspid stenosis is assessed the same way mitral stenosis is assessed (i.e., according to the mean gradient, valve area, and $P_{1/2}$).

Tricuspid regurgitation

List 7 causes of tricuspid regurgitation.

1. Rheumatic fever
2. Tricuspid valve prolapse (may be associated with mitral valve prolapse)
3. Endocarditis (especially in intravenous drug users)
4. Blunt trauma
5. Carcinoid (paraneoplastic syndrome)
6. Annular dilatation (caused by dilatation of the right ventricle)
7. Pulmonary hypertension

What are the signs of tricuspid regurgitation on CXR?

Right atrial enlargement, possibly accompanied by right ventricular enlargement, and decreased pulmonary vasculature

How does one assess the severity of tricuspid regurgitation?

In much the same way as one assesses the severity of mitral regurgitation

Describe the spectral Doppler findings in a patient with severe tricuspid regurgitation.

Early peaking and midsystolic deceleration of the regurgitant jet are seen, owing to rapid equilibration of the left atrial and left ventricular pressures. In addition, one might see systolic reversal of the hepatic venous flow. (These findings correlate with a large v wave on a jugular venous pressure tracing.)

How can the jet of tricuspid regurgitation be used to estimate the pulmonary systolic pressure?

During systole, the pulmonary valve is open. In the absence of pulmonary stenosis, the right ventricular systolic pressure (RVP) is a good representative of the pulmonary systolic pressure. The tricuspid regurgitation jet reflects the pressure gradient (ΔP) between the right ventricle and the right atrium during systole (that is, $\Delta P = RVP - RAP$, where RAP is the right atrial systolic pressure). If we know ΔP, then we can solve for the right ventricular systolic pressure ($RVP = RAP + \Delta P$).

| In order to quantify the pulmonary systolic pressure, it is necessary to estimate the right atrial systolic pressure. How is this done? | Echocardiographers use the size of the right atrium, the tricuspid regurgitation peak velocity, the size and respiratory variation of the IVC, and the characteristics of the hepatic venous flow to estimate the right atrial systolic pressure, which may vary from 5–20 mm Hg. If most of these parameters are normal, then the right atrial systolic pressure is assumed to be 5 mm Hg. |

Pulmonic stenosis

| What is the most common form of pulmonic stenosis? | Congenital pulmonic stenosis owing to fusion of the cusps or incompletely formed raphes |

| Name another cause of pulmonic stenosis. | Metastatic carcinoid tumor |

| What are the echocardiographic characteristics of pulmonic stenosis? | Diminished leaflet excursion with doming of the leaflets and turbulent flow through the valve |

| What other finding may suggest pulmonic stenosis? | Right ventricular hypertrophy (although this finding is not specific) |

Pulmonic insufficiency

| What are the 3 major causes of pulmonic insufficiency? | 1. Pulmonary hypertension
2. Endocarditis
3. Iatrogenic (following balloon valvulotomy to treat pulmonic stenosis) |

| What finding is seen in chronic pulmonic insufficiency? | As with tricuspid regurgitation, right ventricular volume overload can be a sequelae of chronic pulmonic insufficiency. |

ENDOCARDITIS

| What is the best way of diagnosing endocarditis? | Patient history, physical examination, and laboratory studies |

| What are the clinical manifestations of endocarditis? | Persistent fever, positive blood cultures, changing murmur |

What is the role of echo-cardiography in the assessment of endocarditis?

Echocardiography can be used to:
Aid in diagnosis and management
Evaluate hemodynamic sequelae
Follow the functional course of the
    disease
Assess for complications
Assist in determining indications for, and
    timing of, surgery

What is the echocardiographic hallmark of endocarditis?

Vegetations on one or more leaflets

What is the typical appearance of a vegetation on 2DE?

Vegetations appear as discrete, independently mobile, echo-dense masses on a leaflet.

What is the differential diagnosis of a mass on a valve leaflet?

Vegetation
Thrombus
Tumor
Myxomatous degeneration
Rheumatic changes with discrete
    calcification
Artifact

Name 3 ways one can differentiate a vegetation from the other possible causes of a mass on a valve leaflet.

1. The clinical picture, including the course of the illness, can offer valuable clues as to the cause of a mass on a valve leaflet. Following the course of the disease may be the only way to distinguish between thrombus, tumor, and vegetation.
2. Unrestricted movement of the leaflets is often an important clue because in rheumatic valvular disease, leaflet movement is restricted. However, vegetations often coexist with rheumatic valvular disease.
3. Myxomatous degeneration involves the entire leaflet and is associated with leaflet redundancy, whereas vegetations are discrete.

Which is more sensitive for detecting vegetations, TEE or TTE?

TEE

What is the sensitivity of TEE for detecting vegetations?

Approximately 30%–50% (echocardiography will not detect small vegetations)

List 6 complications of endocarditis.

1. Valve regurgitation as a result of valvular disruption and perforation; flail leaflet may be associated with severe hemodynamic consequences
2. Abscess (aortic root, mitral ring, perivalvular, septal)
3. Conduction abnormalities (as a result of septal abscess)
4. Intracardiac fistulas
5. Purulent pericarditis
6. Aneurysm (mycotic or mitral valve)

What are the possible routes of extension of an aortic root abscess?

From the **left coronary cusp,** the infection may extend to the anterior mitral leaflet, the left atrium, and the interatrial septum.

From the **right coronary cusp,** the infection may spread to the membranous and muscular portions of the interventricular septum.

From there, it may invade the right ventricle and the right ventricular outflow tract.

From the noncoronary cusp, the infection may extend into the interventricular septum or right atrium.

Prosthetic valves

What is the primary difficulty encountered when using echocardiography to evaluate a patient with an artificial prosthetic valve?

Acoustic artifacts (e.g., shadowing, reverberation artifacts, and large numbers of echoes within the prosthesis that are difficult to distinguish from pathologic lesions)

Name the 3 common types of prosthetic valves.

Ball-cage, tilting disk (single or dual), and porcine

On 2DE, what are the characteristics of a:

Ball-cage prosthesis?

The cage is often seen protruding into the left ventricle if the prosthesis is in the mitral position, and into the ascending aorta if it is in the aortic position. The ball is seen as a vertical line moving back and forth inside the cage. There is significant shadowing deep to the valve.

Tilting disk prosthesis?

Echo-dense prosthetic leaflets can be seen opening during diastole (if the prosthesis is in the mitral position) or systole (if it is in the aortic position). There is a linear shadowing behind the open leaflets.

Porcine prosthesis?

Echo-dense struts are visible around the annulus and the leaflets can be visualized.

Describe 4 common difficulties associated with using Doppler echocardiography to assess prosthetic valve function.

1. All prosthetic valves are somewhat stenotic; therefore, velocities across the valves are always elevated.
2. Because a single prosthetic valve has orifices of varying sizes, one may easily see varying gradients at different locations along the prosthesis.
3. Color flow Doppler may underestimate a regurgitant jet owing to acoustic shadowing.
4. Prosthetic valves can cause eccentric jets.

Name 4 complications of prosthetic valves.

1. Prosthetic valve stenosis
2. Paravalvular leak
3. Pseudoaneurysm
4. Fistula

How can one rule out prosthetic valve stenosis?

Knowledge of the valve type and size is necessary in order to rule out prosthetic valve stenosis. Normal references for each valve are available.

What are common causes of prosthetic valve stenosis?

Vegetation, thrombus, pannus ingrowth

Name the 2 most common causes of a paravalvular leak.

Endocarditis and torn suture

What measure can be taken to simplify future echocardiographic evaluation of a patient with a prosthetic valve?

After surgery, obtain an echocardiogram of the normally functioning valve to serve as a baseline for later comparison.

CONGENITAL HEART DISEASE (CHD)

See also Chapter 11,
"Pediatric Imaging"

Atrial septal defect (ASD)

**What are the 3 types of
ASD?**

A = Sinus venosus defect
B = Ostium secundum defect
C = Ostium primum defect

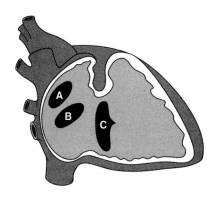

**What is the appearance of
ASD on CXR?**

Increased pulmonary vascularity as a
result of increased pulmonary blood flow

**Identify the type of ASD on
each of the 2DE images
below:**

A = Ostium secundum defect
B = Ostium primum defect
C = Sinus venosus defect

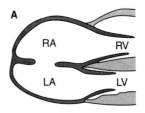

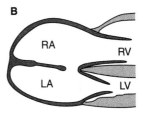

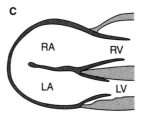

What finding on 2DE increases suspicion for an ASD?

A dilated right ventricle with signs of volume overload (i.e., flattening of the interventricular septum during diastole)

What 3 defects can be associated with an ostium primum defect?

1. Endocardial cushion defect
2. Cleft mitral valve
3. Insertion of the anterior mitral leaflet into the septum

What information about the ASD may be gained by Doppler interrogation?

The shunt fraction (Q_p/Q_s) can be determined by calculating the flow across the pulmonary and aortic valves (Q_p and Q_s, respectively). In addition, the pulmonary systolic pressure can be estimated from the tricuspid regurgitation jet using the modified Bernoulli equation.

How might contrast echocardiography aid in the evaluation of an ASD?

A negative contrast effect in the right atrium confirms the presence of a left-to-right shunt. Contrast may also enhance

Doppler detection of a right-to-left shunt across the defect.

Does a right-to-left shunt always suggest pulmonary hypertension?

No. The shunt direction depends on pressure differences between the two atria. Various situations can cause the atrial pressures to change. For example, a Valsalva maneuver increases the right atrial pressure, increasing right-to-left flow.

Does demonstration of a patent foramen ovale signify the definite presence of an ASD?

No.

Ventricular septal defect (VSD)

Identify each type of VSD on the figure below:

A = Outlet (supracristal)
B = Perimembranous
C = Outlet (infracristal)
D = Inlet
E = Trabecular (muscular)

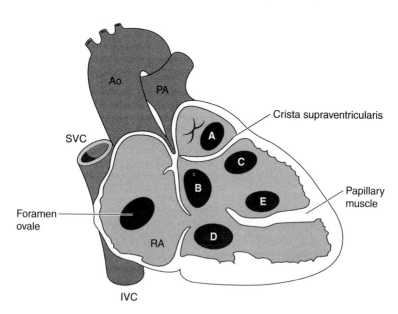

Describe the pathophysiology of VSD.

In VSD, oxygenated blood is shunted from the left ventricle to the right ventricle, causing volume overload of the right ventricle and the pulmonary circuit. The arterial oxygen tension (Pao_2) of the right side of the heart is also elevated.

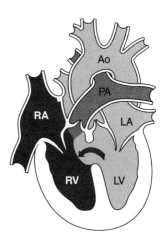

List 6 radiographic findings in VSD with a marked left-to-right shunt.

1. Cardiomegaly, including left atrial enlargement
2. Enlarged pulmonary arteries (diameter of the right pulmonary artery greater that of the bronchus intermedius)
3. Changes consistent with CHF (if the shunt is severe)
4. Signs of recurrent pneumonia
5. Hyperexpanded lungs
6. Small aorta

Which 2DE echocardiographic views are best for visualizing a:

Perimembranous VSD?

Parasternal long-axis, apical four-chamber, and apical five-chamber

Outlet VSD?

Parasternal short-axis

Inlet VSD?

Apical four-chamber or parasternal short-axis (mid-papillary level)

Trabecular VSD?

Any view; depends on the location of the defect

**What are the color flow
Doppler characteristics of:**

A small VSD?   Small, turbulent jet across the defect,
with high velocities

A large VSD?   Less turbulent jet across the defect, with
lower velocities

**Name 3 other ways in which
Doppler echocardiography
is useful in the assessment
of a VSD.**

1. One can demonstrate Eisenmenger's
   physiology.
2. The size of the shunt (Q_p/Q_s)can be
   determined.
3. The right ventricular systolic pressure
   (RVP) can be derived, giving an
   accurate estimate of the pulmonary
   systolic pressure (assuming there is no
   pulmonary stenosis). The modified
   Bernoulli equation is used to calculate
   ΔP. The left ventricular systolic
   pressure (LVP) can be obtained by
   measuring the systolic cuff pressure
   (assuming there is no outflow tract
   gradient). Because $\Delta P = LVP - RVP$,
   $RVP = LVP - \Delta P$. (Alternatively, the
   tricuspid regurgitant jet can be used to
   calculate the pulmonary systolic
   pressure.)

**What is Eisenmenger's
physiology?**   Eisenmenger's physiology develops when
long-standing left-to-right shunting
causes pulmonary hypertension and right
ventricular hypertrophy. The right ventricular pressure exceeds the left ventricular pressure and the shunt reverses,
becoming a right-to-left shunt and resulting in a decreased systemic Pao_2 (i.e.,
cyanosis).

Patent ductus arteriosus (PDA)

**What is the typical location
of a PDA?**   The lesion is usually located left of the
pulmonary trunk, adjacent to the left pulmonary artery. The aortic connection may
be seen opposite and just beyond the left
subclavian artery.

**What echocardiographic
findings may be associated
with PDA?**   A left-to-right shunt, provided Eisenmenger's physiology has not yet
developed

Volume overload of the left ventricle
Findings consistent with pulmonary
hypertension (e.g., a bidirectional
shunt or a right-to-left shunt; right
ventricular failure)

Coarctation of the aorta

What is coarctation of the aorta?

A local narrowing of the descending aorta near the origin of the ductus arteriosus

What are the echocardiographic findings of coarctation of the aorta on:

2DE?

A ridge-like indentation of the posterolateral wall of the aorta is seen.

Doppler?

A turbulent, high-velocity jet through the defect is seen. The ascending aorta may be dilated.

How does one judge the severity of the coarctation?

The pressure gradient can be determined using the modified Bernoulli equation.

What other defect is associated with a coarctation of the aorta?

Bicuspid aortic valve

CORONARY ARTERY DISEASE (CAD)

What signs of CAD can be seen on a CXR?

Plain films have very low sensitivity for detecting lesions; occasionally, coronary artery calcifications can be seen (however, these are neither sensitive nor specific for coronary artery stenosis). Angiography is the gold standard.

Is resting echocardiography sensitive for detecting CAD? Why or why not?

No, for 3 reasons:
1. Many coronary plaques do not diminish resting myocardial blood flow and thus do not produce wall motion abnormalities at rest.
2. Because the movement of one myocardial segment is influenced by adjacent segments (as a result of the tethering effect), abnormal thickening may be masked.

3. Abnormal myocardial thickening may be secondary to a nonischemic etiology, such as cardiomyopathy or valvular disease.

How can the sensitivity of resting echocardiography for detecting CAD be improved?

By using exercise or pharmacologic stress testing to produce myocardial ischemia, thereby inducing abnormal wall motion

What are the 2DE findings of acutely ischemic myocardium?

Abnormal thickening of the ischemic myocardium may be seen. Depressed global left ventricular function can be present in some cases.

How does one differentiate between acute and chronic ischemia by 2DE?

This distinction is very difficult. Both acute and chronic ischemia can be characterized by hypokinesis and akinesis and severe left ventricular dysfunction. However, a few clues may be discerned:
1. In acute ischemia, the unaffected segments may reveal hyperkinesis as a compensatory mechanism (although in multivessel disease, the unaffected segment may not be hyperkinetic.)
2. Secondary findings, such as thinned, hyperechoic myocardium and myocardial aneurysms, usually indicate old infarction.

What CXR changes are seen in acute myocardial infarction?

In 50% of patients, the CXR is normal. Pulmonary venous hypertension or pulmonary edema with a normal-sized heart may be seen if the infarction is severe or accompanied by mitral regurgitation or VSD.

List 8 complications of myocardial infarction.

1. Infarct expansion
2. Ventricular aneurysm
3. Ventricular pseudoaneurysm
4. VSD
5. Free wall rupture
6. Acute papillary muscle rupture and mitral regurgitation
7. Papillary muscle dysfunction
8. Mural thrombus

How can post-infarct complications be diagnosed?

Because most post-infarct complications cause signs of pulmonary edema, a non-specific finding, echocardiography or cardiac catheterization is necessary for definitive diagnosis.

What signs of post-infarct complications can be seen on CXR?

Abnormal evagination along the left heart border (indicative of left ventricular aneurysm)

Severe pulmonary edema without left atrial enlargement or cardiomegaly (indicative of papillary muscle rupture)

Diffusely enlarged cardiac silhouette [as a result of pericardial effusion (Dressler's syndrome)]

Signs of tamponade, hemothorax, or hemomediastinum (as a result of rupture of the free wall)

Acute pulmonary edema pattern (as a result of septal rupture)

What distinguishes a true ventricular aneurysm from a pseudoaneurysm on 2DE?

A true aneurysm has a wide mouth and is dyskinetic, and thinning of the myocardium is gradual. A pseudoaneurysm has a narrow neck and the transition from the myocardium to the aneurysm border is abrupt.

List 3 2DE findings associated with right ventricular infarction.

1. Right ventricular dilatation
2. Abnormal thickening of the right ventricular free wall
3. Pseudorestrictive physiology

CARDIOMYOPATHY

List the 3 general types of cardiomyopathy.

1. Dilated (congestive)
2. Restrictive (obliterative)
3. Hypertrophic

Dilated cardiomyopathy

What symptoms and CXR findings are associated with a decompensated dilated cardiomyopathy?

Symptoms include shortness of breath, edema, paroxysmal nocturnal dyspnea, and orthopnea (as a result of pulmonary congestion) and fatigue (as a result of a low output state).

CXR findings include cardiomegaly and signs of left ventricular failure; right ventricular failure may also be present.

Restrictive cardiomyopathy

What qualities characterize restrictive cardiomyopathy?

Restriction of ventricular filling and decreased compliance

List 4 causes of restrictive cardiomyopathy.

1. Amyloidosis (most common)
2. Hemochromatosis (usually causes dilated cardiomyopathy, but may cause restrictive cardiomyopathy as well)
3. Transplant
4. Idiopathic

What CXR findings are associated with restrictive cardiomyopathy?

CXR findings are uncommon and nonspecific. Biatrial enlargement is usually seen; increased pulmonary vascularity may also be noted.

What 2DE finding suggests restrictive cardiomyopathy?

Biatrial enlargement in the presence of normal-sized ventricles

Describe the 2DE characteristics of amyloidosis.

The myocardium, all four cardiac valves, and the interatrial septum are thickened.
The myocardium may show a fine, speckled pattern.
Small pericardial effusions may be seen.

What Doppler findings are seen in patients with restrictive cardiomyopathy?

Rapid mitral inflow, demonstrated by a tall, narrow E wave
No significant respiratory variation of the mitral or tricuspid inflow patterns
Reversal of flow in the mitral inflow pattern during mid-diastole (may cause diastolic mitral regurgitation)
Diminished systolic hepatic venous flow with flow reversal during inspiration

Hypertrophic cardiomyopathy

What causes hypertrophic cardiomyopathy?

Idiopathic hypertrophic subaortic stenosis is a primary type of hypertrophic cardiomyopathy. Secondary causes include aortic stenosis and hypertension.

Are there other variants of primary hypertrophic cardiomyopathy?

Yes. The obstruction may be of variable severity and location. For example, in Japan, an apical variant is found. The obstruction with this variant is apical and not subaortic.

What are the symptoms of hypertrophic cardiomyopathy?

Impaired diastolic function and potentially, left ventricular outflow tract obstruction may lead to shortness of breath, pulmonary congestion, angina, syncope or sudden death.

What conditions may mimic idiopathic hypertrophic subaortic stenosis clinically?

Concentric left ventricular hypertrophy, hypovolemia, and anemia are three conditions that can result in mid-ventricular cavity obstruction and cause symptoms similar to those of idiopathic hypertrophic subaortic stenosis.

What are the CXR findings of hypertrophic cardiomyopathy?

Radiographic findings may be few until late in the disease, at which time massive cardiomegaly with rounding of the cardiac apex or left atrial enlargement may be seen. Cardiomegaly is often accompanied by increased pulmonary vascularity and pulmonary edema.

List 3 classic 2DE findings of idiopathic hypertrophic subaortic stenosis.

1. Disproportionate hypertrophy of the septum (septum-to-posterior wall ratio of 1.5:1)
2. Systolic anterior motion of the mitral valve
3. Midsystolic closure of the aortic valve

What are the Doppler findings of idiopathic hypertrophic subaortic stenosis?

On color flow Doppler, the obstruction is manifested as a turbulent jet in the outflow tract. On spectral Doppler, increased velocity across the outflow tract gives a "saber tooth" shape to the spectral tracing of the left ventricular outflow tract. Other findings include signs of diastolic dysfunction, a "spike and dome" appearance to the aortic pressure wave form, and mitral regurgitation as a result of systolic anterior motion of the mitral valve.

"Saber tooth"   "Spike and dome"

CONGESTIVE HEART FAILURE (CHF)

What are the 4 common causes of left-sided CHF?

1. Ischemia (acute or chronic)
2. Multiple infarcts
3. Cardiomyopathy
4. Valvular heart disease

What are 5 signs of left-sided CHF on CXR?

1. Enlarged cardiac silhouette (suggests a more chronic cause)
2. Increased pulmonary vascularity with redistribution
3. Interstitial or alveolar edema
4. Pleural effusions
5. Azygos vein enlargement

Name 6 causes of right-sided CHF.

1. Left-sided CHF
2. PE
3. Pulmonary hypertension [primary, or as a result of obstructive sleep apnea or chronic obstructive pulmonary disease (COPD)]
4. Valvular pathology (tricuspid and pulmonary)
5. Right ventricular dysplasia
6. Intracardiac shunts (i.e., ASD, VSD, TAPVR)

What are the signs of right-sided CHF on CXR?

1. Right ventricular enlargement (on a lateral CXR)
2. Azygos vein enlargement
3. Enlargement of the SVC or IVC and elevated right hemidiaphragm as a result of hepatomegaly (in advanced disease)

HYPERTENSION

Describe the signs of hypertension on CXR.

Usually, only long-standing hypertension results in radiographic signs, which may include concentric left ventricular hypertrophy in response to an increased afterload, aortic dilatation (convexity of the upper right cardiac border and enlargement of the aortic knob), and calcification of the aorta and coronary arteries (in patients with arteriosclerosis).

VENTRICULAR ANEURYSM

What causes a ventricular aneurysm?

Necrosis and remodelling of the myocardium

What are the 2 major types of ventricular aneurysm and how do they differ?

1. True ventricular aneurysm: A thin wall of myocardium bulges outward.
2. False ventricular aneurysm: The wall consists of only the pericardium; rupture is pending.

What is the appearance of a true ventricular aneurysm on CXR?

Bulge along the left heart border (usually post-infarction)
Calcification in the wall

What percentage of true ventricular aneurysms are associated with contour abnormalities?

Only approximately 33%!

What is the appearance of a false ventricular aneurysm?

Located at the diaphragmatic surface, narrow neck

BUNDLE BRANCH BLOCK

How might a left bundle branch block be evidenced echocardiographically?

Left bundle branch block causes asynchronous motion of the interventricular septum. This finding is non-specific for bundle branch block and may be seen with hemodynamic abnormalities as well.

PERICARDIAL DISEASE

What is the differential diagnosis of pericardial thickening or effusion?

ATN MIIIICU
Aortic dissection
Trauma
Neoplasm (melanoma, lymphoma, metastasis from breast or lung)
Metabolic disorder (e.g., myxedema)
Inflammatory disorder [e.g., post-myocardial infarction (Dressler's syndrome), post thoracotomy]
Infection (e.g., viral, fungal, bacterial, tuberculous)
Iatrogenic (radiation, isoniazid, hydralazine, procainamide)

m

Idiopathic
Collagen vascular disease
Uremia

What echocardiographic findings are associated with constrictive disease?

Spectral Doppler reveals increased respiratory variation of the mitral and tricuspid inflow patterns. 2DE shows biatrial enlargement, small ventricular chambers, dilation of the IVC, and possibly, thickening of the pericardium.

Can one differentiate restrictive and constrictive disease using echocardiography?

It is difficult, but with constrictive disease, no variation is seen in the mitral and tricuspid inflow patterns with respiration.

Pericardial effusion

List 2 signs of a pericardial effusion on CXR.

1. Enlarged heart shadow, often with a globular shape (i.e., the transverse diameter is disproportionately increased)
2. "Fat pad" sign (i.e., a soft tissue stripe wider than 2 mm between the epicardial fat and the anterior mediastinal fat is noted on a lateral view)

What clue on serial films is particularly suggestive of pericardial effusion?

Rapid changes in the size of the heart shadow

How much fluid must be in the pericardium to lead to a change in the heart shadow on CXR?

400–500 ml

How can pericardial effusion be definitively diagnosed?

Echocardiography (highly sensitive for detecting pericardial fluid) or CT (also quite sensitive)

How can one differentiate between a pericardial effusion and a pleural effusion using 2DE?

In the parasternal long axis, a pericardial effusion is anterior to the descending aorta, while a pleural effusion is posterior to the descending aorta.

What is the appearance of a pericardial effusion on CT?

Fluid filling the pericardial space

List 5 echocardiographic findings associated with cardiac tamponade.

1. Right atrial diastolic inversion or collapse
2. Right ventricular diastolic inversion or collapse
3. Increased respiratory variation of tricuspid inflow velocities (i.e., the E wave velocity increases by more than 40% with inspiration)
4. Increased respiratory variation of mitral inflow velocities (i.e., the E wave velocity decreases by more than 25% with inspiration)
5. Fixed, dilated IVC

How might echocardiography be used to facilitate a pericardiocentesis?

The echocardiogram may be used to locate the effusion, determine the feasibility of performing a pericardiocentesis, and guide needle placement. Furthermore, a post-procedure study can be used to demonstrate efficacy.

Pericarditis

What does pericardial calcification seen on CXR suggest?

Chronic pericarditis, usually postinfective (e.g., following tuberculosis)

Other than pericardial calcifications, what are the other signs of chronic pericarditis on CXR?

Dilation of the SVC or IVC (if the pericarditis is constrictive)
Enlarged heart silhouette—or, it may be normal

Describe the utility of 2DE in the evaluation of pericarditis.

2DE is neither sensitive nor specific for detecting pericarditis, per se. Thickened pericardium is difficult to appreciate but can be more readily seen when pericardial fluid is present.

What is the best radiologic study for the diagnosis of chronic pericarditis?

CT

How is chronic pericarditis definitively diagnosed?

Biopsy

CARDIAC MASSES

What is the most common area for a fatty deposition in the heart?	Lipomatous hypertrophy of the inter-atrial septum. The lesion appears as a dumbbell-shaped echodensity, sparing the fossa ovalis.
What is the most common primary cardiac neoplasm?	Myxoma
What are the most common locations of cardiac myxomas?	The left atrial septum is most common, although a myxoma can occur on any wall. The right atrium is the next most common location. Myxomas may also be seen on the ventricles.

List 5 other tumors found in the heart.

1. Papillary fibroelastoma (often found on the ventricular side of heart valves; often pedunculated)
2. Rhabdomyoma and rhabdomyosarcoma (most commonly found in the ventricles)
3. Fibroma (often involves the intraventricular septum)
4. Lymphoma
5. Metastatic tumors

CARDIAC TRAUMA

When should one suspect blunt cardiac injury in a trauma patient.

When there is evidence of sternal fracture or precordial soft tissue injury

List 4 cardiac manifestations of blunt cardiac trauma.

1. Cardiac contusion, the most common manifestation of blunt cardiac trauma, may mimic myocardial infarction clinically and biochemically.
2. Traumatic rupture of the chordae or papillary muscles may lead to acute valvular insufficiency and pulmonary edema.
3. Disruption of the tricuspid valve leads to tricuspid regurgitation and is fairly common.
4. Aortic dissection leads to aortic insufficiency, and possibly pericardial effusion.

DISEASES OF THE AORTA

What diseases of the aorta may be diagnosed by echocardiography?	Dissection, aneurysm, pseudoaneurysm, intramural hematoma, athersosclerosis, thrombi, perforation
What echocardiographic technique is the most useful for assessing diseases of the aorta?	TEE

5

Vascular Imaging

Clinton R. Nichols

ANATOMY

Describe the general structure of the arterial wall.

Tunica intima: Luminal (innermost) layer consisting of a single thickness of endothelial cells

Internal elastic lamina: Separates the tunica intima and the tunica media

Tunica media: Thickest layer of the vessel wall, consisting of smooth muscle cells

External elastic lamina: Separates the tunica media and the tunica externa

Tunica adventitia: Outermost layer, connective tissue sheath

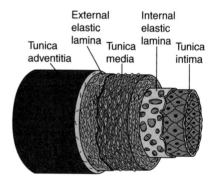

Tunica adventitia | External elastic lamina | Tunica media | Internal elastic lamina | Tunica intima

THORACIC REGION

Identify the following structures:

A = Root of the aorta
B = Ascending aorta
C = Superior vena cava (SVC)
D = Right brachiocephalic vein
E = Right brachiocephalic artery
F = Right subclavian artery
G = Right common carotid artery

H = Left common carotid artery
I = Left subclavian artery
J = Left brachiocephalic vein
K = Arch of the aorta
L = Ligamentum arteriosum
M = Main pulmonary artery

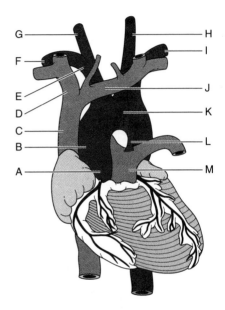

What are the dilatations at the root of the aorta called?

The sinuses of Valsalva

At what level (anterior and posterior) is the arch of the aorta?

Anterior: At the sternal angle
Posterior: Vertebrae T4–T5

What percentage of people have variant aortic arch anatomy?

30%

What is the most common arch variant?

Bovine arch (i.e., common origin of the left common carotid and left subclavian arteries)

What are the branches of the descending thoracic aorta?

The bronchial, intercostal, and aortic esophageal arteries

At what levels do the inferior vena cava (IVC), esophagus, and descending aorta cross the diaphragm, respectively?

Vertebrae T8, T10, and T12, respectively

ABDOMINAL AND PELVIC REGIONS

Identify the branches of the abdominal aorta:

A = Celiac artery
B = Superior mesenteric artery (SMA)
C = Left renal artery
D = Lumbar arteries
E = Inferior mesenteric artery (IMA)
F = Median sacral artery
G = Common iliac artery
H = Gonadal artery

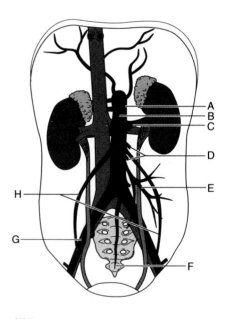

What percentage of people have accessory renal arteries?

35%

Label the branches of the celiac artery:

A = Left gastric artery
B = Splenic artery
C = Common hepatic artery
D = Proper hepatic artery
E = Gastroduodenal artery

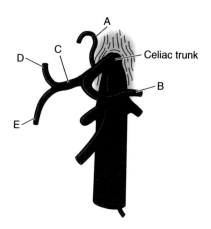

What are the branches of the SMA?

A = Inferior pancreaticoduodenal artery
B = Right colic artery
C = Ileocolic artery
D = Jejunal and ileal branches
E = Marginal artery of Drummond
F = Middle colic artery

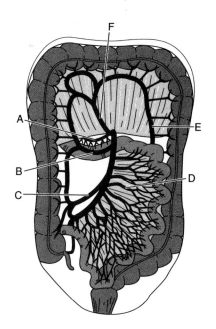

What are the branches of the IMA?

A = Left colic artery
B = Sigmoid arteries
C = Superior rectal artery

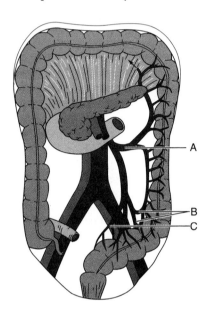

Which area of the bowel is particularly susceptible to injury from ischemia?

Infarcts are likely to involve watershed areas (i.e., areas at the borders of arterial territories), such as the area of the transverse colon and splenic flexure supplied by the marginal artery of Drummond. The marginal artery of Drummond is formed by anastomosis of the branches of the SMA and IMA.

What arteries supply the stomach?

The lesser curvature of the stomach is supplied by the left gastric artery (B), a branch of the celiac artery (A), and the right gastric artery (C), a branch of the hepatic artery (G).

The greater curvature of the stomach is supplied by the short gastric arteries (D); the left gastroepiploic artery (E), a branch of the splenic artery; and the right gastroepiploic artery (F), a branch of the gastroduodenal artery.

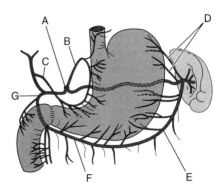

What vessel is most likely the source of bleeding from a duodenal ulcer?

The gastroduodenal artery, which courses posterior to the duodenum

What arteries supply the liver?

Right and left hepatic arteries, branches of the proper hepatic artery

What percentage of people have a variant arterial supply to the liver?

Approximately 50%

What are the most common variants of the hepatic arterial vasculature?

Right hepatic artery (or the accessory right hepatic artery) branching off the SMA (so-called "replaced" right hepatic artery)

Left hepatic artery (or the accessory left hepatic artery) branching off the left gastric artery

What percentage of blood supply to the liver comes from the hepatic artery and the portal vein, respectively?

25% and 75%, respectively

Label the portal venous anatomy:

A = Portal vein
B = Superior mesenteric vein
C = Inferior mesenteric vein
D = Splenic vein
E = Left gastric vein
F = Gastroepiploic vein
G = Short gastric veins

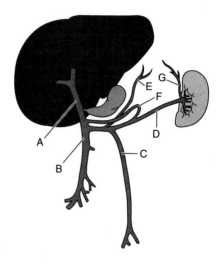

Label the pelvic vasculature:

A = Abdominal aorta
B = IMA
C = Common iliac artery
D = Median sacral artery
E = Internal iliac artery
F = External iliac artery
G = Inferior gluteal artery
H = Superior gluteal artery
I = Deep femoral artery (profunda femoris)
J = Superficial femoral artery

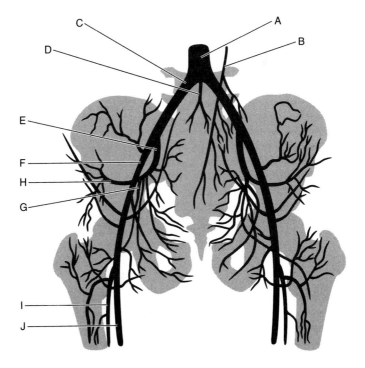

**What are the variants of the
left renal vein (LRV) and
the IVC?**

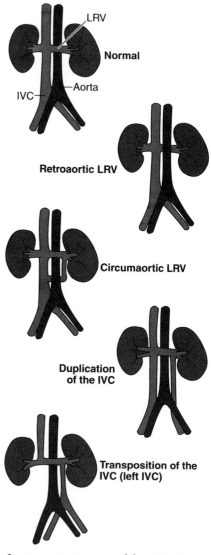

**How does blood return to
the heart in patients with
azygos continuation of the
IVC?**

In azygos continuation of the IVC, the
IVC terminates at the renal veins and no
intrahepatic segment is present. Blood
flows from the IVC to the dilated azygos
system and returns to the SVC through
the azygos arch.

**Why is it important to
recognize anomalies of the
LRV and IVC?**

1. Vessels have a rounded appearance on
   axial images and simulate the
   appearance of lymph nodes, especially

on unenhanced and early-phase computed tomography (CT) scans. One would not want to plan a biopsy of the left IVC.

2. Anomalous configuration of the IVC changes the approach to placement of IVC filters.

EXTREMITIES

Label the arterial supply of the upper limb:

A = Thyrocervical trunk
B = Subclavian artery
C = Thoracoacromial artery
D = Axillary artery
E = Deep brachial artery
F = Brachial artery
G = Radial recurrent artery
H = Radial artery
I = Interosseous artery
J = Ulnar recurrent artery
K = Ulnar artery
L = Superficial palmar arch
M = Deep palmar arch
N = Common digital arteries

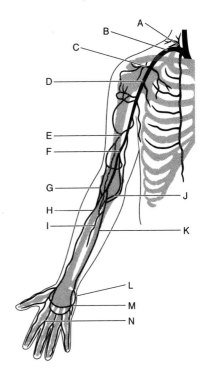

What artery courses through the "anatomic snuff box"?   The radial artery

Label the venous drainage of the upper extremity:

A = Median cubital vein
B = Basilic vein
C = Cephalic vein
D = Brachial vein
E = Axillary vein
F = Subclavian vein
G = External jugular vein
H = Internal jugular vein
I = Brachiocephalic vein
J = SVC

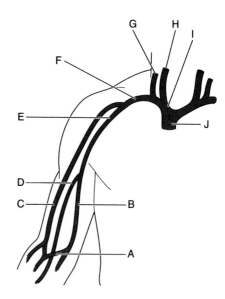

How are the femoral vessels and nerve oriented below the inguinal ligament?

To remember the orientation of the femoral vessels and nerve from lateral to medial, think **NAVEL:** Nerve, **A**rtery, **V**ein, **E**mpty space with **L**ymphatics

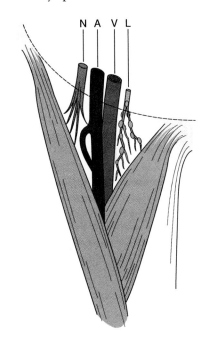

What are the three arteries below the knee?

Anterior tibial, posterior tibial, and peroneal arteries

What is an easy way to memorize the vessels below the knee as they appear on an anterior angiogram?

LAMP: Lateral = **A**nterior tibial, **M**edial = **P**osterior tibial

Label the arterial supply of the lower extremity:

A = External iliac artery
B = Common femoral artery
C = Deep femoral artery (profunda femoris)
D = Superficial femoral artery
E = Popliteal artery
F = Tibial-peroneal trunk
G = Peroneal artery
H = Anterior tibial artery (becomes the dorsalis pedis)
I = Posterior tibial artery
J = Dorsalis pedis

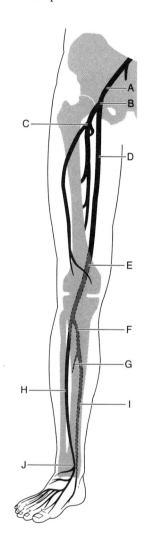

What veins constitute the superficial veins of the lower extremity and where do they drain into the deep system?

The dorsal venous arch drains to the popliteal vein, which enters the deep system. The dorsal venous arch also drains into the lesser saphenous and accessory saphenous veins, which flow to the greater saphenous vein (medial) to drain into the femoral vein.

Label the deep veins of the lower extremity:

A = Plantar venous arch
B = Posterior tibial veins
C = Peroneal veins
D = Anterior tibial veins
E = Popliteal vein
F = Femoral vein
G = Deep femoral vein
H = Common femoral vein

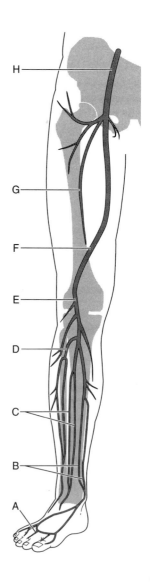

IMAGING STUDIES

ANGIOGRAPHY

What is angiography?

The study of blood vessels (arteries = arteriography, veins = venography), traditionally performed by injecting contrast into the vessels and visualizing them fluoroscopically; now also performed with computed tomography (CT) and magnetic resonance imaging (MRI)

What are the indications for angiography?

Diagnostic: Vascular disease, neoplasia, hemorrhage, dissection, trauma
Therapeutic: Angioplasty, embolization, selective drug therapy

What are the absolute and relative contraindications for angiography?

Absolute: None
Relative: Coagulopathy, allergy to contrast agents, renal insufficiency, dehydration, metformin use within 48 hours, congestive heart failure (CHF), recent myocardial infarction (MI)

What aspects of the patient history are important to discern prior to performing angiography?

Symptoms that would indicate a need for angiography:
History of prior radiographic studies, including exposure to contrast and any history of contrast reaction
Medication history (e.g., use of aspirin, warfarin, heparin, metformin, drugs that contribute to renal toxicity)
History of surgery (especially vascular)
History of prior interventions (e.g., angioplasty, stent placement)
Past medical history (e.g., allergies, asthma, diabetes, coagulopathy, cerebro- or cardiovascular disease, renal disease, hypertension)

What should be the focus of the physical examination prior to the procedure?

Vital signs: Is the patient stable? Uncontrolled hypertension increases the risk of complications.
Pulse examination: Documenting the pulses prior to performing the procedure enables you to choose a site for vascular access and provides a baseline for the evaluation of complications.

Ankle to brachial index (ABI): Blood pressure ratios should be obtained if the need for peripheral vascular intervention is anticipated.

What laboratory studies should be ordered?

Prothrombin time (PT) and partial thromboplastin time (PTT)

Blood urea nitrogen (BUN) and creatine levels

Hemoglobin, hematocrit, white blood cell (WBC) count, platelet count

What 2 tasks are imperative prior to performing angiography?

1. Obtain and document informed consent.
2. Review all pertinent imaging studies in order to develop a clear idea of the ultimate goal of the procedure.

What orders need to be followed prior to the procedure?

1. Withhold aspirin prior to the procedure.
2. Withhold warfarin approximately 3–4 days prior to the procedure.
3. Withhold metformin following the parenteral administration of iodinated contrast.
4. Correct coagulopathy using fresh frozen plasma.
5. Correct thrombocytopenia; platelet level should exceed 100,000/mm³.
6. Keep patient on clear liquids approximately 8 hours prior to the procedure.
7. Administer intravenous fluids to maintain hydration.
8. Initiate antibiotic therapy if entry into a contaminated or infected area is suspected.
9. Initiate contrast reaction prophylaxis if indicated.
10. Shave and prep each groin for standard common femoral approach.

How can heparin be reversed emergently?

Administer 1 mg protamine sulfate per 100 U heparin.

How can warfarin be reversed?

Administer vitamin K (may take at least 6 hours to reverse the warfarin) or fresh frozen plasma

Why is it important to withhold metformin after the parenteral administration of iodinated contrast?

Metformin, an oral hypoglycemic agent used in the treatment of type II non-insulin dependent diabetes mellitus, is excreted solely through the kidneys. Patients who take metformin and have impaired renal function are at risk for developing a potentially fatal lactic acidosis. Radiographic contrast may lead to acute renal failure, and therefore places patients taking metformin at risk for developing a severe lactic acidosis.

What types of anesthesia may be used during the procedure?

Local: Lidocaine without epinephrine is used to numb the puncture site.

Conscious sedation: Usually a benzodiazepine is used in combination with a narcotic; close monitoring is required.

General anesthesia may be required for some procedures [e.g., transjugular intrahepatic portosystemic shunt (TIPS)] or for pediatric patients.

Why is the skin at the entry site numbed using lidocaine without epinephrine?

To avoid vessel spasm caused by epinephrine

What precautions are taken during the procedure to ensure patient safety?

Monitoring (blood pressure, heart rate, respiratory rate, pulse oximetry, cardiac monitoring)

Systemic heparinization (to prevent thrombosis in certain cases)

Catheter flushing (i.e., intermittent flushing with heparinized saline to prevent clot formation within or at the tip of the catheter)

What specific care is required post-procedure?

Puncture site

Straighten and remove catheters over a guidewire to avoid arterial injury.

Apply firm manual compression to prevent oozing without fully obstructing distal blood flow. Compression should be held for at least 15 minutes, longer if the patient has complicating medical conditions (e.g., coagulopathy, hypertension).

Apply a sterile dressing and a compression bandage.

Patient must lie flat and the limb used for vascular access must be kept straight for 6–8 hours.

Distal pulses. Evaluate and document the distal pulses prior to releasing the patient to return to the floor.

Medical management. Coagulopathy must be corrected and blood pressure controlled.

Nursing. Evaluate the following at regular intervals to detect any complications: vital signs, distal pulses, puncture site (for hematoma), and motor and neurologic function of the punctured and/or treated extremity.

Achieving vascular access

What is the name of the common technique used to achieve arterial access?

Seldinger technique

Describe the steps in the Seldinger technique of percutaneous arterial catheterization.

1. A needle (usually 18-gauge) with a stylet is advanced through both walls of the vessel.
2. The stylet is removed and the needle is withdrawn slowly into the vessel lumen. Pulsatile blood will flow out the back of the needle.
3. A guidewire is advanced into the vessel using fluoroscopic guidance.
4. The guidewire is held in place and the needle is removed over the wire while firmly compressing the puncture site.
5. A catheter is passed over the wire into the vessel lumen.
6. The guidewire is removed, leaving the catheter in the vessel ready for the injection of contrast material.
(See figure on next page)

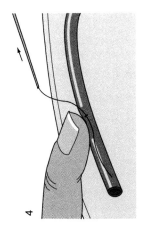

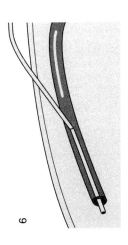

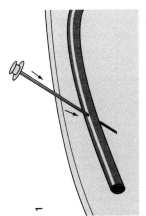

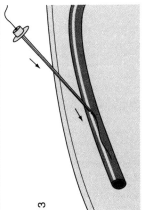

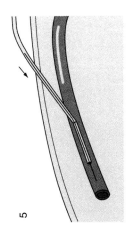

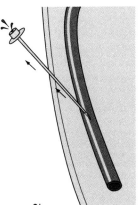

Is it always necessary to use fluoroscopy while advancing the guidewire?

Yes.

What should you do if you meet resistance with the guidewire?

Stop! A contrast injection may be needed to show the lumen.

What should you do if the arterial puncture is unsuccessful?

Remove the Seldinger needle, flush with saline, and replace the central stylet before attempting the procedure again.

What are the 2 most common approaches for percutaneous arterial catheterization?

Common femoral artery approach
Brachial artery approach

List 2 advantages of the common femoral artery approach.

The common femoral artery is superficial and easily palpated, and hemostasis can be achieved by applying pressure over the femoral head.

What is the ideal entry site when using the common femoral artery approach?

Below the inguinal ligament at the level of the mid-femoral head; position should be confirmed using fluoroscopy

Why is it important to accurately place the needle?

If the artery is punctured above the inguinal ligament or below the femoral head, control of hemostasis may be difficult or impossible.

Under what circumstances is the brachial artery approach used?

When a femoral artery approach cannot be performed safely (e.g., in a patient with absent femoral pulses, recent femoral artery surgery, hematoma, or infection)

What is the main advantage of the brachial artery approach?

Permits easier manipulation for selective splanchnic arteriography or intervention.

What are the disadvantages of the brachial artery approach?

Poorer control of hemostasis, possible nerve injury

Is the left or right side preferred with the brachial artery approach?

Left

Why?	Approaching from the left side allows access to the descending aorta without crossing the right brachiocephalic and left common carotid arteries, reducing the risk of stroke
When is the right brachial artery used?	When the left is compromised by vascular disease or when studying the ascending aorta, right subclavian, or right vertebral arteries
What is seen in images following arterial contrast injection?	Sequential opacification of the down-stream vascular bed (i.e., arterial, capillary, and venous phases)
What approaches are used for venography?	Venipuncture of a distal peripheral vein, venous catheterization (usually of the common femoral vein), and selective contrast injection

Catheters, guidewires, and pharmacologic agents

What is the conversion between the metric system and "French" sizes?	1 mm = 3 French (Fr)
How are the outer diameter (OD), inner diameter (ID), and length of a catheter measured?	OD measured in French, ID measured in 1/1000 of an inch, length measured in centimeters
What are the advantages of multiple-hole and side-hole catheter configurations?	These configurations: 1. Reduce the resistance to flow; used for high volume injection 2. Minimize trauma to the vessel wall from forceful injections 3. Reduce the recoil of the catheter 4. Improve distribution of contrast within the lumen of large vessels
What is the disadvantage of the side-hole catheter configuration?	Clots tend to form in the lumen of the side-hole catheter if the catheter is not flushed vigorously.
What is the primary use for single end-hole catheters?	Selective arteriography

What is the main disadvantage of an end-hole catheter?

The risk of causing a dissection is increased.

What is meant by catheter "memory?"

The ability of a catheter to maintain its shape during manipulations

How are the size and length of a guidewire measured?

Size measured in 1/1000 of an inch (for instance, 0.038 inch is a common size)
Length measured in centimeters (standard length is 145 cm; exchange length is 220+ cm for use with long catheters)

What is a "J" and how is it measured?

"J" refers to the radius of the curvature at the end of a shaped wire and is measured in millimeters.

What are the disadvantages of straight guidewires?

Straight wires tend to injure vessel walls and undermine atherosclerotic plaques, leading to dissection and embolization.

What are the advantages of straight guidewires?

They are more easily advanced into a small vascular orifice.

What factors influence the dose of contrast?

The dose of contrast for a study depends on the size and flow rate of the vessel to be studied, as well as the type of study. Lower volumes are needed when using digital subtraction angiography (DSA).

Why might vasodilators be administered during angiography?

To improve visualization of vasculature
To treat vasospasm and mesenteric ischemia
To augment flow during intra-arterial pressure measurements

List 3 potential complications of vasodilator administration.

Hypotension, tachycardia, arrhythmias

What vasodilators are commonly used for angiography?

Intra-arterial administration: Verapamil, tolazoline hydrochloride, nitroglycerin, papaverine hydrochloride
Oral administration: Nifedipine

Why might vasoconstrictors be administered during angiography?

To control hemorrhage and to differentiate normal vessels from tumor vessels

How can vasoconstrictors help distinguish normal vessels from tumor vessels?	Tumor vessels do not vasoconstrict in response to medications and will stand out in contrast to normally constricted vessels.
What complications are associated with vasoconstrictor administration?	Vasoconstrictors may precipitate angina, myocardial infarction, or arrhythmias and can cause ischemia if infused into end-arteries.
What vasoconstrictors may be used?	Epinephrine or vasopressin
What side effect is unique to vasopressin?	Water retention [owing to the antidiuretic hormone (ADH) effect]

Complications of angiography

What age groups are at higher risk than the rest of the population for catheter-related complications?	Children are at higher risk owing to the higher catheter to vessel ratio, while the elderly are at higher risk owing to cardiovascular insufficiency and atherosclerotic vessel walls.
What are the possible complications of angiography, related to:	
Use of contrast? (List 2)	Anaphylactoid reaction, nephrotoxicity
Achieving vascular access? (List 8)	Hemorrhage, hematoma, pseudoaneurysm, arteriovenous (AV) fistula, thrombosis, dissection, infection, nerve damage
The distal vasculature? (List 5)	Thrombosis, embolism, dissection, perforation, hemorrhage
What is the death rate attributable to angiography?	Less than 0.05%
List 4 factors that predispose patients to the development of puncture site complications.	Suboptimal technique, hypertension, obesity, coagulopathy
List 8 ways the angiographer can minimize puncture site complications.	1. Choose the proper vascular access site (femoral artery: mid-femoral head, below the inguinal ligament).

2. Minimize the catheter size.
3. Use a vascular sheath if pericatheter leak occurs.
4. Straighten catheters and guidewires on removal.
5. Apply firm manual compression for a minimum of 15 minutes.
6. Correct coagulopathy prior to the procedure.
7. Control hypertension.
8. Decrease procedure time.

What percentage of patients develop a hematoma after:

Femoral catheterization?   Approximately 5%

Femoral catheterization that requires surgical intervention?   Less than 0.5%

Brachial catheterization that requires surgical intervention?   3%

What is the mechanism of injury that leads to AV fistula formation?   Inadvertent simultaneous puncture of an artery and vein

What is a pseudoaneurysm?   Dilatation of a vessel wall that involves 0, 1, or 2 tunics, usually saccular (true aneurysms involve all three tunics)

List 8 factors that contribute to arterial thrombosis at the puncture site.

1. Catheter tip thrombosis (vessel stripped by the tip of the catheter as it is withdrawn, forming a nidus for thrombosis)
2. Multiple puncture attempts
3. Use of large catheters or sheath
4. Repeated catheter/guidewire exchanges
5. Hypotensive patient
6. Contrast reaction resulting in hypotension and stasis
7. Lengthy procedure
8. Poor manual compression

List 4 factors that increase the likelihood of embolism.

1. Thrombosis within or around the catheter

2. Dislodged atherosclerotic plaque or cholesterol embolism
3. Introduction of air into the vessel via the catheter or flushing
4. Introduction of foreign material into the vessel

List 7 ways the angiographer can minimize the risk of thrombosis or embolization.

1. Minimize the procedure time.
2. Minimize vessel wall damage by using floppy curved-tip or steerable guidewires.
3. Institute systemic heparinization.
4. Flush the catheter frequently with heparinized saline.
5. Always use a guidewire to advance the catheter.
6. Use a "J"-shaped guidewire to avoid undermining atherosclerotic plaques.
7. Use catheters with side holes whenever possible.

How is a dissection created at the puncture site?

Dissection occurs when the bevel of the needle used for vascular access lies only partially within the lumen, causing the guidewire to pass between the layers of the vessel wall.

How is a dissection created in distant vessels?

The guidewire may pass underneath an atherosclerotic plaque and into the vessel wall. A pressure injection through a single end-hole catheter positioned against a vessel wall can also result in dissection.

ULTRASOUND

What are the advantages of ultrasound for imaging vascular structures?

Contrast not required, noninvasive, relatively inexpensive

When is color Doppler ultrasound indicated?

When it is necessary to determine the patency of vessels of grafts or demonstrate the physiological significance of atherosclerotic plaques or stenoses

COMPUTED TOMOGRAPHY (CT)

What type of vascular contrast is used for CT?

The same iodinated contrast agents used in conventional angiography

List 3 advantages of CT for evaluating the vascular system.

Noninvasive, excellent for measuring lesions, easily demonstrates intraluminal clots and extravascular hematoma

What is a CT angiogram (CTA) and how is it created?

A CTA is a 3-dimensional computer reconstruction of blood vessels, created from a thin-slice helical CT scan taken with intravascular contrast. The surrounding structures may be "subtracted" (removed).

MAGNETIC RESONANCE IMAGING (MRI)

What are the advantages of MRI for the study of vascular structures?

MRI is noninvasive, does not require the use of radiation or contrast, and images can be reconstructed in any plane. When contrast is used, the MRI contrast agents are not as nephrotoxic or allergenic as conventional iodinated contrast agents.

How is the 3-dimensional image of an MR angiogram (MRA) made?

A computer program "stacks" the flow voids or contrast-enhanced vessel images from sequential MRIs to render a 3-dimensional image.

What are the advantages of MRA over standard angiography?

It is noninvasive, and because iodinated contrast is not needed, MRA can be used safely in patients with renal insufficiency.

What are the disadvantages of MRA over standard angiography?

Sensitivity to motion limits use in the thoracic region (owing to ventilation) and the abdomen (owing to peristalsis).

How is MRA different from conventional angiography or CTA?

MRA depicts both anatomy and flow rate (i.e., physiology), whereas other techniques show only flow.

DIGITAL SUBTRACTION ANGIOGRAPHY (DSA)

What is DSA?

Serial images are stored electronically. The initial image (without contrast) is subtracted from the postinjection images to eliminate nonvascular structures from the image.

List 4 advantages of DSA.

1. Improved contrast resolution of opacified vascular structures
2. Uses less contrast agent

3. Permits the use of smaller catheters, leading to a lower incidence of puncture site complications
4. May allow computer "correction" for some movement artifacts

What are 2 disadvantages of DSA?

Lower spatial resolution and movement create subtraction artifacts

THERAPEUTIC PROCEDURES

PERCUTANEOUS TRANSLUMINAL ANGIOPLASTY (PTA)

What is PTA?

Mechanical recanalization of an occluded or stenotic vessel segment using a balloon catheter

Identify the components of a balloon catheter:

A = Distal lumen
B = Balloon
C = Opaque marker
D = Distal end hole
E = Opening for contrast
F = Inflation lumen

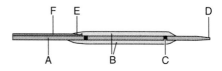

What are the indications for PTA?

Vaso-occlusive disease (i.e., athero-sclerosis, Takayasu's arteritis, fibro-muscular dysplasia, surgical bypass graft failure)

What are the 7 steps in performing PTA?

1. Diagnostic angiogram
2. Cross the lesion (i.e., place the wire and then the catheter beyond the lesion)
3. Systemic heparinization after the lesion is crossed
4. Pressure measurements proximal and distal to the stenosis
5. Balloon inflation
6. Balloon deflation
7. Post-procedure angiogram and pressure measurements

On what basis is the PTA balloon selected?

The balloon diameter is chosen by measuring the diameter of the normal segment adjacent to the narrow or occluded segment.

What gradient is physiologically significant?

A gradient of more than 10 mm Hg

What is a sign that the angioplasty balloon has been fully inflated?

A "waist" is seen as the balloon inflates adjacent to the plaque. This waist disappears when the balloon is fully inflated.

How does PTA achieve recanalization?

Inflation of the balloon leads to compression of the soft elements of the plaque, fissuring and fracture of the atherosclerotic plaque and tunica intima, and stretching of the tunica media and adjacent normal vessel.

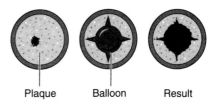

Plaque   Balloon   Result

List 3 factors that favorably affect the outcome of PTA.

Single, short segment of stenosis; large- to medium-sized vessel; patent vessel proximal and distal to the stenosis

List 9 factors that unfavorably affect the outcome of PTA.

1. Diffuse, multifocal stenoses
2. Small vessel
3. Compromised inflow or outflow
4. Occluded lumen
5. Diabetic patient
6. Heavily calcified plaque
7. Inability to cross the lesion
8. Inability to dilate the segment
9. Long area of stenosis

What short-term complications are associated with PTA?

Arterial rupture, balloon rupture, complications of arterial catheterization (e.g., spasm, dissection, thrombosis, embolism)

What long-term complications are associated with PTA?

Intimal hyperplasia and progression of atherosclerotic disease

What is intimal hyperplasia?

Intimal hyperplasia, an exaggerated reparative response to vessel injury, results when damage to the vessel elements leads to migration of smooth muscle cells from the tunica media to the tunica intima, causing intimal thickening and narrowing of the vessel lumen.

What percentage of patients develop intimal hyperplasia at the site of PTA?

100%. All patients develop intimal hyperplasia to some degree following PTA.

List 4 options if the results of PTA are unfavorable.

1. Repeat PTA with a different size of balloon
2. Stent placement
3. Percutaneous atherectomy
4. Surgical bypass

What is a stent?

An expandable tube, often made of metal, that is introduced percutaneously and deployed across an area of stenosis to help maintain vessel patency

List 4 indications for stent placement in the treatment of atherosclerotic stenosis.

1. Long segments of stenosis or occlusion
2. Ulcerated plaque
3. Unsuccessful PTA [i.e., residual stenosis ($> 30\%$), residual pressure gradient (> 10 mm Hg), dissection
4. Recurrent stenosis

THERAPEUTIC EMBOLIZATION

List 7 indications for therapeutic embolization.

1. Hemorrhage
2. Aneurysm
3. Organ ablation (alternative to surgery)
4. Neoplasia (decrease tumor bulk, palliation of pain)
5. Adjunct to surgery (performed prior to surgery to decrease intra-operative bleeding)
6. Arteriovenous malformation (AVM) or AV fistula
7. Varicocele

When are temporary embolic agents used?	Gastrointestinal bleed
What types of temporary embolic agents are used?	Gelfoam, autologous blood clot, cellulose
When is it favorable to use permanent embolic agents?	Tumors, AVM, AV fistula
What types of permanent embolic agents are used?	Detachable balloon, ethyl alcohol, polyvinyl alcohol, steel coils, cyanoacrylate
What is meant by the term "proximal" embolization?	Large particles are used to occlude feeding arteries or arterioles
What is meant by the term "distal" embolization?	Small particles or chemicals are used to occlude the capillary bed
What are the complications of embolization therapy?	Postembolization syndrome (fever, elevated WBC count, nausea, vomiting, pain), inadvertent embolization of other vascular beds, infection, recurrent hemorrhage

THROMBOLYSIS

What are the indications for thrombolysis?	Arterial, venous, or graft thrombosis
What are the absolute and relative contraindications for thrombolysis?	**Absolute:** Active bleeding, pregnancy, intracranial pathology **Relative:** Recent major surgery; postpartum status; cardiac thrombus; coagulopathy; history of gastrointestinal bleeding, varices, or ulcer
What factors predispose to a favorable outcome?	Fresh clot, catheter positioned within clot, preservation of inflow (proximal) and outflow (distal) to the clot
List 3 complications of thrombolytic therapy.	Bleeding (at puncture site or distant site), embolization, reperfusion syndrome
What percentage of patients undergoing thrombolysis experience a major hemorrhage?	7%

What thrombolytic agents are available?	Streptokinase, recombinant tissue plasminogen activator (rTPA)
Why is streptokinase no longer used?	It is antigenic (patient makes antibodies to streptokinase)

TRANSJUGULAR INTRAHEPATIC PORTOSYSTEMIC SHUNT (TIPS)

What is TIPS?	A procedure used in the treatment of chronic liver disease whereby a shunt is created between branches of the portal vein (*porto-*) and the hepatic (*systemic*) veins
What are the established indications for TIPS?	Acute variceal bleeding refractory to other treatment options Recurrent variceal bleeding in candidates for liver transplant Recurrent variceal bleeding requiring frequent endoscopy Gastric varices (difficult to treat endoscopically)
What are the possible indications for TIPS?	Budd-Chiari syndrome, refractory ascites, refractory hepatic hydrothorax, hepato-renal syndrome, transplant (in order to reduce portal pressures prior to the procedure)
List 8 contraindications to TIPS.	Bile duct dilatation, cholangitis, hepatic abscess, hepatic tumor, severe coagu-lopathy, polycystic liver disease, severe encephalopathy
What needs to be done prior to performing the TIPS procedure?	History and physical examination, endos-copy (to confirm varices as the source of gastrointestinal bleeding), Doppler ultra-sound or MRI (to confirm patency of the portal vein and evaluate vascular anat-omy), correction of coagulopathy or thrombocytopenia
How is TIPS performed?	1. Vascular access is achieved via the right internal jugular vein.

2. A catheter is advanced into a branch of the hepatic vein.
3. The wedged hepatic pressure is obtained.
4. An image of the portal vein is attained via reflux of contrast through the sinusoids.
5. A Colapinto needle is advanced into the hepatic vein and passed through the liver parenchyma.
6. Suction is placed on the needle as it is slowly withdrawn. When there is blood return, a contrast injection is made to confirm that the needle tip is in a branch of the portal vein.
7. A guidewire is passed into the portal vein.
8. A balloon is used to dilate the tract in the parenchyma.
9. A stent is placed, creating a shunt between the branches of the portal vein and the hepatic veins.

How can graft patency be examined noninvasively?

Doppler ultrasound or CT

What is the primary graft patency rate at 1 year?

50%

What is the recurrence rate for gastrointestinal hemorrhage following TIPS?

10%

List 4 advantages of TIPS over surgical creation of a portocaval shunt.

1. Decreased periprocedural morbidity and mortality
2. Stent can be placed under local anesthesia
3. Vascular anatomy is preserved for liver transplantation
4. Decreases portal pressures and blood loss during liver transplantation

List 7 complications of TIPS.

1. Encephalopathy (as many as 24% of patients)
2. Stenosis or occlusion (caused by shunt thrombosis or intimal hyperplasia)
3. Puncture of the liver capsule or intra-abdominal hemorrhage

4. Volume overload leading to right-sided heart failure
5. Contrast nephrotoxicity
6. Accelerated liver failure
7. Infection

PERIPHERALLY INSERTED CENTRAL CATHETER (PICC)

What is the advantage of a PICC line over a subclavian or internal jugular central venous catheter?

Placement of a PICC line into the veins of the arm avoids the procedure-related complications associated with placement of a standard central line (e.g., pneumothorax, arterial injury, central venous stenosis at the puncture site).

List 4 indications for PICC line placement.

1. Absence of peripheral venous access
2. Need for short-term venous access (generally less than 3–6 months)
3. Need for frequent blood draws
4. Outpatient intravenous therapy

List 7 contraindications to PICC line placement.

1. Need for frequent transfusions (blood products have high viscosity and therefore do not infuse reliably through a PICC)
2. Need for long-term intravenous access (longer than 3–6 months)
3. Severe coagulopathy
4. Central venous occlusion (relative contraindication)
5. Thrombophlebitis
6. Bacteremia
7. Insufficient patient support for the safe use of a PICC line

What are the sites of venous access routinely used for PICC line placement?

Veins of the upper arm (basilic, brachial, or cephalic veins)
Veins of the antecubital fossa or forearm (when done at bedside without fluoroscopy)

What are the disadvantages of placing lines in the veins of the antecubital fossa and forearm?

Longer catheter limits the flow rates, catheter prone to kinking with elbow flexion, decreased patient satisfaction

List 3 sites for venous access in the upper arm.

Cephalic vein (superficial, lateral)
Basilic vein (superficial, medial)

Brachial veins (deep, paired veins that follow the path of the brachial artery)

What are the common modalities used for obtaining venous access in the upper arm?

Direct visualization: Rarely, a superficial vein in the upper arm can be visualized and punctured directly.

Intravenous contrast: Intravenous access is achieved peripheral to the intended puncture site and contrast is injected. The vein is then accessed under fluoroscopic guidance.

Ultrasound: The needle is advanced under direct visualization of both arteries and veins.

How is a PICC line placed?

1. Double wall puncture of a vein in the upper extremity
2. Needle is withdrawn under fluoroscopy as a guidewire is probed for the vein (the guidewire will follow a linear course without resistance when introduced into the lumen of a vessel)
3. Guidewire advanced into the vein under fluoroscopy
4. Introducer sheath is advanced over the guidewire, stiffner and guidewire are removed simultaneously leaving introducer sheath behind
5. Catheter is advanced until the tip lies in the SVC, adjacent to the right atrium, sheath is removed
6. Catheter sutured in place with nonresorbable suture
7. Semipermeable transparent dressing placed over the site
8. Chest radiograph (CXR) taken to document tip position

List 4 early potential complications of PICC line placement.

Arrhythmia (catheter or guidewire advanced into heart), nerve injury, hematoma, arterial injury

List 6 late potential complications of PICC line placement.

Occlusion of catheter (best avoided with frequent flushing), loss of position in cavoatrial junction, line fracture, local infection at puncture site, thrombophlebitis (3%–10%), sepsis (1%–3%)

How should patients be instructed to care for the PICC line?	Flush the catheter frequently (after each use and every 12 hours) with 10 ml saline followed by 2 ml of heparin (100 U/ml) in each lumen. Change the dressing frequently. Keep the line clamped and capped. Seek medical attention if problems develop.

PATHOLOGY

ATHEROSCLEROSIS

What is a stenosis?	Narrowing of a vessel lumen
What are the causes of arterial stenoses?	Atherosclerosis, congenital defects, external compression (e.g., from a mass or fibrous band), vasculitis
Describe the characteristic lesions of atherosclerosis.	**Fatty streak:** Lipid accumulation within the tunica intima leads to the formation of elevated linear lesions. **Fibrous plaque:** Accumulation of smooth muscle cells and lipid-filled macrophages leads to the development of a central atheroma. **Complicated plaque:** A fibrous plaque undergoes calcification, ulceration, hemorrhage, or necrosis and becomes susceptible to thrombosis.
What vessels are commonly affected by atherosclerotic disease?	Aorta (abdominal > thoracic), coronary artery, carotid artery, circle of Willis, peripheral arteries (especially in the lower extremities)
Where does atherosclerosis most commonly affect vessels?	Areas of tortuosity and bifurcations
List 4 complications of atherosclerotic disease.	Stenosis and occlusion (leading to ischemia and infarction), thrombosis, embolization, aneurysm formation

ANEURYSM

What is an aneurysm?	A localized dilatation of all 3 layers of the wall of a vessel

List 7 causes of aneurysm formation.

1. Atherosclerosis
2. Congenital weakness of vessel wall
3. Bacterial infection
4. Cystic medial necrosis
5. Trauma
6. Vasculitis
7. Stenosis (aneurysm can form distal to it)

What modalities are used to study aneurysms, and when is each best used?

Angiography: Best for delineating branch vessel involvement and for preoperative assessment

Ultrasound: Ideal for following the progress of aneurysm size over time

CT: Most accurate means of measuring aneurysms; identifies mural thrombus and extraluminal hematoma

MRI: Can image aneurysms in any plane; especially useful in patients allergic to iodinated contrast

What is the shape of most atherosclerotic aneurysms?

Fusiform (occasionally saccular)

Where are atherosclerotic aneurysms most commonly found?

Proximal descending thoracic aorta; abdominal aorta; iliac, femoral, and popliteal arteries

Where are most congenital aneurysms found?

Intracranial vessels (congenital berry aneurysm)

What is the cause of most congenital aneurysms?

Weakness of the muscular arterial wall at points of bifurcation

What is a mycotic aneurysm?

Weakening of the arterial wall and dilatation owing to bacterial infection

What is the typical shape of most mycotic aneurysms?

Saccular

List 5 conditions that predispose to the formation of mycotic aneurysms.

Bacterial endocarditis, sepsis, intravenous drug abuse, immunocompromise, adjacent tissue infection

Where are mycotic aneurysms likely to be found?

Aorta, cerebral vasculature, mesentery, splenic vasculature, renal vasculature

Why is it important to recognize a mycotic aneurysm?

They are prone to rapid expansion and rupture and often require emergency surgery.

EMBOLUS

What is embolization?	Intraluminal material flows downstream and lodges in the vasculature

List the 9 most common sources of arterial emboli.

1. Atrial fibrillation (leads to left atrial clot)
2. Myocardial infarction (leads to mural thrombus in the left ventricle)
3. Valvular vegetations
4. Myxoma
5. Aneurysms with mural thrombus
6. Ulcerated atherosclerotic plaque
7. Dislodged atherosclerotic plaque owing to angiographic manipulation
8. Air
9. Foreign bodies

What is the most common cause of venous emboli?	Dislodged clot from the deep venous system of the pelvis and lower extremities
What is a paradoxical embolus?	A venous embolus that travels through a right-to-left cardiac shunt, resulting in arterial embolization

What is the angiographic appearance of an embolus?

Abrupt vessel occlusion
Intraluminal filling defect ("tram-track" sign)
Convex outline of the intraluminal clot ("meniscus" sign)
Poor collateral flow around the obstruction (owing to acute obstruction of the vessel)

ARTERIAL TRAUMA

What is the gold standard for the evaluation of arterial injury in the setting of trauma?	Angiography

List 8 angiographic signs of arterial injury.

1. Hemorrhage (extravasation of contrast)
2. Occlusion of distal segment
3. Dissection (longitudinal intimal tear, true and false lumens)
4. Pseudoaneurysm
5. Derangement of normal anatomy

(e.g., displacement by hematoma or bone)
6. Arterial spasm (narrowing and delayed filling)
7. Thrombosis
8. AV fistula

VASCULITIS

What is vasculitis?

Inflammation of the walls of blood vessels, cause may be infectious, immune, or idiopathic

What is the characteristic arteriographic appearance of vasculitis?

Occlusion and irregular stenoses of the distal vessels, often giving a beaded appearance
Long, smooth narrowings
Aneurysms

How can one distinguish between arteriography-induced vasospasm and vasculitis?

Vasospastic segments dilate following the intra-arterial administration of a vasodilator

ARTERIOVENOUS MALFORMATION (AVM)

What is an AVM?

A congenital connection between an arterial and a venous structure, without an intervening capillary bed

What is the angiographic appearance of an AVM?

Hypertrophic feeding arteries (often multiple)
Dilated, tortuous draining veins (thickened "arterialized" veins)
Rapid flow of contrast through the lesion without visualization of a capillary phase
Nidus (small connecting arterioles and venules)

How are AVMs treated?

Surgically or with embolization

How effective is emboliza-tion therapy for AVMs?

Variable. Large AVMs with multiple feeding vessels or rapid arteriovenous shunting often require multiple emboliza-tion sessions, which are often only par-tially successful. Results are better with small AVMs if a superselective catheter can be placed directly in the feeding vessel.

ARTERIOVENOUS (AV) FISTULA

What is an AV fistula?	An acquired arteriovenous communication with a single feeding vessel
List 4 causes of AV fistula.	1. Penetrating or blunt trauma 2. Rupture of an aneurysm (e.g., aortocaval fistula following rupture of an abdominal aortic aneurysm into the IVC) 3. Iatrogenic (e.g., created for dialysis access, surgical arterial injury, inadvertent simultaneous puncture of an artery and a vein during angiography) 4. Renal biopsy
What studies are used in the preoperative assessment of AV fistula?	Ultrasound is excellent for detecting the fistula initially. Angiography localizes the fistula for surgical therapy (the site may be difficult to find at surgery owing to thickened, tortuous draining veins).
What is the primary complication of embolization therapy in patients with a large AV fistula?	Pulmonary embolus (PE) can occur if the embolization device fails to remain in the fistula and flows directly into the venous circulation, lodging in the pulmonary vasculature.
How can the risk of PE be minimized?	By selecting a coil of the appropriate size or a detachable balloon as the embolic device, and by positioning the device using fluoroscopic guidance
What is a dialysis fistula or graft?	A surgically created connection between an artery and vein to allow for repeated vascular access for dialysis [may be direct (fistula) or involve an intervening vein or Gortex (graft)]
What are the common causes of dialysis graft or fistula failure?	Stenosis (most commonly at the venous anastomosis) Thrombosis (within the graft)
What methods are used to study the patency of grafts?	**Doppler ultrasound** can provide information on the flow dynamics of a graft, allowing identification of patients that may need angiography. **Angiography** is diagnostic and therapeutic.

What are the advantages of using ultrasound for the evaluation of grafts?	Ultrasound can reveal stenoses and thromboses, detect extraluminal hematomas, and provide a measurement of flow volume/unit time
What is the hallmark of stenosis on ultrasound?	Elevated peak systolic velocity
What is considered a significant stenosis of a graft (on Doppler ultrasound)?	$\geq$ 4 meters/sec flow velocity
If an angiogram reveals graft failure, what are the therapeutic options?	Thrombolysis or percutaneous thrombectomy of acutely thrombosed grafts, PTA of stenotic segments

TUMOR

Why is angiography indicated in the work-up of tumors?	The angiogram provides a "road map" of the vascular supply and drainage of a tumor to guide the surgeon. (Angiography was once widely used for the characterization of tumors, but has since been replaced by CT, ultrasound, and MRI.)
What therapeutic options are available in the angiography suite for the treatment of tumors?	Embolization (small particle or distal embolization employed to cause tumor necrosis) Selective intra-arterial chemotherapy
What are the 6 arteriographic characteristics typical of a tumor?	**BEDPAN** **m** **B**lush **E**ncasement of vessels by the tumor (abnormal-appearing vessels with irregular narrowings or dilatations) **D**isplacement of normal vascular structures by a hyper- or hypovascular mass **P**ooling of contrast **A**rteriovenous shunting **N**eovascularity
Is hypervascularity pathognomonic for malignancy?	No. Benign lesions (e.g., hemangioma, osteoid osteoma) and infectious processes may also appear hypervascular.

What often is the cause of arteriographically demonstrated hypovascular areas within a tumor?	Tumor necrosis and cystic tumors

DISORDERS OF THE THORACIC VASCULATURE

PULMONARY EMBOLUS (PE) [SEE ALSO CHAPTER 3]

What are the indications for pulmonary arteriography in a patient with suspected PE?	Indeterminate ventilation-perfusion (V/Q) scan (intermediate probability) Low-probability V/Q scan with high clinical suspicion High-probability V/Q scan in a patient at high risk of complications if begun on anticoagulation therapy High clinical suspicion in a patient who is hemodynamically unstable and may need immediate therapy High clinical suspicion in a patient with a high likelihood of having an indeterminate V/Q scan owing to preexisting lung disease
What are the steps in performing a pulmonary arteriogram?	1. Venous access obtained (usually via the common femoral vein) 2. Injection in the common femoral vein to rule out IVC thrombosis 3. Guidewire and catheter manipulated into the right ventricle, across the pulmonic valve 4. Pulmonary artery pressures measured 5. Selective contrast injection of the right and left pulmonary arteries
What are typical arteriographic findings of:	
Acute PE?	Sharply demarcated intraluminal filling defect, abrupt vessel cutoff, underperfused area distal to the suspected embolus, "tram tracking" of contrast outlining embolus
Chronic PE?	Eccentric mural filling defects, irregular arterial luminal narrowing or tapering (owing to remodeling of the clot), webs, concave vessel occlusion

What are the risks associated with pulmonary arteriography?	Arrhythmia (especially right bundle branch block) and bleeding at the puncture site
What are contraindications to pulmonary arteriography?	Left bundle branch block, coagulopathy, significantly elevated pulmonary artery pressure (added volume may lead to right-sided heart failure)
What is normal pulmonary artery pressure?	Less than or equal to 25/10 mm Hg (mean = 15 mm Hg)

THORACIC AORTIC ANEURYSM

What are the 5 most common causes of thoracic aortic aneurysm?	1. Atherosclerosis (75% of patients) 2. Trauma (pseudoaneurysm) 3. Infection 4. Cystic medial necrosis (connective tissue disease, hypertension, syphilis) 5. Aortitis (Takayasu's arteritis, giant cell arteritis, collagen vascular disease)
What modalities are used to evaluate thoracic aortic aneurysms?	Angiography, CT, MRI, transesophageal echocardiography

In thoracic aortic aneurysm, what are the:

Advantages of angiography?	Better demonstrates involvement of branch vessels and the aortic valve
Disadvantages of angiography?	Poor modality for measuring aneurysm Does not reveal mural thrombus or extravascular hematoma
Advantages of CT?	Sensitive and specific for diagnosis Ideal for measuring and following the size of the aneurysm Can detect mural thrombus or extravascular hematoma Can reveal complications of aneurysm (e.g., bone erosion, compression of venous structures or airways)
Disadvantages of CT?	Does not reliably delineate involvement of branch vessels

Which study is used for the preoperative assessment of thoracic aortic aneurysms?

Angiography (to determine the extent of the aneurysm and the presence of branch involvement)

What is the angiographic finding most predictive of impending rupture?

Focal dilatation, size greater than 6 centimeters

Where are most thoracic atherosclerotic aneurysms found?

Descending aorta, near the isthmus

What is cystic medial necrosis?

Focal degeneration of the muscular and elastic elements of the media

Where are aneurysms caused by cystic medial necrosis usually found?

Ascending aorta

What is the radiographic appearance of an aneurysm caused by cystic medial necrosis?

"Tulip bulb" symmetric dilatation of the proximal aorta and aortic sinuses; not usually calcified

List 3 complications of an aneurysm of the ascending aorta.

Aortic valvular insufficiency, rupture into the pericardium resulting in tamponade, dissection

Where are most syphilitic aneurysms found?

Ascending aorta and aortic arch

In what stage of syphilis do patients develop syphilitic aortic aneurysms?

Tertiary syphilis (decades after contracting the disease)

What is the mechanism of vessel wall damage leading to a syphilitic aneurysm?

Obliterative endarteritis (i.e., inflammation of the vasa vasorum and adventitial lymphatics)

What is the radiographic appearance of a syphilitic aneurysm?

Asymmetric dilatation of the proximal aorta and aortic sinuses; "tree bark" calcification

Where are most thoracic mycotic aneurysms found?

Ascending aorta and the isthmus of the aorta

Which 5 organisms most commonly cause mycotic aneurysms?

Staphylococcus, Streptococcus, Salmonella, Neisseria gonorrhoeae, Mycobacterium tuberculosis

What evidence on CT scan would lead to the diagnosis of a mycotic aneurysm?

Perianeurysmal inflammation

AORTIC DISSECTION

What occurs during an aortic dissection?

A tear in the tunica intima allows blood to enter and "track down" the vessel wall, creating a "false lumen" within the wall

Aortic arch

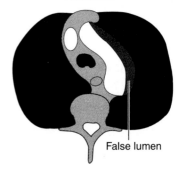

Ascending and descending aorta

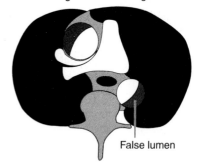

Abdominal aorta

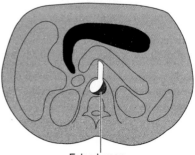

An aortic dissection normally occurs in which plane of the vessel wall?

The outer third of the media

List 6 causes of aortic dissection.

Hypertension, atherosclerosis, Marfan's syndrome, bicuspid aortic valve, coarctation of the aorta, cystic medial necrosis

What is the classic clinical presentation of a dissecting aortic aneurysm?

"Tearing" chest pain that radiates to the back; unequal pulses in the arms and legs

What is the:

De Bakey classification schemes for aortic dissection?

BAD: Both, **A**scending, **D**escending
I: Ascending and descending aorta (approximately 45%)
II: Ascending aorta only (approximately 10%)
III: Descending aorta only (approximately 45%)

$\boldsymbol{m}$

Stanford classification schemes for aortic dissection?

A: Any aneurysm involving the ascending aorta (proximal to the takeoff of the left subclavian artery)
B: Any aneurysm involving the descending aorta (distal to the takeoff of the left subclavian artery)

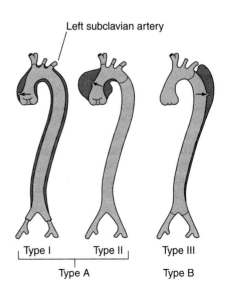

Left subclavian artery

Type I   Type II   Type III

Type A   Type B

How do the treatments of types A and B aortic dissection differ?	Type A is treated surgically (owing to the high risk of aortic insufficiency, cardiac tamponade, stroke, or rupture) and type B is treated medically (i.e., by managing hypertension), unless the patient develops complications.
List 8 complications of aortic dissection.	Rupture, myocardial infarction, cardiac tamponade, aortic valvular insufficiency, stroke, mesenteric ischemia, renal insufficiency, paraplegia
What are the plain film findings of aortic dissection?	1. Widened mediastinum 2. Thickened wall sign (> 8 mm; normal wall is 2–3 mm) 3. Localized dilatation of the aortic knob or proximal descending aorta 4. Displacement of the trachea 5. Medial displacement of the calcified tunica intima 6. Pleural effusion or hemothorax 7. Cardiomegaly
What modalities are used to evaluate aortic dissection?	CT, MRI, transesophageal echocardiography, angiography, plain film radiography
What percentage of patients with documented aortic dissection have a normal CXR?	25%
What is the gold standard for evaluation of aortic dissection?	Angiography
What is the angiographic feature diagnostic of aortic dissection?	A longitudinal intimal flap that separates true and false lumens
What would be seen if the catheter were accidentally advanced into the false lumen and a contrast injection were performed?	Slow flow and an absence of branch vessels
What is the angiographic characteristic of a dissecting aneurysm with a thrombosed false lumen?	"Twisted tape" sign (i.e., compression of a narrowed true lumen filling with contrast by the thrombosed false lumen)

Which vessels typically originate from the false lumen and are therefore at risk for thrombosis?

Right coronary, left renal, and left iliac

List 4 reasons an arteriogram is performed pre-operatively.

To determine if the ascending aorta is involved, which in turn influences treatment (surgical versus medical)

To visualize the entry site (i.e., the site of the intimal tear) and the re-entry site (i.e., sites of fenestration, or holes connecting the true and false lumens)

To determine involvement of the branch vessels (especially the coronary and cerebral arteries)

To evaluate complications (e.g., hemorrhage, aortic insufficiency)

When is transesophageal echocardiography indicated?

As an initial evaluation to see if the ascending aorta is involved

List 3 advantages of CT in the evaluation of aortic dissection.

Allows determination of patency (versus thrombosis) of the false lumen

Allows detection of extra-aortic hematoma

High sensitivity

What are the disadvantages of CT in the evaluation of aortic dissection?

Less helpful for the determination of branch vessel and aortic valve involvement, poor visualization of the entry and re-entry sites

What is the appearance of aortic dissection on CT?

The false lumen is usually lateral and may be filled or partially filled with clot

What type of CT should be performed for the evaluation of aortic dissection?

A spiral CT scan during long injection of contrast is needed to image the late filling and slow flow of the false lumen.

AORTIC TRAUMA

What is the cause of most traumatic aortic injuries?

Sudden decelerating accidents (e.g., high speed motor vehicle accident, fall)

What sites are involved most often?

Aortic root, aortic isthmus, aortic hiatus of diaphragm

Which site is most often involved?	Injury at the aortic isthmus is seen in 95% of patients. (Most patients with aortic root tear die at the scene.)
List 9 plain film findings suggestive of aortic injury.	1. Abnormally contoured aortic arch and loss of the aortic knob 2. Loss of anterior-posterior (AP) window concavity 3. Widened mediastinum 4. Apical capping (blood accumulation over the apices) 5. Left mediastinal stripe 6. Widened right paratracheal area 7. Pleural effusion 8. Broken ribs (1 and 2) 9. Trachea or nasogastric tube deviation to the right
What are the indications for aortography?	Clinical suspicion owing to mechanism of injury, with or without an abnormal CXR
List 3 angiographic findings of traumatic aortic injury.	Pseudoaneurysm, intimal tear or linear defect, irregular aortic contour
What is the most likely cause of a false-positive arteriogram?	Ductus bump or diverticulum (i.e., an embryologic remnant that appears as a smooth area of dilatation at the aortic isthmus)
What helpful information can be provided by CT?	Whether mediastinal widening is caused by mediastinal hematoma or fat

COARCTATION OF THE AORTA

What is coarctation of the aorta?	A congenital shelf of tissue or narrowing within the aorta that can cause varying degrees of obstruction
Where is the most common location for a coarctation?	Juxtaductal, just distal to the left subclavian artery
What other vascular pathology is often associated with a coarctation?	Bicuspid aortic valve (50%-80% of patients), aortic stenosis, atrial septal defect, ventricular septal defect, idiopathic hypertrophic subaortic stenosis
What percentage of patients have an associated post-stenotic aneurysm?	4%

What are the characteristic physical findings of a coarctation?	Hypertension in the upper extremities with decreased blood pressure or absent pulses in the lower extremities Systolic murmur at the left sternal border, radiating to the back
List 4 findings of a coarctation on a CXR.	"3" sign (indentation at the site of the coarctation), dilated ascending aorta, rib notching, enlarged left ventricle
What would be seen with aortography?	Collateral channels, poststenotic dilatation, associated vascular pathology
Which modality has recently become the study of choice for imaging a coarctation?	MRI

TAKAYASU'S ARTERITIS ("PULSELESS DISEASE")

What is Takayasu's arteritis?	An idiopathic (possibly autoimmune) inflammatory disease affecting the arterial walls
What vessels are primarily affected?	Aorta, brachiocephalic vessels, and pulmonary arteries
How is the wall of the aorta affected?	Intimal thickening and destruction of (or granuloma formation within) the tunica media leads to fibrosis of the vessel wall, resulting in stenoses and occlusions of major branch vessels.
What are the clinical manifestations of the disease?	Ischemia owing to stenosis or occlusion of the branch vessels
What demographic set of patients is characteristically affected?	Young women
List 5 features seen on angiographic examination.	1. Smooth segmental narrowing 2. Marked irregularity of the aorta (resembling severe atherosclerotic disease) 3. Stenosis or occlusion of the aorta and branch vessels (brachiocephalic vessels involved most often) 4. Thickened aortic wall 5. Aneurysms

What therapeutic option is available in the angiography suite?	PTA (with or without stent placement); should not be performed during the active phase of the disease

THORACIC OUTLET SYNDROME

What is thoracic outlet syndrome?	Compression of the subclavian artery or vein or the brachial plexus that results in upper extremity ischemia, embolism, or Raynaud's phenomenon.
List 5 causes of thoracic outlet syndrome.	1. Costoclavicular syndrome (compression of the neurovascular structures between the clavicle and first rib), most common cause 2. Cervical rib or anomalous first rib 3. Fibrous band 4. Scalenus tunnel syndrome (i.e., compression in the scalene triangle by muscle) 5. Neoplasia
When would plain film examination be helpful?	Only in the case of a cervical rib or anomalous first rib
What percentage of people have a cervical rib?	0.5%
What percentage of people with a cervical rib are symptomatic?	5%
What study would best show subclavian arterial obstruction?	Angiography shows the obstruction regardless of cause.
What is done to accentuate the obstruction during angiography?	Adson's maneuver (i.e., abduction of the arm with the head turned to the opposite side)
What is the characteristic finding on the angiogram?	Subclavian stenosis with poststenotic dilatation and dilated collateral channels

SUBCLAVIAN STEAL SYNDROME

What is subclavian steal syndrome?	Stenosis or occlusion of the first part of the subclavian artery means that the affected upper extremity receives its

blood supply from retrograde flow through the ipsilateral vertebral artery. In other words, it "steals" blood from the posterior circulation of the brain.

How would subclavian steal syndrome appear on an angiogram?	**Initial images:** Proximal subclavian stenosis, no contrast filling of the affected upper extremity **Delayed images:** Retrograde flow through the ipsilateral vertebral artery and subsequent filling of the distal subclavian vessels

SUPERIOR VENA CAVA (SVC) SYNDROME

What is SVC syndrome?	Thrombosis or external compression leads to occlusion of the SVC and edema of the face, neck, and arms.
What is the most likely cause of:	
SVC thrombosis?	Long-term indwelling catheter
SVC compression?	Bronchogenic carcinoma
What studies are appropriate if SVC obstruction is clinically suspected?	Venography, CT, magnetic resonance venogram (MRV)
List 3 characteristic findings on a venogram in a patient with SVC obstruction?	Peripheral venous distention, proximal occlusion, collateral venous flow
List 3 therapeutic options for patients with external compression of the SVC.	PTA with stent placement, surgical bypass, radiation therapy (to shrink the tumor and palliate symptoms)

DISORDERS OF THE ABDOMINAL AND PELVIC VASCULATURE

ABDOMINAL AORTIC ANEURYSM (AAA)

Where are most AAAs located?	Below the renal arteries (95% are infrarenal)
What is the most common cause of AAA?	Atherosclerosis

What are the physical findings of an AAA?	Palpable, midline, supraumbilical, pulsatile abdominal mass
List 4 risk factors for rupture.	Large diameter (> 4–5 cm), recent rapid expansion, hypertension, chronic obstructive pulmonary disease (COPD)
What are the plain film findings in a patient with AAA?	Eggshell calcifications (best seen on lateral projection)
What diameter is used to define an AAA?	> 3 cm
What studies best measure the diameter of an AAA?	CT (most accurate) and ultrasound
What study is used to follow the size of an AAA over time and why?	Ultrasound, because it is inexpensive, noninvasive, and provides images in multiple planes
How should a person be evaluated if an AAA leak is suspected?	CT (if the patient is stable and the diagnosis is in doubt) allows most accurate evaluation of the retroperitoneum for hemorrhage.
What is the CT finding characteristic of a slow-leaking aneurysm?	Perianeurysmal fibrosis with a thickened, irregular, enhancing aortic wall ("inflammatory aneurysm")
When is an angiogram indicated to study an AAA?	Preoperatively (best study for determining the involvement of the origins of the renal, mesenteric, or iliac arteries)
Why is angiography NOT used to study the diameter of an AAA?	Angiography gives an image of the functional lumen. Because AAAs often have large mural thrombi visualized only as filling defects, angiography underestimates the true diameter of the aneurysm.
What is the classic triad of a ruptured AAA?	Abdominal pain, hypotension, pulsatile abdominal mass
When is surgery indicated?	Rupture, recent rapid expansion, size > 4–5 cm, symptoms

INFERIOR VENA CAVA (IVC) OBSTRUCTION

What are the causes of IVC obstruction?	Thrombosis, external compression or invasion by tumors

What imaging modalities are used to evaluate the IVC?	Venography, ultrasound, MRI, CT
What type of tumor is the most likely cause of IVC invasion?	Renal cell carcinoma
What is a common cause of IVC thrombosis?	DVT of the lower extremity or pelvis with proximal propagation of the clot
What are the therapeutic options for patients with IVC thrombosis?	Systemic anticoagulation, IVC filter placement, thrombolysis
What are the indications for placement of an IVC filter?	Documented PE or DVT in patients with contraindications to anticoagulation therapy, or recurrent PE while on optimal anticoagulation therapy
How is an IVC filter placed?	Percutaneously, through a catheter under fluoroscopic guidance
What study must be performed prior to IVC filter placement and why?	An IVC venogram: to detect femoral or iliac IVC intraluminal clots, to measure the IVC diameter, and to localize renal veins
What approach is most often used to insert the filter if:	
The femoral or iliac IVC does not have a thrombus?	Femoral approach
The femoral or iliac IVC does have a thrombus?	Brachial or internal jugular approach (to avoid dislodging the clot and causing PE)
Where is the optimal position for an IVC filter?	Below the renal veins (to reduce the risk of thrombosis)

RENOVASCULAR HYPERTENSION

What is the cause of:	
Acute renovascular hypertension?	Renal arterial embolus, thrombosis, or stenosis owing to involvement by aortic dissection

Chronic renovascular hypertension?

Atherosclerosis (70%), fibromuscular dysplasia (25%), miscellaneous causes [e.g., polyarteritis nodosa (PAN), Takayasu's arteritis]

What is the mechanism leading to increased blood pressure?

Refractory hypertension results when renal artery obstruction causes the juxtaglomerular apparatus to sense a decrease in blood pressure, which in turn leads to the production of renin and the activation of the renin-angiotensin-aldosterone axis.

Renal artery stenosis is the cause of renovascular hypertension in what percentage of hypertensive patients?

Approximately 5%

What is the pathologic appearance of the affected kidney?

Small kidney with a smooth contour

What is the shrunken ischemic kidney of renal artery stenosis called?

"Goldblatt kidney"

What would be seen on an intravenous pyelogram (IVP) of a patient with unilateral renal artery stenosis?

The delayed appearance of a nephrogram on the affected side
Decreased kidney size in a chronically affected organ

What studies are appropriate for the diagnosis of renal artery stenosis?

Angiography, ultrasound, MRA, CTA

What study is used to definitively prove renal artery stenosis as the cause of refractory hypertension?

Venography with sampling of blood from both renal veins (the renin level will be more than 1.5 times higher in venous blood from the affected kidney)

What is fibromuscular dysplasia (FMD)?

An idiopathic process characterized by alternating areas of intimal and medial thickening (stenosis) and medial destruction (aneurysmal dilatation)

Does FMD affect arteries other than the renal arteries?

Yes, but the renal arteries are affected most often.

What demographic set of patients is more likely to have FMD?	Young women
What is the classic angiographic appearance of FMD?	"String of beads," more commonly of the distal renal artery, bilateral in 50% of patients
What are the therapeutic options for patients with renal artery stenosis?	PTA (with or without stent placement), surgical bypass, organ ablation or nephrectomy
What is the 5-year patency rate for PTA when the procedure is performed on patients with:	
Renal artery stenosis caused by atherosclerotic narrowing?	70%–90%
Renal artery stenosis caused by FMD?	95%
What type of lesion responds poorly to PTA?	Ostial lesion (within 1 cm of origin)

POLYARTERITIS NODOSA (PAN)

What is PAN?	Necrotizing vasculitis, mainly of the small vessels
What is the result of inflammation or necrosis of the arterial wall?	Aneurysm formation (nodose lesions)
What areas of the vascular tree are particularly prone to damage from PAN?	Regions of bifurcation
What vessel is most often affected?	Renal artery (70% of patients)
What evidence of PAN is seen on the angiogram?	Multiple small aneurysms

RENAL TRANSPLANT

Why is arteriography used for preoperative assessment of renal donors?	To evaluate the arterial supply and identify multiple renal arteries

GASTROINTESTINAL HEMORRHAGE

List 7 major causes of upper gastrointestinal bleeding.	Duodenal ulcer (25%), gastric ulcer (20%), acute gastritis (20%), esophageal varices (20%), Mallory-Weiss tear (10%), esophagitis, esophageal or gastric tumors
List 9 major causes of lower gastrointestinal bleeding.	Diverticular disease, angiodysplasia, colorectal carcinoma, hemorrhoids, intussusception, volvulus, mesenteric ischemia, inflammatory bowel disease, anticoagulation
What is the landmark that separates upper bleeds from lower bleeds?	The ligament of Treitz (located between the fourth portion of the duodenum and the proximal jejunum)
What imaging modalities are used to localize gastrointestinal bleeding?	Angiography, radiolabeled sulfur colloid (SC) nuclear medicine scan, radiolabeled red blood cell (RBC) nuclear medicine scan
What nuclear medicine scan is used for evaluation of acute gastrointestinal hemorrhage and why?	An SC scan is used more often because it is more sensitive than an RBC scan.
How is an RBC scan performed?	The patient's RBCs are collected, labeled with a radioisotope, and returned to the patient's circulation, and sequential images are obtained. Active bleeding is seen as pooling of radioactivity outside of the major blood vessels.
When is an RBC scan helpful?	For patients with intermittent bleeding or bleeding from an upper gastrointestinal source
What are the advantages of angiography?	It can be used for both localization and therapy.

In a patient with gastro-intestinal bleeding, when is angiography indicated?

When there is active hemorrhage refractory to other therapies

How is acute bleeding confirmed?

Upper gastrointestinal bleeding:
Active bleeding above the ligament of Treitz can be confirmed by esopha-gogastroduodenoscopy (EGD) or ice water lavage (continuous finding of aspirate with bright red blood after lavage indicates active bleeding).
Lower gastrointestinal bleeding:
Active bleeding below the ligament of Treitz is difficult to confirm even by angiography.

At what rate can the bleeding be visualized by:

Angiography?

Faster than 0.5 ml/min

Radiolabeled SC or RBC scan?

Faster than 0.1 ml/min

What angiographic finding is diagnostic of gastrointes-tinal hemorrhage?

Extravasation of contrast into the bowel lumen

Which source of bleeding will NOT be visualized by angiography?

Venous bleeding caused by esophageal or gastric varices

What is the gastric "pseu-dovein" sign?

Extravasation of contrast into the stomach and pooling within the rugae gives the appearance of a vein

What therapeutic options does angiography offer?

Vasoconstrictor infusion or embolization (upper gastrointestinal bleed)

What drug is infused selectively to stop gastro-intestinal bleeding?

Vasopressin

What embolic material is used most commonly in the setting of gastrointestinal hemorrhage and why?

Gelfoam particles—temporary proximal embolization allows for control of hemorrhage without causing bowel ischemia (i.e., the collateral circulation is not affected)

Why is embolization NOT used routinely for lower gastrointestinal hemorrhage?	Poorer collateral circulation leads to a much higher rate of bowel wall infarction
What needs to be performed after achieving hemostasis and why?	Diagnostic studies (e.g., EGD, colonoscopy, CT), because angiography is used to localize and treat—not characterize—the lesion

MESENTERIC ISCHEMIA

What is mesenteric ischemia?	Reduction in the arterial supply provided by the mesenteric arteries may lead to bowel infarction
When does chronic mesenteric ischemia become evident clinically?	Only with significant stenoses of all 3 mesenteric arteries (because of the rich collateral network in the area)
What are the causes of:	
Acute mesenteric ischemia?	Embolus, thrombosis, dissection, expanding aneurysm, mesenteric venous occlusion or thrombosis, non-occlusive mesenteric ischemia (NOMI; caused by hypotension or hypoperfusion)
Chronic mesenteric ischemia?	Atherosclerosis
What is the classic clinical presentation of chronic mesenteric ischemia?	Abdominal angina (i.e., severe abdominal pain after meals), weight loss, and fear of food
What is the gold standard for the evaluation of mesenteric ischemia?	Selective mesenteric arteriography
How does an infarcted bowel appear on CT scan?	Gas in the bowel wall, thickening of the bowel wall, and gas in the portal venous system (a late sign suggestive of a poor prognosis)
What therapeutic options does angiography provide?	PTA, selective vasodilator infusion (usually papaverine hydrochloride) for NOMI

PORTAL VENOUS HYPERTENSION

What is portal venous hypertension?	Pressures that exceed 10 mm Hg in the portal vein owing to increased resistance through the hepatic vasculature
What is the normal portal venous pressure?	Less than 5 mm Hg
What are the causes of portal hypertension?	**Presinusoidal:** Portal vein occlusion (thrombosis, invasion) **Sinusoidal:** Cirrhosis (most common), metastatic disease **Postsinusoidal:** Budd-Chiari syndrome, IVC occlusion
What is the Budd-Chiari syndrome?	Hepatic vein thrombosis
What are the routes of venous drainage seen with portal hypertension?	Left gastric vein to esophageal veins to azygos system Superior rectal vein to middle or inferior rectal veins to IVC Paraumbilical veins to epigastric veins Colic veins to systemic retroperitoneal veins
What studies are indicated for the evaluation of portal hypertension?	Ultrasound and angiography
What features of portal hypertension are seen on ultrasound?	Hepatic parenchymal or vascular pathology, retrograde flow in the portal vein, collateral venous flow, recanalized umbilical vein, ascites, splenomegaly
How can portal hypertension be diagnosed using angiography?	Retrograde portal venous flow and collaterals visualized Measurement of the pressure gradient across the hepatic sinusoids [a corrected sinusoidal pressure (CSP)> 10 mm Hg is diagnostic]
How is the CSP calculated?	CSP = wedged hepatic pressure − IVC pressure
What is the normal CSP?	Less than 5 mm Hg

DISORDERS OF THE PERIPHERAL VASCULATURE

PERIPHERAL VASCULAR DISEASE (PVD)

What are the symptoms of PVD?	Intermittent claudication (i.e., leg pain occurring with exercise and alleviated on resting), rest pain (usually foot pain that awakens the patient and is alleviated by hanging the leg over the side of the bed or standing up), ischemic ulcer, non-healing wound or infection, sensorimotor loss, impotence
What are the physical examination findings associated with PVD?	Decreased peripheral pulses, bruits, muscular atrophy, decreased hair growth, thick toenails, ischemic ulcers, non-healing wound or infection
What is Leriche's syndrome?	Vascular disease of the distal aorta or iliac arteries
What is the classic triad seen with Leriche's syndrome?	Buttock or thigh claudication, gluteal atrophy, impotence (in men)
What noninvasive test would be performed to evaluate PVD?	ABI
What would the ABI be in a:	
Healthy person?	1.0
Person with claudication?	Less than 0.9
Person with rest pain?	Less than 0.5
In what group of patients are ABIs inaccurate?	Patients with diabetes, owing to often heavily calcified arteries
What are the characteristics of PVD in patients with diabetes?	Diffuse, multilevel disease Small vessels affected to a greater extent, more frequently have disease in the arteries below the popliteal trifurcation Onset at a younger age
How is ultrasound used in the study of PVD?	Doppler ultrasound, a noninvasive means of characterizing arterial flow and pathology, will delineate intraluminal pathology (e.g., stenoses, aneurysm) as well as extraluminal pathology (e.g., external compression, hematoma).

What is the normal Doppler waveform in the femoral or popliteal arteries?

A triphasic waveform that varies with the cardiac cycle:
Forward flow during systole
Retrograde flow during the first part of diastole
Low-velocity forward flow late in diastole

How is this waveform affected by stenosis?

Changes to a monophasic waveform–retrograde flow and low-velocity forward flow (previously seen during diastole) are no longer a part of the waveform

What invasive test is used to plan intervention for PVD?

Aortogram with runoff

What is an aortogram with runoff?

A bolus of contrast is injected into the distal aorta and films are taken sequentially from the pelvis to the feet as the contrast flows into the distal vessels of the lower extremities.

In relation to the lower extremity arteries, what is:

  Inflow?

Iliac arteries, left femoral artery

  Outflow?

Superior femoral artery, popliteal artery

  Runoff?

Trifurcation and distal

What is the arteriographic characteristic of a chronic arterial stenosis or occlusion?

Eccentric, irregular plaque and vessels that taper to occlusion; collateral flow with distal reconstitution

What information can arteriography provide about the physiologic significance of a stenosis?

The pressure gradient across the stenosis (anything greater than 10 mm Hg is physiologically significant)

What are the therapeutic options for PVD?

Exercise, smoking cessation, hypertension control, diet modification
PTA or atherectomy with stent placement
Surgical bypass
Endarterectomy
Amputation

List 6 advantages of treating vaso-occlusive disease with PTA.

1. Minimally invasive
2. High initial success rate
3. Does not distort anatomy in case

future surgical bypass becomes
necessary
4. Patency rates in properly selected
patients are as good as with surgical
bypass
5. Low rate of complications requiring
additional surgery (3%, same as for
surgical bypass)
6. Low mortality rate (less than 1%, as
opposed to 1%-4% with surgical
bypass)

What angiographic findings suggest the best chance of successful treatment with PTA?

Single, short area (< 5 cm) of stenosis in large vessels with preserved inflow and outflow

When PTA is used to treat PVD, what is the:

Initial success rate?

Approximately 90%

Long-term success rate?

Variable (70% for iliac, less for more distal vessels)

DEEP VENOUS THROMBOSIS (DVT)

What is DVT?

A clot within the vessels of the deep venous system of the upper or lower limbs

What can cause DVT?

Venous stasis resulting from prolonged immobilization, congestive heart failure, obesity
Hypercoagulable states resulting from oral contraceptives, pregnancy, neoplasia, coagulopathy (e.g., protein C or S deficiency, antithrombin III deficiency, lupus anticoagulant)

What imaging modalities may be used to detect DVT?

Ultrasound, venography, magnetic resonance venography, CT

What is the gold standard modality for the diagnosis of DVT?

Venography

**What is the veno-
graphic appearance
of thrombus?**

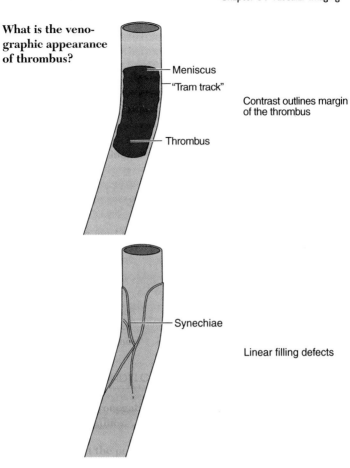

— Meniscus

—"Tram track"

Contrast outlines margin
of the thrombus

— Thrombus

— Synechiae

Linear filling defects

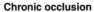

Chronic occlusion

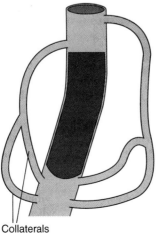

Blood and contrast rerouted
through the superficial
venous system

Collaterals

How is ultrasound used to evaluate for thrombus?

Ultrasound permits detailed examination of the deep venous system using a combination of gray-scale, compression, and color Doppler imaging. The ultra-sound transducer is held to show the vein in cross-section or longitudinally at 1- to 2-centimeter intervals along the entire length of the vein. Compression is performed while imaging the vein in cross-section.

What is the appearance of healthy deep veins on gray-scale imaging?

Normal vessels appear as thin-walled, tubular structures with an anechoic or hypoechoic lumen.

Why is gray-scale imaging alone inadequate for the diagnosis of DVT?

Because acute thrombus can appear anechoic (i.e., the same as flowing blood) on gray-scale imaging

How is the compression exam done?

Normal artery remains round owing to high internal pressure and its rigid muscular wall

Normal vein collapses ("winks") owing to low internal pressure and flexible, thin wall

(See figure on next page)

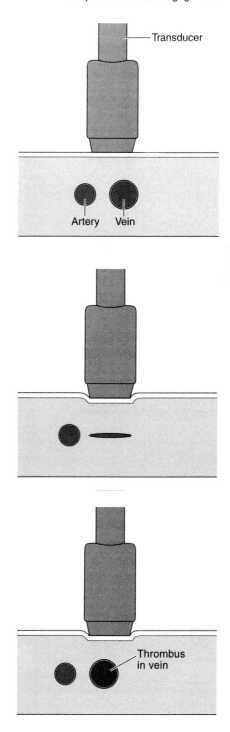

How is Doppler ultrasound different from gray-scale ultrasound?	With Doppler ultrasound, flowing blood creates a signal, while static blood does not. The flowing blood is assigned one of two colors depending on the direction of flow; static blood is not colored.

What is the appearance of a thrombosed vein on:

Gray-scale ultrasound evaluation?	**Chronic thrombus:** intraluminal echogenicity and collaterals **Acute thrombus:** distended venous structures, with or without internal echoes
Compression ultrasound?	Internal echoes, failure to "wink"
Doppler ultrasound?	Absence of spontaneous flow, loss of respiratory variation in the waveform, vein remains hypoechoic
How can you differentiate the deep veins from collateral venous structures?	Deep veins are usually paired and follow a course paralleling an artery
What are the advantages of color Doppler ultrasound?	Provides useful information when compression technique yields ambiguous results Easily identifies arteries, which can then be used as landmarks for their accompanying veins (particularly useful in the evaluation of the deep veins of the calf)
What are treatment options for DVT?	Anticoagulation, IVC filter placement, thrombolysis

RAYNAUD'S PHENOMENON

What is Raynaud's phenomenon?	Intermittent, transient vasoconstriction of the small vessels of the hand
What are the clinical signs?	Hand becomes sequentially pale, cyanotic, and then red Hand feels painful, numb, or tingling Exacerbated or precipitated by cold, emotions

List 9 causes of Raynaud's phenomenon.	Raynaud's disease, repeated trauma, neurovascular compression syndromes, atherosclerosis, Buerger's disease, vasculitis, embolism, ergotism, collagen vascular disease
What is Raynaud's disease?	Idiopathic disease, most common in young women, bilateral involvement, no arteriographic evidence of occlusion

BUERGER'S DISEASE (THROMBOANGIITIS OBLITERANS)

What is Buerger's disease?	Vaso-occlusive disease of the small arteries of the peripheral vasculature
What groups of patients are at high risk for developing Buerger's disease?	Heavy smokers, young people, males, Caucasians or Asians
What is the pathologic lesion of Buerger's disease?	Intimal proliferation and vessel occlusion by thrombus or granulation tissue
How does Buerger's disease differ from atherosclerosis angiographically?	Lesions appear as occlusions or long string-like narrowings Upper extremity most likely to be involved Lesions start distally and progress proximally without skipping areas (smaller distal vessels severely occluded with collateral flow; larger proximal vessels spared) No calcifications in the arterial wall

6

Musculoskeletal Imaging

Brent K. Milner

ANATOMY

What are long bones?

The bones of the extremities; their length is greater than their width

Identify the parts of the long bone before fusion of the epiphysis:

A = Epiphysis
B = Physis (growth plate)
C = Metaphysis
D = Diaphysis
E = Medullary cavity
F = Diaphyseal cortex
G = Periosteum
H = Articular cartilage

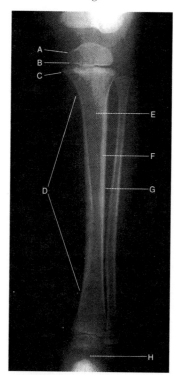

What are short bones?

The bones of the wrist, ankle, and foot (i.e., the carpals and tarsals); they are roughly cuboidal in shape

What are flat bones?

The diploic bones of the vault of the skull (e.g., the parietal and frontal bones) and the iliac bone

What are sesamoid bones?

Small bones located in tendons (e.g., the sesamoid bones of the great toe meta-tarsophalangeal joint)

SPINE ANATOMY

How many vertebrae make up each region of the spine?

Cervical: 7
Thoracic: 12
Lumbar: 5
Sacral: 5 (fused)

Identify the parts of a lumbar vertebra:

A = Body
B = Pedicle
C = Superior articulating facet
D = Inferior articulating facet
E = Transverse process
F = Spinous process
G = Lamina

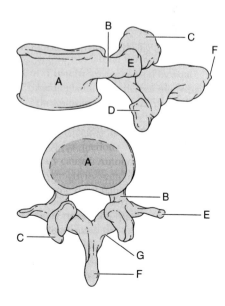

What are the posterior elements?	The pedicle, lamina, and spinous process
What is the unique articulation found in the cervical spine?	The uncovertebral joint
What is the uncovertebral joint?	The articulation of the inferior posterior and lateral vertebra with the uncal process of the vertebra below
What is the main determinant of spinal stability?	The integrity of the ligamentous structures
What are the 4 major ligaments that contribute to spinal stability?	Anterior longitudinal ligament Posterior longitudinal ligament Ligamentum flavum Interspinous ligaments
What is the posterior ligament complex?	The interspinous ligament, ligamentum flavum, posterior longitudinal ligament, and supraspinous ligament

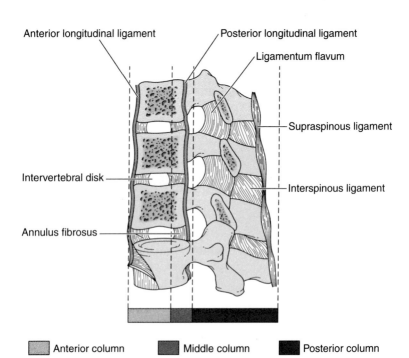

How many cervical nerve roots are there?

8

Where do they exit the neural foramen?

They exit from the lower portion of the neural foramen of the level above (e.g., C4 root exits at C3-C4 foramen)

How many lumbar nerve roots are there?

5

Where do they exit the neural foramen?

They exit from the upper portion of the neural foramen of the level below (e.g., L4 root exits at L4–L5 foramen)

Identify the structures of the lumbar spine on the following magnetic resonance imaging (MRI) sagittal views:

A = L1 vertebra
B = L4–L5 intervertebral disc
C = L5 vertebra
D = S1 vertebra
E = Conus
F = Thecal sac
G = Cauda equina

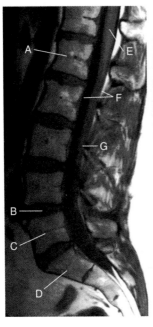
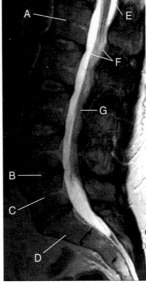

T$_1$–Weighted   T$_2$–Weighted

SHOULDER ANATOMY

Which bones comprise the shoulder girdle?	The scapula, clavicle, and humerus
What are the parts of the scapula?	The glenoid fossa, coracoid process, acromion, body, and spine
Is the coracoid process anterior or posterior?	Anterior
Is the acromion anterior or posterior?	Posterior (and lateral)
What 3 ligaments comprise the acromioclavicular joint?	Coracoacromial, coracoclavicular, acromioclavicular
What 3 structures comprise the shoulder joint?	The fibrous joint capsule, the rotator cuff, and the glenohumeral joint
Describe the glenohumeral joint.	The humeral head articulates with the glenoid labrum, the cartilaginous covering of the bony glenoid fossa of the scapula. Three glenohumeral ligaments hold the humeral head in apposition.
Describe the rotator cuff.	The rotator cuff is comprised of four muscles that originate on the scapula and insert into the anatomic neck and tuberosities of the humerus to convey structural stability to the glenohumeral joint. The rotator cuff surrounds the joint capsule.

Name the muscles of the rotator cuff.

SITS:
Supraspinatus muscle
Infraspinatus muscle
Teres minor muscle

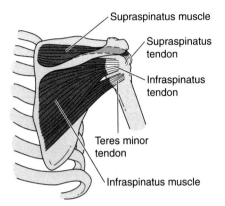

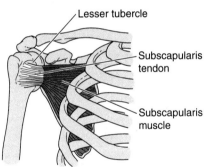

Where is the subacromial bursa?

Deep to the deltoid muscle and superficial to the rotator cuff

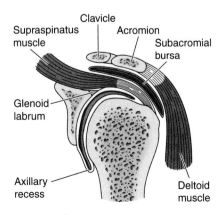

Subscapularis muscle

ELBOW ANATOMY

What bones articulate at the elbow?

Radius, ulna, and humerus

How do the ulna and humerus articulate?

The olecranon process of the ulna articulates with the trochlea and olecranon fossa of the humerus.

How do the radius and humerus articulate?

The radial head articulates with the capitellum.

What are the key anatomic relationships in the elbow?

1. The anterior humeral line (i.e., a line drawn parallel to the anterior humerus should pass through the middle third of the capitellum)
2. Radial head-capitellum alignment (i.e., the radial head should align with the capitellum in all projections)

WRIST ANATOMY

m

What are the bones of the wrist?

Some **L**overs **T**ry **P**ositions **T**hat **T**hey **C**an't **H**andle
Proximal row:
Scaphoid
Lunate
Triquetrum
Pisiform
Distal row:
Trapezium
Trapezoid
Capitate
Hamate

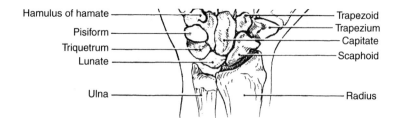

Hamulus of hamate — Trapezoid
Pisiform — Trapezium
Triquetrum — Capitate
Lunate — Scaphoid
Ulna — Radius

What 4 joints are in the wrist? Distal radioulnar joint
Radiocarpal joint
Midcarpal joints
Carpometacarpal joints

What are the key anatomic relationships in the wrist:

On the lateral view? Alignment of the radius, lunate, and capitate bones from proximal to distal

On the anterior-posterior (AP) view? 3 carpal rows:
Proximal aspect of proximal row
Distal aspect of proximal row
Proximal aspect of distal row

What is ulnar variance? The length of the distal ulna in comparison with the radius

What is:

Normal ulnar variance? Zero (i.e., the ulna and radius articulating surfaces are in continuity)

Negative ulnar variance? Ulnar articulating surface is proximal to that of the radius (i.e., ulna is short relative to the radius)

Positive ulnar variance? Ulnar articulating surface is distal to that of the radius (i.e., ulna is long relative to the radius)

Why is ulnar variance important to report? Positive ulnar variance predisposes the patient to ulnar impaction syndrome
Negative ulnar variance predisposes the patient to avascular necrosis of the lunate (Kienböck's disease)

What 4 structures are housed in the carpal tunnel?	The median nerve, superficial flexor tendons (4), flexor profundus tendons (4), and flexor pollicis longus tendon

HAND ANATOMY

What are the parts of a metacarpal?	Base, shaft, neck, head
What are the joints in the thumb called?	Carpometacarpal, metacarpophalangeal, interphalangeal
In terms of joints, how is the thumb unique?	It has one less joint; all of the other digits have a proximal interphalangeal and a distal interphalangeal joint

PELVIS AND HIP ANATOMY

What are the bones of the pelvis?	The **ilium, ischium,** and **pubis** (fused), the **sacrum,** and the **coccyx**
What are the pelvic columns?	The anterior (iliopubic) column runs obliquely inferoanteriorly and medially from the anterior part of the superior iliac crest to the pubic symphysis. The posterior (ilioischial) column runs inferiorly from the angle of the greater sciatic notch to the ischial tuberosity. (See figure next page)

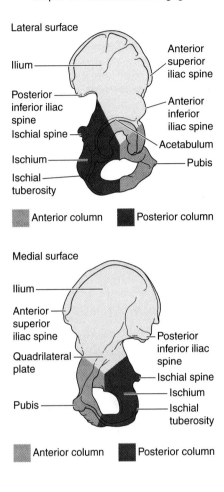

Lateral surface

Ilium

Anterior superior iliac spine

Posterior inferior iliac spine

Ischial spine

Anterior inferior iliac spine

Acetabulum

Ischium

Pubis

Ischial tuberosity

Anterior column   Posterior column

Medial surface

Ilium

Anterior superior iliac spine

Quadrilateral plate

Posterior inferior iliac spine

Ischial spine

Ischium

Pubis

Ischial tuberosity

Anterior column   Posterior column

Why are these columns important clinically?

The location of the fracture (i.e., anterior or posterior) determines the surgical approach to repair.

What is Shenton's line?

A smooth, curved line drawn along the medial border of the femoral metaphysis and superior border of the obturator foramen

Identify the radiographic lines of the hip joint:

A = Iliopubic (iliopectineal) line
B = Ilioischial line (posterior quadrilateral plate of ilium)
C = Anterior rim of the acetabulum
D = Acetabular teardrop (radiographic overlap of the anterior quadrilateral plate, the medial acetabular wall, and the acetabular notch)
E = Shenton's line
F = Posterior rim of the acetabulum
G = Acetabular roof

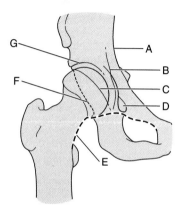

What is the acetabular angle and what is its normal measurement?

The angle that the acetabular roof makes with the horizontal, normally 15°–35°

What are the 5 parts of the proximal femur?

Head, neck, shaft, greater trochanter, lesser trochanter

How does the femoral head receive blood?

Retrograde arterial supply via the branches of the circumflex arteries

KNEE ANATOMY

What are the three articulations of the knee?

Medial tibiofemoral, lateral tibiofemoral, and patellofemoral

Which ligaments provide stability for the knee?

Medial collateral ligament complex
Lateral collateral ligament complex
Anterior cruciate ligament
Posterior cruciate ligament

What are the components of the:

Lateral collateral ligament complex?

From posterior to anterior, **BLT:** **B**iceps femoris, **L**ateral collateral ligament, and ilio**T**ibial band

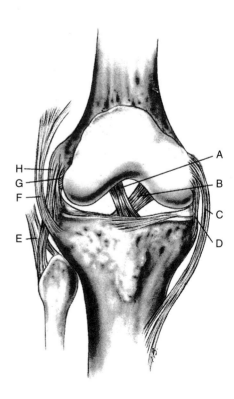

Medial collateral ligament complex?

Superficial and deep portions of the medial collateral ligament

Identify the following structures of the knee joint:

A = Anterior cruciate ligament
B = Posterior cruciate ligament
C = Medial collateral ligament
D = Deep head of the medial collateral ligament
E = Attachment of the biceps femoris
F = Iliotibial band
G = Tendon of the popliteus muscle
H = Lateral collateral ligament

Identify the structures on this superior view of the knee joint with the femur removed:

A = Patellar tendon
B = Joint capsule
C = Transverse meniscal ligament
D = Iliotibial band
E = Lateral meniscus
F = Popliteus muscle tendon
G = Biceps femoris attachment
H = Ligament of Wrisberg
I = Ligament of Humphrey
J = Posterior cruciate ligament
K = Semimembranosus muscle
L = Deep head of the medial collateral ligament
M = Medial collateral ligament
N = Medial meniscus
O = Anterior cruciate ligament

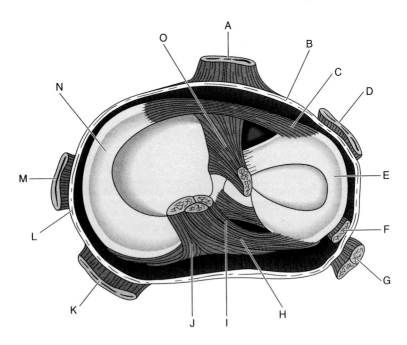

What are the menisci?

The semilunar fibrocartilages between the femoral condyles and the tibial plateau

ANKLE ANATOMY

What are the joints of the ankle?

Tibiotalar, tibiofibular, talocalcaneal

AP view

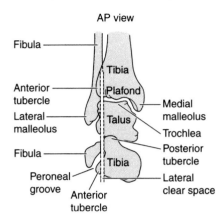

Lateral view

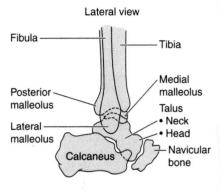

What is the lateral malleolus?	The distal fibula
What is the medial malleolus?	The distal medial tibia ending in the colliculus
What is the tibial plafond?	The distal tibia at the tibiotalar joint
What is the trochlea?	The proximal talus at the tibiotalar joint
What are the ligaments of the ankle?	**Laterally:** Anterior talofibular, posterior talofibular, and calcaneofibular ligaments **Medially:** Deltoid ligament

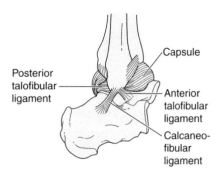

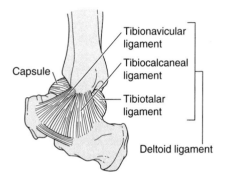

What structures cross behind the medial malleolus of the ankle?	**T**om, **D**ick, **A**nd **H**arry: **T**ibialis posterior, flexor **D**igitorum, **A**rtery and nerve, flexor **H**allucis From medial to lateral

FOOT ANATOMY

What are the bones of the:

Hindfoot?	Talus, calcaneus
Midfoot?	Cuboid bone, navicular bone, cuneiform bones (3)
Forefoot?	Metatarsals, phalanges

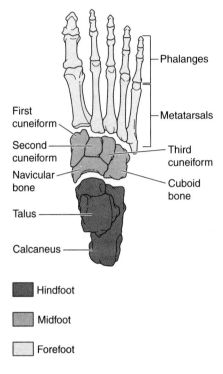

First cuneiform

Second cuneiform

Navicular bone

Talus

Calcaneus

Phalanges

Metatarsals

Third cuneiform

Cuboid bone

Hindfoot

Midfoot

Forefoot

What is Boehler's angle?   The angle formed by lines drawn tangent to the superior and inferior aspects of the calcaneus; normally 20°–40°

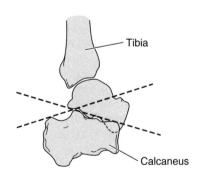

Tibia

Calcaneus

IMAGING STUDIES

When are the following studies used to image the musculoskeletal system?

Plain film radiography	To evaluate trauma, arthritides, bone alignment, and bone tumors
Computed tomography (CT)	To evaluate complex fractures (e.g., wrist, acetabular, and tibial plateau fractures), to evaluate tumor matrix, and to guide biopsies
MRI	To evaluate tendons, ligaments, cartilage, and soft tissue abnormalities (e.g., infection) and to stage tumors

ARTHROGRAPHY

What is arthrography?	Imaging evaluation of a joint following the injection of contrast agent into a joint space; may be performed with plain films, CT, or MRI
What 2 steps must be taken prior to performing arthrography?	1. Plain films must be obtained prior to the arthrogram. 2. Joint fluids should be aspirated and sent for culture or other tests as indicated.
Name 4 indications for arthrography.	1. Ligament and tendon tears 2. Cartilage injuries 3. Masses and intra-articular loose bodies (i.e., "joint mice") 4. Implant loosening
List 2 contraindications to arthrography.	1. Previous severe reaction to contrast media (relative contraindication) 2. Skin infection overlying injection site (absolute contraindication)
Name 4 complications that can result from arthrography.	Pain (most common), allergic reaction to contrast agent, infection, sterile synovitis
Which joints are commonly studied by arthrography?	Shoulder, elbow, wrist, hip, knee, ankle

NUCLEAR MEDICINE BONE SCAN

How is a bone scan performed, and why?	A radioactive compound is injected intravenously to detect abnormal areas of

bone metabolism; often performed in three phases to yield perfusion, blood pool, and delayed images

What are the primary uses of bone scans?

Early detection of osteomyelitis, stress fractures, osteonecrosis, reflex sympathetic dystrophy (RSD), prosthetic loosening, malignancy

Focal osseous abnormalities

List 6 causes of single or multiple focal areas of increased osseous uptake (i.e., "hot" lesions).

1. Arthritis
2. Metastatic disease (activity may increase in treated lesions for weeks to months secondary to the "flare" phenomenon)
3. Fracture or other trauma
4. Stress injury
5. Infection
6. Paget's disease

Other causes include fibrous dysplasia, benign and malignant primary bone tumors, infarction (subacute phase owing to bone remodeling), and increased blood flow.

List 5 causes of single or multiple focal areas of decreased osseous uptake (i.e., "cold" lesions).

1. Radiation therapy
2. Early osteonecrosis
3. Infarction (very early or late)
4. Anaplastic tumor (e.g., renal cell carcinoma, thyroid carcinoma, neuroblastoma, multiple myeloma)
5. Artifact from overlying attenuating material (e.g., a metal prosthesis or other dense object)

Extraosseous (i.e., soft tissue) abnormalities

List 6 causes of:

Focal extraosseous uptake

1. Poor radiopharmaceutical preparation [free technetium 99m (Tc-99m) seen in salivary glands, thyroid gland, and stomach]
2. Reduced, hydrolyzed technetium colloid (activity in liver and bone marrow)
3. Recent nuclear medicine examination (location depends on agent)

4. Primary tumors (e.g., osteosarcoma, neuroblastoma, breast carcinoma, meningioma) in the absence of metastatic disease
5. Metastatic deposits from breast tumors, ovarian tumors, gastrointestinal tumors, lung tumors, or osteosarcoma
6. Myositis ossificans

Diffuse (widespread) extraosseous uptake

1. Poor radiopharmaceutical preparation (free Tc-99m seen in the salivary glands, thyroid gland, and stomach)
2. Recent nuclear medicine examination (location depends on agent)
3. Renal failure
4. Metastases from breast tumors, ovarian tumors, lung tumors, or osteosarcoma
5. Lymphedema
6. Myositis ossificans

List 7 causes of increased renal uptake.

1. Urinary tract obstruction (unilateral or bilateral)
2. Chemotherapy
3. Nephrocalcinosis
4. Hypercalcemia
5. Radiation nephritis
6. Acute tubular necrosis
7. Thalassemia

List 6 causes of decreased renal uptake.

1. Renal failure
2. Superscan
3. Paget's disease
4. Osteomalacia
5. Hyperthyroidism
6. Nephrectomy (unilateral or bilateral)

BONE DENSITOMETRY

What is bone densitometry?
A technique that uses radionuclide or dual energy x-ray (DEXA) to measure the density of bone (most often, the hip and vertebral bones)

When is bone densitometry used?
To identify and assess the degree of osteoporosis and to monitor the effectiveness of treatment by evaluating disease progression

PATHOLOGY

What 5 questions should you ask yourself when assessing bones?	What is the alignment? (fractures, subluxations) What is the bone density? (osteopenia, sclerosis) Are the soft tissues normal? (swelling, effusion) Are the joint spaces normal? (widened, narrowed) Is the cortex normal? (intact, thickened)

STRESS FRACTURES

What is a stress fracture?	A fracture not caused by trauma
What is a fatigue fracture?	A stress fracture caused by repetitive stress that overloads the healing mechanisms of normal bone
What is an insufficiency fracture?	A stress fracture caused by normal stresses imposed on abnormally weakened bone
List the 7 common sites of fatigue fractures.	1. Metatarsals 2. Tibial shaft 3. Midfibula 4. Patella 5. Calcaneus 6. Pars interarticularis 7. Pubic ramus
List 5 conditions that can predispose to an insufficiency fracture.	1. Osteoporosis 2. Osteomalacia 3. Fibrous dysplasia 4. Paget's disease 5. Hyperparathyroidism
When will a stress fracture become visible on a plain film?	7–14 days after the injury
What is the radiographic appearance of a stress fracture?	Transverse fractures of the shaft of the bone Subtle, thin radiolucent lines (if visible at all) that usually do not extend through the cortex; some fractures may not be apparent until signs of healing (e.g., callus formation) arise

May also appear as a linear density owing to bone impaction

What is the best imaging modality for early diagnosis of a stress fracture?

Bone scan or MRI; MRI is more specific

What are the MRI features of stress fracture?

A linear area of decreased signal on T_1-weighted MRI surrounded by edema (high signal on T_2-weighted MRI)

OSTEOPENIA

Define the following terms:

Osteopenia

Decreased bone density as a result of decreased bone production, increased bone resorption, or both

Osteoporosis

Osteopenia as a result of an abnormal bone matrix

Osteomalacia

Osteopenia caused by abnormal mineralization of bone

Rickets

Osteomalacia in children

Can osteoporosis and osteomalacia be distinguished radiographically?

No. Classically, osteoporosis has a "picture frame" appearance, with a sharp cortex and decreased density otherwise, while osteomalacia has decreased density with blurring of the trabeculae and cortex. However, in practice, osteoporosis and osteomalacia are difficult to distinguish from one another, which is why some advocate labeling all such cases by the generic term "osteopenia."

Osteoporosis

When does osteoporosis become radiographically detectable?

When a 30%–50% decrease in bone mass occurs

What is the differential diagnosis of generalized osteoporosis:

In children?

Osteogenesis imperfecta, scurvy, leukemia, steroid therapy, juvenile osteoporosis

In adults?

Postmenopausal status, Cushing's disease, acromegaly, thyrotoxicosis, osteomalacia, multiple myeloma, hyperparathyroidism

What are the findings of osteoporosis on plain radiographs?

1. "Picture framing": Cortex is sharp, trabeculae are decreased
2. "Empty box" sign: Relative increased density of vertebral endplates with resorption of central spongy bone
3. "Codfish vertebrae": Biconcavity of the vertebral bodies owing to bulging of the structurally stronger disk
4. Compression fractures of the vertebrae

What is disuse osteoporosis?

Osteoporosis caused by immobilization

How does disuse osteoporosis differ from senile osteoporosis?

Disuse osteoporosis occurs more rapidly, may be local or regional, and may appear patchy or permeative.

What is reflex sympathetic dystrophy (RSD, Sudeck's atrophy)?

Typically occurring following trauma, RSD is severe osteoporosis and soft tissue swelling owing to hyperemia, thought to result from disordered vasomotor regulation.

What are the plain film radiographic findings associated with RSD?

Diffuse osteopenia

What are the bone scan findings associated with RSD?

Classically, diffusely increased activity in an extremity is seen in all three phases. Several months after the onset of symptoms, blood flow and blood pool return to normal, with only increased late-phase activity. More than 1 year after the onset of symptoms, the delayed phase may show normal or even decreased activity.

Osteomalacia

What are the most common causes of osteomalacia:

In developed countries?	Malabsorption and renal disease (e.g., renal tubular acidosis, proximal tubule disorders that lead to phosphorous loss, dialysis)
In third-world countries?	Vitamin D, calcium, or phosphorus deficiency
Name 2 radiographic characteristics of osteo-malacia.	1. Diffuse osteopenia 2. Looser's zones [i.e., pseudofractures (cortical stress fractures) filled with inadequately mineralized fibrous material that are typically seen at the axillary margin of the scapula, the inferior surface of the femoral neck, the ribs, the iliac wings, and the pubic rami]
What is Milkman's syndrome?	Multiple Looser's zones and osteomalacia
What is renal osteo-dystrophy?	Any bony change seen on radiographs secondary to renal failure
What radiographic findings are associated with renal osteodystrophy?	Osteomalacia, osteoporosis, "rugger jersey" spine, widened sacroiliac joints, lytic lesions (brown tumors), sub-periosteal bone resorption
What is the pathogenesis of scurvy?	Scurvy is caused by poor collagen production as a result of vitamin C insufficiency. The British navy recognized the cause of this disease and rationed their sailors with limes, which is how some citizens of the crown came to be known as "Limeys."
List 5 radiographic charac-teristics of scurvy.	1. Decreased bone density 2. Lines of Frankel (i.e., dense metaphyseal lines) 3. Wimberger's ring (i.e., sclerotic epiphyseal rim) 4. Periostitis resulting from subperiosteal hemorrhage 5. Pelken's fractures (i.e., metaphyseal corner fractures)

OSTEONECROSIS

What is osteonecrosis?	Bone death caused by a vascular insult (i.e., trauma, emboli, or increased marrow pressure)

What are the other names for osteonecrosis?	Avascular necrosis, ischemic necrosis, aseptic necrosis

What are the common causes of osteonecrosis?

ASEPTIC
Alcohol
Sickle cell disease, **S**ystemic lupus erythematosus (SLE), and **S**cleroderma
Endogenous or **E**xogenous steroids
Pancreatitis
Trauma (fracture of the femoral neck or navicula, dislocation of the talus)
Idiopathic (Legg-Calvé-Perthes disease, Blount disease, Kienböck's disease) and **I**atrogenic (radiation therapy, steroid therapy)
Caisson disease (the "bends")

What are the common sites of osteonecrosis?

Femoral head, humeral head, scaphoid, talus, medial femoral condyle

Describe the following diseases that are characterized by osteonecrosis:

    Legg-Calvé-Perthes's disease

Osteonecrosis of the femoral head in school-aged children

    Kienböck's disease

Osteonecrosis of the lunate, often post-traumatic (most common in men between the ages of 20 and 30 years)

    Preiser's disease

Osteonecrosis of the scaphoid

    Panner's disease

Osteonecrosis of the humeral capitellum

    Freiberg's disease

Osteonecrosis of the distal metatarsal

    Blount disease

Osteonecrosis of the medial tibia

What are the stages of radiographic osteonecrosis?

Stage 0: Normal radiograph and bone scan
Stage I: Normal radiograph, abnormal bone scan or MRI
Stage II: Mottled sclerosis

Stage III: Lucency without loss of bone contour, crescent sign (i.e., radiolucent subcortical fracture in the femoral or humeral head)

Stage IV: Flattening or loss of bone contour without joint space narrowing

Stage V: Loss of bone contour with joint space narrowing [degenerative joint disease (DJD)]

What are the characteristics of osteonecrosis on:

Bone scan?

Decreased area of uptake in the early stages, changing to increased area of uptake in the late stages

T_1-weighted MRI?

Hypointense ischemic areas
"Double line" sign with ring of low signal intensity at the viable-devascularized bone interface
Loss of high-signal intensity subchondral fat

T_2-weighted MRI?

Periarticular edema (early)
High-signal intensity "double line" sign

What is the most sensitive imaging technique for detection of osteonecrosis?

MRI has a sensitivity and specificity of more than 95%.

What is transient osteo-porosis?

A disorder of unknown cause, typically seen in men and characterized by a transient decrease in bone density

Why is transient osteo-porosis important?

It may mimic osteonecrosis, but it is self-limited.

What is OCD?

Separation of fragments of articular cartilage and subchondral bone from the underlying bone, thought to result from chronic trauma

Among which demographic group is OCD most common?

Children and young adults

Where is OCD seen most often?

Lateral aspect of the medial femoral condyle (75% of cases)

Lateral aspect of the lateral condyle (15% of cases)
Medial aspect of the medial femoral condyle (10% of cases)
Talar dome and capitellum

What is the best imaging modality for the diagnosis of OCD?

Early changes are best seen on MRI. In addition, MRI can evaluate the stability of the fragment.

In OCD, what features are seen on:

A plain film radiograph?

Joint effusion is the earliest finding. Radiolucent separation of the osteochondral fragment from the condyle may occur. Multiple calcific intra-articular loose bodies ("joint mice") may be seen later.

MRI?

Low-signal intensity of the necrotic fragment

Which patients are most susceptible to bone infarction?

Those with bone pain and a history of sickle cell disease or SLE

What are the plain film radiographic findings in patients with bone infarction?

Plain film radiographic findings are often equivocal, showing mixed patchy lytic-sclerotic lesions.

What MRI finding is characteristic in patients with bone infarction?

Serpiginous border

What condition may mimic a bone infarct?

Enchondroma

ORTHOPEDIC PROCEDURES

JOINT REPLACEMENT

What materials are used to make prosthetic joints and are they radiolucent or radiopaque?

Polyethylene: Radiolucent; usually backed by metal
Silastic: Mixed with a radiopaque material during manufacture
Metal alloys (e.g., **titanium, chromium**): Radiopaque

Methylmethacrylate cement: Made radiopaque by the manufacturer

What are the types of prosthetic implants?

Cemented (methylmethacrylate) prostheses are usually used in older patients. Usually, in the hip, the acetabular component is fixed with screws while the femoral component is cemented.

Sintered prostheses are designed to allow bony ingrowth into the porous, coated implant, obviating the need for cement. These prostheses are used for younger patients.

Name 2 problems that are commonly associated with joint replacement.

Infection and loosening

What is prosthetic loosening?

Abnormal movement of the prosthesis

Is prosthetic loosening acute or chronic?

It can be either: acute loosening is infection until proven otherwise; chronic loosening is wear-related and the incidence increases with the age of the prosthesis.

Describe the 2 types of hip replacements.

Total hip replacement involves implantation of acetabular and femoral head components.

Partial hip replacement involves a simple hemiarthroplasty or Austin-Moore procedure, or placement of a bipolar prosthesis

What are the best modalities for evaluating prostheses?

Plain radiographs and bone scans

List 4 radiographic features of prosthetic loosening.

1. Widening of the radiolucent line at the bone-cement or metal-bone interface by more than 2 mm
2. Migration of components or dislocation of the prosthesis
3. Periosteal reaction and bone destruction
4. Cement fracture

What type of bone scan is used to evaluate prosthetic joints and what are the indications?

A three-phase bone scan is usually used and is indicated when it is necessary to differentiate loosening from infection.

What are the patterns seen with loosening and infection?

Loosening demonstrates abnormal **late-phase activity** around the proximal femur and tip of the device.

Infection demonstrates increased activity on **all three phases,** with late-phase activity that surrounds the prosthesis.

For how long can one expect to see bone scan activity following implantation of the device?

For as long as 6 months following surgery for a non-porous (cemented) device, and for 1 year or more following implantation of a porous (non-cemented) prothesis

Where is activity most likely to be seen around hip prostheses after implantation?

At the tip of the device and in the trochanteric region

Is a bone scan effective for evaluating all types of prostheses?

Bone scans are most likely effective only for evaluating hip prostheses; knee and shoulder prostheses demonstrated variable increased late-phase uptake long after surgery.

OTHER PROCEDURES

What is arthrodesis?

Fusion of a joint achieved by removal of articular cartilage and fixation of the ends of articulating bones

What is osteotomy?

Surgical correction of bone shape; may involve bone cuts or interposition of wedges for alignment, removal of bone for length discrepancy, or interposition of bone for lengthening procedures

What is a bone graft?

The placement of bone in bony defects to stimulate bone growth and to provide mechanical stability; may be either autografts (i.e., the patient's own bone) or allografts (i.e., cadaveric bone)

How long does it take for a bone graft to become fully incorporated?

Approximately 1 year

What is spinal fusion?

Placement of a mechanical prosthesis or a bone graft to provide spinal stability following fracture or surgical resection; the hardware provides short-term stability while bony fusion provides long-term stability

TRAUMA

GENERAL CONSIDERATIONS

Common terms

Define the following terms:

Dislocation

Total loss of congruity between the articular surfaces of a joint

Subluxation

Anything less than total loss of congruity between articular surfaces

Closed fracture

Intact skin over the fracture site

Open fracture

Open wound overlying the fracture; fracture fragments are in continuity with the wound

Periarticular fracture

Fracture close to, but not involving, a joint

Intra-articular fracture

Fracture through the articular surface of a bone

Pathologic fracture

Fracture at sites weakened by neoplasm, metabolic disease, infection, or other bone abnormalities

Impending fracture

A lytic lesion larger than 2 cm in diameter or involving more than 50% of the cortex of a weight-bearing bone

Occult fracture

A fracture not visible on a standard plain film

Fracture evaluation

What are the minimum required radiographic views with any fracture?

1. A view that includes the joints immediately above and below the fracture

2. Two views of the fracture site taken at 90° to each other, usually an AP view and a lateral view

Which 3 radiographs are mandatory in the initial evaluation of a patient with multiple trauma?

1. Lateral cervical spine film
2. Chest film (to exclude mediastinal hematoma, pneumothorax, hemothorax, rib fracture, and pulmonary contusion)
3. AP pelvic film

Which 4 pieces of information obtained from the radiograph are essential for describing a fracture?

1. Anatomic site
2. Fracture pattern
3. Alignment
4. Associated soft tissue injuries

Anatomic site

How is the anatomic site of a fracture described?

Bone or bones injured
Location on the bone (distal or proximal)
Intra- or extra-articular involvement

Fracture patterns

Identify the following fracture patterns:

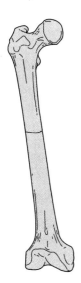

Simple transverse fracture (2 fracture fragments, fracture line perpendicular to the long axis of the bone)

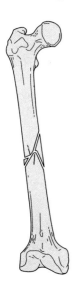

Comminuted fracture (fracture resulting in more than 2 fracture fragments)

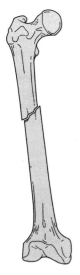

Oblique fracture (fracture line at an oblique angle to the long axis of the bone)

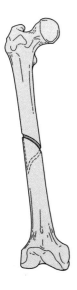

Spiral fracture (severe oblique fracture in which the fracture plane rotates along the long axis of the bone; occurs secondary to rotational force)

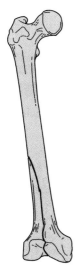

Longitudinal fracture (fracture line nearly parallel to the long axis of the bone, essentially a long oblique fracture)

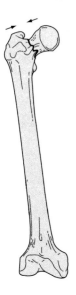

Impacted fracture (i.e., the end of the bone is driven into the contiguous metaphyseal region without displacement; occurs secondary to axial or compressive force)

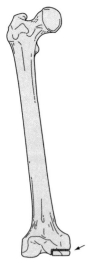

Depressed fracture (i.e., an impacted fracture that involves the articular surface of a bone, resulting in joint incongruity)

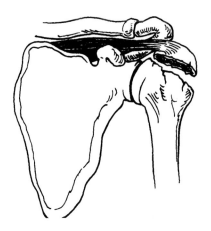

Avulsion fracture (i.e., the tendon is pulled away from the bone, carrying a bone fragment with it)

Fracture alignment

How is fracture alignment specified?

Displacement, angulation, rotation, length discrepancy

What are medial and lateral displacement?

Cortices out of alignment; described according to the direction of movement of the distal fragment relative to the proximal fragment

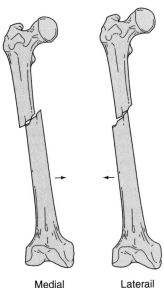

| Medial displacement | Laterail displacement |

How is angulation described?

According to the direction of the apex or the direction in which the distal fragment is angled

What is a varus deformity?

Apex of angulation away from the midline (i.e., "bowleggedness"); distal structure moves medially

What is a valgus deformity?

Apex of angulation toward the midline (i.e., "knock-kneed"); distal structure moves laterally

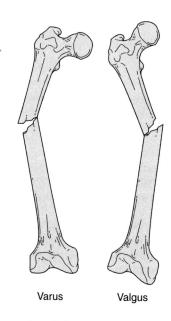

Varus   Valgus

In valgus deformity, the distal bone angles laterally.

How are internal and external rotation described?

According to the direction of movement of the distal fragment

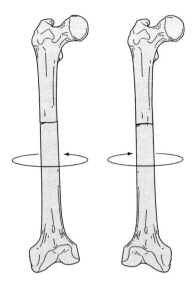

Internal rotation   External rotation

What is:

Bayonet apposition?   Overlap of fracture fragments

Distraction?   Longitudinal separation of fracture fragments

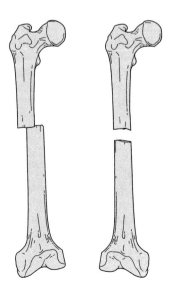

Fracture repair and healing

Define the following terms:

Reduction
A maneuver that restores proper alignment to a fracture or joint

Closed reduction
Reduction done without surgery

Open reduction
Surgical reduction

Fixation
Stabilization of a fracture after reduction by means of surgical placement of hardware, either externally or internally

Ex-fix
External fixation

ORIF
Open reduction, internal fixation

Malunion
Healing of a fracture in nonanatomic alignment

Delayed union
Slower-than-expected fracture healing (e.g., 16–18 weeks)

Nonunion
Failure of fracture healing; usually diagnosed when healing takes longer than 6 months (the fracture is not expected to heal completely without intervention)

Pseudoarthrosis
Type of nonunion characterized by the formation of a false joint cavity with a synovial-like capsule

Nonreactive nonunion
Atrophic nonunion characterized by an absence of bone reaction at the fracture site

Reactive nonunion
Hypertrophic, exuberant bone reaction characterized by flaring and sclerosis at the bony ends

Infected nonunion
Nonunion as a result of chronic, inactive osteomyelitis (characterized by an irregular, thick cortex and sclerosis) or an acute, active osteomyelitis (characterized by soft tissue edema, cortical destruction, and sequestration)

Myositis ossificans	Post-traumatic heterotopic bone formation in a chronic hematoma within a muscle
What is the radiographic appearance of myositis ossificans?	Peripheral calcification with a radiolucent center
What condition can mimic myositis ossificans?	Juxtacortical osteosarcoma, but this condition has central, not peripheral, calcification

FACIAL TRAUMA

What is the most common type of facial fracture?	Nasal fractures
What are the radiographic characteristics of facial fractures?	Cortical disruption Fragment displacement Asymmetry Opacification or air-fluid levels in sinuses Orbital emphysema Soft tissue swelling

Nasal fractures

What are the best radiographic views for evaluating nasal fractures?	Waters' view Nasal lateral view (exposure decreased to visualize the thin nasal bone) Occlusal view (for demonstrating the anterior nasal spine)
List 3 of the most common radiographic findings.	1. Transverse fracture 2. Anterior nasal spine avulsion 3. Depressed or displaced fracture fragments
What normal anatomic landmark may be confused with fracture lines on radiographs?	Normal longitudinal nasociliary grooves may be mistaken for fracture lines. Vessels do not cross the nasal bone; fractures do.
How are cartilaginous injuries best evaluated by imaging?	CT

Mandible fractures

What areas of the mandible are most prone to fracture?	Areas of structural weakness (e.g., the neck of the coronoid process, the incisive

foramen, the mandibular angle, the
mental foramen, and the ramus)

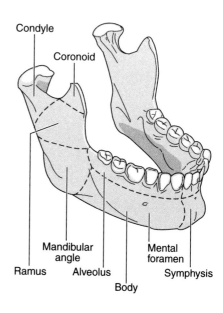

Condyle
Coronoid
Mandibular
angle
Ramus   Alveolus
Body
Mental
foramen
Symphysis

**What is the most common
fracture pattern of the
mandible?**

Fracture of the parasymphyseal region
(around the mental foramen), with a
contralateral ramus fracture

Zygomatic fractures

**What is the best view for
evaluating fractures of the
zygomatic arch?**

The "jug handle" view taken superior to
inferior at 90° to the arch

**Which are more common,
simple or comminuted arch
fractures?**

Comminuted fractures are much more
common

**What is the most common
complex arch fracture?**

The tripod (zygomaticomaxillary, FIZL)
fracture
FIZL fracture
Frontozygomatic suture
Infraorbital rim
Zygomatic arch
Lateral maxillary wall

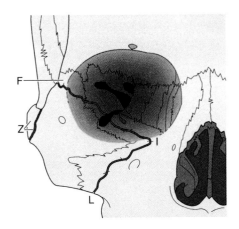

Le Fort fractures

What structure is involved in all Le Fort fractures?

The pterygoid plate

Which 3 structures are fractured in a Le Fort I fracture?

Nasal septum, maxilla, and the pterygoid plate; also known as the **"floating palate"**

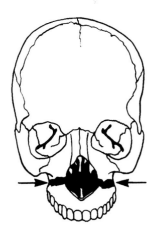

Which 6 structures are fractured in a Le Fort II fracture?

Nasal bones, frontal process of the maxilla, the medial orbital wall, the inferior orbital wall, the maxillary sinus, and the pterygoid plate; also known as the **"floating maxilla"**

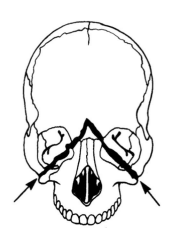

Which 7 structures are fractured in a Le Fort III fracture?

Nasal bones, frontal process of the maxilla, the medial orbital wall, the inferior orbital wall, the lateral orbital wall, the zygomaticofrontal suture, and the pterygoid plate; also known as the **"floating face"**

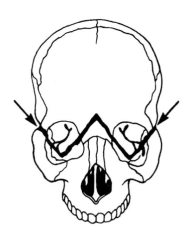

SPINAL TRAUMA

Which vertebra is fractured most often?

C7

List the next 3 most common sites of vertebral fracture, in order of decreasing frequency.

C1–C2 (upper cervical), C5–C6 (lower cervical), and T10–T12 (thoracolumbar)

What percentage of spinal fractures are multiple?	Approximately 20%
What percentage of multiple spinal fractures are at nonadjacent levels?	Only 5%. Most multiple spinal fractures occur at contiguous levels.
In patients with spinal trauma, does most spinal cord damage occur at the time of injury or as a late complication?	In most patients, the most spinal cord damage occurs at the time of injury (85% of cases).
What are the 3 most common causes of spinal fracture?	Motor vehicle crash (MVC; 50%), falls (25%), sports injuries (10%)
What imaging studies are required for all patients with suspected spinal cord injury?	Plain film AP and lateral views CT (to characterize fractures and identify bony compromise of the vertebral canal) MRI (to evaluate the soft tissues, including the ligaments, intervertebral disks, and spinal cord)

Cervical spine trauma

What radiographs are usually obtained in patients with a suspected cervical spine fracture?	A cross-table lateral view, an AP view, and an AP open-mouth odontoid view
What is the best way to approach radiographic examination of the patient?	A cross-table lateral view is usually examined first, in order to avoid moving the spine of a patient with a cervical fracture. If the lateral film is normal, then the rest of the C-spine series is obtained.
What additional film may be needed if the lower cervical spine is not imaged well on lateral views?	Swimmer's view (i.e., one arm up, one down)
When are flexion and extension lateral films obtained?	When no fracture is seen on initial films and pain is present
What other imaging modality is useful in evaluating cervical spine fractures?	CT can be used to better define the fracture and evaluate associated fractures, and to detect fracture fragments in the spinal canal.

How should a lateral cervical spine film be read?

1. All 7 cervical vertebrae should be well visualized—count down to vertebra T1.
2. Check the thickness of the retropharyngeal/retrotracheal space.
3. Assess the 4 parallel lines for discontinuity or step-off.
4. Examine the atlantodental interval (i.e., the distance from the anterior arch of C1 to the odontoid process of C2).
5. Scrutinize the disk spaces for narrowing or widening caused by acute injury.

What are the 4 parallel lines?

1. Anterior vertebral line
2. Posterior vertebral line
3. Spinolaminar line
4. Posterior spinous line

In addition, it is also important that the odontoid process of C2 aligns with the clivus.

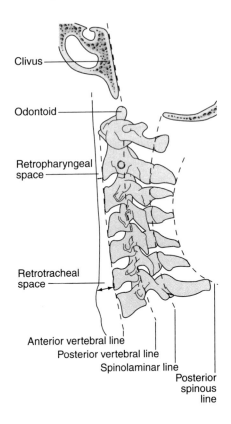

When looking at the posterior vertebral line, how far away should the soft tissue be from:

Vertebrae C1–C3?	< 5 mm
Vertebrae C4–C7?	< 20 mm
How wide is the atlantodental interval normally?	< 3 mm in adults or < 5 mm in children
What does widening of the atlantodental interval suggest?	Disruption of the transverse ligament
What are the 3 major mechanisms of cervical spine trauma?	Hyperflexion, hyperextension, compression

What are 6 common injuries associated with flexion?	1. Subluxation 2. Locked ("jumped") facets (unilateral or bilateral) 3. Odontoid fractures 4. Wedge fracture 5. Clay shoveler's fracture 6. Teardrop fracture
What are 3 common injuries associated with extension?	1. C1 posterior arch fracture 2. Hangman's fracture 3. Extension teardrop fracture
What are 2 common injuries associated with extension compression?	Jefferson's fracture and burst fracture
Which 6 cervical spine injuries are considered unstable?	1. Bilateral locked facets 2. Type II odontoid fracture 3. Teardrop fracture 4. Hangman's fracture 5. Jefferson's fracture 6. Burst fracture
What is a Jefferson's fracture?	Jefferson's fracture is a compression fracture of the bony ring of vertebra C1, characterized by splitting of the lateral masses and tearing of the transverse ligament. As with any bony ring, fracture always occurs in two or more places (try breaking a hard pretzel in one place only).

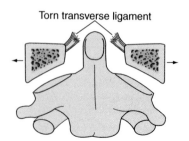

Torn transverse ligament

What is the mechanism of injury?

Axial force applied to the vertex of the head (commonly seen in diving injuries)

What are the radiographic features?

Displacement of the lateral masses of vertebra C1 beyond the margins of the body of vertebra C2 (displacement of < 2 mm or unilateral displacement may be indicative of a fracture or an artifact caused by head tilt)

Describe the 3 types of odontoid fracture.

Type I: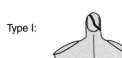

Fracture of the superior odontoid (rare); usually stable

Type II: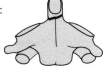

Fracture through the base of the odontoid; unstable

Type III: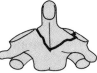

Fracture through the base of the odontoid into the body of the axis (vertebra C2); stable with a good prognosis

What is a hangman's fracture?

Traumatic spondylolisthesis of the axis resulting from hyperextension and distraction; seen with hanging and in MVCs when the chin strikes the dashboard

Name 4 radiographic hall-marks of a hangman's fracture.

1. Bilateral pars interarticularis (or less frequently, pedicle) fractures of vertebra C2

2. Anterior dislocation of the C2 vertebral body
3. Anterior inferior avulsion fracture associated with rupture of the anterior longitudinal ligament
4. Prevertebral soft tissue swelling

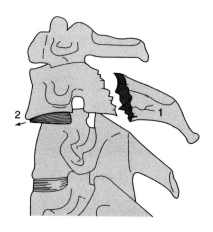

What is a flexion teardrop injury?

Severe flexion injury (such as occurs with neck injuries caused by diving into shallow water) results in posterior ligament disruption and an anterior compression fracture of the vertebral body

What is the prognosis for patients with this type of fracture?

Flexion teardrop injuries are the most severe and unstable spinal fractures. Remember **"teardrop"** for the **sad outcomes** associated with this fracture.

Describe 5 radiographic features of flexion teardrop injuries.

1. Anterior vertebral body avulsion fracture (teardrop body)
2. Posterior vertebral body subluxation or displacement into the spinal canal
3. Fracture of the spinous process
4. Prevertebral hematoma associated with anterior longitudinal ligament tear
5. Cord compression from fragments or vertebral body displacement

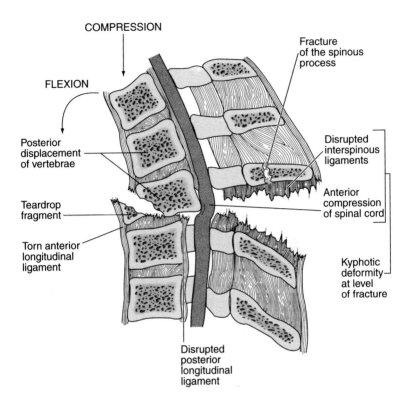

COMPRESSION

FLEXION

Fracture
of the spinous
process

Posterior
displacement
of vertebrae

Disrupted
interspinous
ligaments

Teardrop
fragment

Anterior
compression
of spinal cord

Torn anterior
longitudinal
ligament

Kyphotic
deformity
at level
of fracture

Disrupted
posterior
longitudinal
ligament

What is a clay shoveler's fracture?	Fracture of a spinous process, often seen in the lower cervical spine (i.e., vertebrae C6–T1)
What is the mechanism of injury?	Workers shoveling red Virginia clay (some people may say the workers were in North Carolina, England, or Australia, but don't be fooled!) sustained these fractures when they tried to toss a heavy shovelful of clay over their shoulders and the clay stuck to the shovel.
Describe 2 radiographic characteristics of a clay shoveler's fracture.	1. Spinous process fracture, best visualized on the lateral view 2. Ghost sign (i.e., "double" spinous process of C6 or C7 resulting from caudal displacement of the fractured spinous process; seen on the AP view)
Describe the 2 types of locked facet injuries.	**Unilateral:** Rotation injury of the upper cervical vertebrae resulting in rupture

of the apophyseal joint ligaments and facet joint dislocation; the facet joint may "lock" in an overriding position

Bilateral: Injury resulting from extreme hyperflexion and leading to complete anterior dislocation of the vertebral body; associated with a very high risk of cord damage

Which type of locked facet injury is considered unstable?

Bilateral

What is the radiographic appearance of:

    Unilateral locked facets?

Widening of the disk space
"Bow tie" or "bat wing" appearance of the overriding locked facets

    Bilateral locked facets?

Complete anterior dislocation of the vertebra
Disturbance of the posterior ligament complex and detachment of the anterior longitudinal ligament
"Bow tie" or "bat wing" appearance of the locked facets

What is the mechanism for anterior subluxation?

Anterior subluxation occurs with disruption of the posterior ligamentous complex following hyperflexion. The injury may be stable or unstable.

What radiographs are required for patients with anterior subluxation?

In addition to the basic cervical spine films, flexion and extension views are usually necessary.

What are the radiographic features of anterior subluxation?

Fanning or widening of the interspinous distance
Loss of normal cervical lordosis or hyperkyphosis
Anterior displacement of the vertebral body with flexion

Describe 4 radiographic indications of an unstable injury.

1. Changes in normal disk space (widening or narrowing)
2. Fanning or widening of the interspinous distance

3. Associated compression fracture of more than 25% of the affected vertebral body
4. Anterior subluxation of more than 4 mm

What are 8 common causes of C1–C2 subluxation?

1. Rheumatoid arthritis
2. Juvenile rheumatoid arthritis
3. Psoriasis
4. Ankylosing spondylitis
5. SLE
6. Down syndrome
7. Morquio's syndrome
8. Trauma

What is the most common cause of lower cervical spine subluxation?

Degenerative osteoarthritis of the facet joints

What imaging technique should be used if disk herniation, epidural hematoma, or spinal cord contusion is suspected?

MRI. A CT myelogram may be obtained if MRI is not available or the patient has contraindications to MRI (e.g., a pacemaker).

Thoracolumbar spine trauma

How are thoracolumbar spinal fractures classified?

By mechanism of injury:
Compression fractures are caused by anterior or lateral flexion
Burst fractures are caused by axial loading and acute flexion injuries of the spine

What is a compression fracture?

Anterior wedging of the affected vertebral body

Is the prognosis for patients with compression fractures good or bad?

Compression fractures are typically stable and not associated with neurologic injury.

What is a burst fracture?

A burst fracture is a fracture through the anterior and posterior cortex of the vertebral body, usually extending into the posterior elements. Retropulsion of fracture fragments into the spinal canal, leading to spinal cord injury, is common.

What radiographic signs are associated with:

Compression fracture?	Wedge-shaped deformity of the vertebral body and loss of vertebral body height
Burst fracture?	Comminution of the vertebral body Retropulsion of fracture fragments into the spinal canal Widening of the interpedicular distance on the AP view
What is a Chance fracture?	A Chance fracture is characterized by transverse splitting of the vertebra and spinous process, often with associated rupture of the intervertebral disk and posterior complex ligaments. The anterior, middle, and posterior columns are involved. Neurologic deficits occur only with dislocation. These fractures are often associated with significant intra-abdominal pathology.
What is the mechanism of injury?	Hyperflexion. Chance fractures (also called "seat belt injuries") are often seen in MVC passengers who were restrained with a lap belt only.
What is a spinal fracture-dislocation?	Anterior compression, distraction, and rotation injury; an extremely unstable fracture pattern that is associated with neurologic deficit and intra-abdominal injury
What is a spinal dislocation?	A highly unstable injury caused by rotation, distraction, and sheer forces and characterized by disruption of all three columns; almost always associated with neurologic deficit
What views are required for evaluation of acute low back pain?	AP and lateral views
When are oblique views helpful?	When a pars interarticularis injury is suspected
What is the Scotty dog?	The outline formed by the elements of

the vertebral arches of the lumbar spine on an oblique film such that if the patient is turned to the right, the left neural foramen is visualized

What are the anatomic landmarks found in the Scotty dog?

Nose: *transverse process*

Eye: *pedicle*

Neck: *pars interarticularis*

Front leg: *inferior articular process*

Ear: *superior articular process*

Tail: *contralateral superior articular process*

Body: *lamina*

Rear leg: *contralateral inferior articular process*

What is spondylolysis?

A bony defect of the pars interarticularis

What is the radiographic appearance of spondylolysis?

The bony defect forms a "collar" on the neck of the Scotty dog:

Spondylolytic defect

What is a common cause of spondylolysis?

Spondylolysis is believed to be a chronic stress fracture and is seen most often in adolescent athletes.

Where does spondylolysis usually occur?

L5 Vertebra , most commonly

What is spondylolisthesis?

Anterior slippage of a vertebral body relative to its inferior adjacent vertebra

What can cause spondylolisthesis?

Spondylolisthesis is most often caused by bilateral spondylolysis or degenerative disease of the facets. Rarely, it is caused by disk pathology (e.g., infection) or is congenital.

Where does spondylolisthesis usually occur?

95% of cases occur at the L4–L5 or L5–S1 levels

What percentage of patients with spondylolisthesis also have spondylolysis?

100%; true spondylolisthesis is always associated with spondylolysis. All other causes of spondylolisthesis result in "pseudo" spondylolisthesis.

What percentage of patients with spondylolysis also have spondylolisthesis?

Approximately 50%

How is spondylolisthesis graded?

I–IV, according to the degree of anterior translation of the affected vertebra:
Grade I: < 25% displacement
Grade II: 25%–50% displacement
Grade III: 50%–75% displacement
Grade IV: > 75% displacement

What is retrolisthesis?

Posterior subluxation of a vertebra onto its inferior adjacent neighbor

What is pseudospondylolisthesis?

Pseudospondylolisthesis (degenerative spondylolisthesis) is anterior displacement of a vertebral body that occurs secondary to degeneration and subluxation of the apophyseal joints.

In a patient with pseudospondylolisthesis, what are the:

Plain film findings? (List 4)

1. Anterior subluxation of superior vertebrae onto inferior vertebrae
2. Facet hypertrophy
3. Disk space narrowing
4. Osteophytes

CT findings? (List 2)

1. Vacuum disk sign (i.e., gas in the disk space caused by degeneration of the disk)
2. Facet disease

MRI finding?

Hourglass-shaped thecal sac compression

How is pseudospondylolisthesis differentiated from true spondylolisthesis?

In true spondylolisthesis, the step-off in the line formed by the tips of the spinous processes is above the level of the slip. In pseudospondylolisthesis, the step-off is below the level of the slip. This is called the **spinous process sign.**

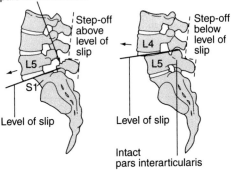

List 3 instances where it would be appropriate to obtain an MRI for a patient with low back pain.

1. Failure of conservative therapy
2. Symptoms of cord compression or cauda equina symptoms
3. History of cancer

What are the imaging modalities of choice for detecting lumbar disk herniation?

MRI is best for identifying disk changes and evaluating the extent of injury. In addition, MRI provides direct sagittal imaging. CT is also sensitive and is less expensive. Discography, which entails the injection of contrast into the disk under fluoroscopic guidance, reproduces pain if the disk is the cause of the patient's symptoms.

SHOULDER TRAUMA

What radiographic views are most useful for evaluation of shoulder problems?

A true AP view of the shoulder (taken with the patient inwardly rotated 40° so that the scapula is in profile) with the humerus in internal and external rotation, possibly accompanied by either an axillary or transscapular "Y" view

Shoulder fractures and dislocations

What is the most common fracture in the shoulder area?	Clavicular fracture
In which direction is the fracture fragment displaced in most patients with a fractured clavicle?	The distal fragment is displaced medially and caudally relative to the proximal fragment.
What is the frequency of fracture by location along the clavicle?	Middle third (80%), distal third (15%), proximal third (5%)
Which types of clavicular fractures can be easily treated with closed reduction and immobilization?	Proximal and middle third fractures
What are the most difficult fractures to diagnose in the shoulder region?	Scapular fractures
Why is it important to identify scapular fractures?	Scapular fractures are often associated with other injuries, usually thoracic in nature.
What is the best radio graphic view for detecting:	
A scapular fracture?	The transscapular Y view
Occult fractures of the acromion and coracoid?	35° cephalic tilt view
What is an os acromiale?	An unfused acromial apophysis; may be confused with an acromial fracture
What is the most common site of clavicular separation?	The acromioclavicular joint
How is acromioclavicular separation defined?	Disruption of the acromioclavicular ligament with or without injury to the coracoclavicular ligaments
What is the mechanism of injury?	Acromioclavicular separation results from a downward blow to the clavicle and is

usually sports-related. Injury may also be caused by applying traction to the arm or falling on the hand or elbow with the arm flexed at a 90° angle.

How are acromioclavicular separations classified?

According to injury of the acromio-clavicular and coracoclavicular ligaments and the position of the clavicle

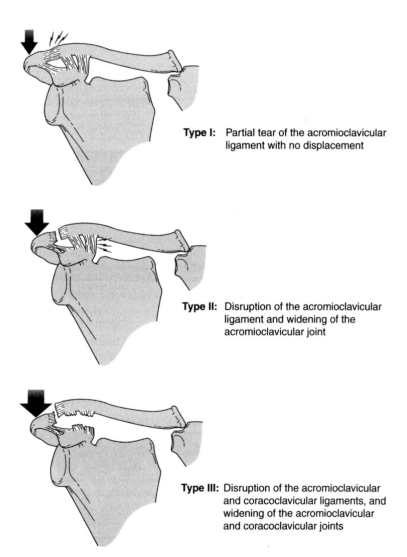

Type I: Partial tear of the acromioclavicular ligament with no displacement

Type II: Disruption of the acromioclavicular ligament and widening of the acromioclavicular joint

Type III: Disruption of the acromioclavicular and coracoclavicular ligaments, and widening of the acromioclavicular and coracoclavicular joints

How is acromioclavicular separation graded radiographically?	**Grade I:** Not detectable by plain film; the acromioclavicular joint space is 0.8–1.0 cm and the coracoclavicular distance is normal **Grade II:** The acromioclavicular joint space is 1.0–1.5 cm and the coracoclavicular distance is increased (by 25%–50%) **Grade III:** The acromioclavicular joint space is greater than 1.5 cm and the coracoclavicular distance is increased (by 50% or more)
What is the best view for evaluating acromioclavicular joint injury?	A stress view of the acromioclavicular joint (obtained with the patient in the upright position with 10–15 pounds suspended from each wrist) is best for differentiating type II and type III sprains. An AP view showing both the affected and nonaffected acromioclavicular joints should also be taken.
What is the most common direction of glenohumeral (shoulder) dislocation?	More than 95% of all shoulder dislocations are anterior.
What are the required radiographic views for suspected shoulder dislocation?	A true AP view (with internal and external rotation of humerus) and either an axillary or a transscapular "Y" view are required to assess the position of the humeral head in the glenoid fossa.
Why is an axillary or transscapular "Y" view required?	More than 60% of posterior dislocations are missed on initial presentation with standard shoulder films alone.
What is the mechanism of injury in anterior glenohumeral dislocation?	External rotation and hyperextension of the shoulder in abduction
What are the radiographic features of anterior glenohumeral dislocation?	In an anterior dislocation, the humeral head is displaced anteromedially and typically slightly inferior to the glenoid fossa.
What are common injuries associated with anterior dislocation?	Hill-Sachs fracture of the humeral head (associated with 50% of anterior dislocations)

Fractures of the greater tuberosity
(associated with 15% of anterior
dislocations)
Bankart fracture

What is a Hill-Sachs fracture?

A defect of the posterior lateral humeral
head that occurs with anterior dislocation
of the shoulder and is caused by contact
between the posterior humeral head and
the anterior inferior glenoid rim

What is a Bankart fracture?

An avulsion fracture of the anterior labrum or glenoid fossa at the inferior aspect

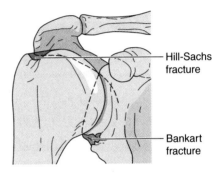

On what view are Hill-Sachs fractures most visible?

AP view of the shoulder with internal
rotation of the humerus

On what view are Bankart fractures most visible?

Axillary view

What MRI findings are associated with anterior glenohumeral dislocation?

Tears of the anterior glenoid labrum,
anterior capsule injury

What is a posterior shoulder dislocation?

The humeral head is displaced posterior
and, usually, superior to the glenoid fossa

What is the mechanism of injury?

Indirectly applied force to the arm while
the shoulder is flexed, adducted, and
internally rotated; often seen in patients
who have had seizures or sustained an
electrical burn (great force required to
cause this injury)

What is a reverse Hill-Sachs lesion?

A compression fracture of the anterior
humeral head that occurs with posterior

dislocation of the shoulder and is caused by contact of the humeral head with the posterior inferior glenoid rim

What are the radiographic features of a reverse Hill-Sachs lesion?

Sharp angle of the scapulohumeral arch

What is pseudodislocation of the humerus?

Wide glenohumeral distance attributable to post-traumatic hemarthrosis

What is the imaging modality of choice for patients with suspected glenoid labral tears?

MRI or MR arthrography have sensitivities of nearly 95%.

What is the common labral tear called?

A **SLAP** lesion: **S**uperior **L**abrum **A**nterior and **P**osterior (to the biceps anchor)

Subacromial syndromes

What defines a subacromial syndrome?

Pain caused by a subacromial process

Name 2 common subacromial syndromes.

Impingement and rotator cuff tears

What is impingement of the shoulder?

Entrapment of the rotator cuff tendons between the humeral head and the coracoacromial arch (i.e., the acromion, acromioclavicular joint, and coracoacromial ligaments)

What 3 anatomic factors play a role in impingement?

1. Morphology of the acromion process (i.e., its shape and slope)
2. Subacromial osteophyte formation
3. Acromioclavicular joint disease

What is the best plain film view for assessing the morphology of the acromion?

A supraspinatus (scapular outlet) view provides an excellent image of the morphology of the acromion and acromioclavicular joint. This lateral scapula film is taken with the x-ray tube angled inferiorly at 10°.

What other imaging modality can be used to assess a patient with a suspected subacromial process?

MRI provides excellent demonstration of the acromion and subacromial space, allowing visualization of the rotator cuff and its relationship to the acromion.

Describe the 3 types of acromial morphology and the associated risk for development of a subacromial syndrome.

Type I: Flat acromion; < 5% of cases
Type II: Curved acromion; 27% of cases
Type III: Hooked acromion; 70% of cases

Which rotator cuff tendon is most commonly torn?

Supraspinatus tendon

Name the 2 primary causes of rotator cuff tears.

Repetitive microtrauma from impingement and acute trauma

What is the imaging study of choice for patients with a suspected rotator cuff tear?

MRI has approximately 95% sensitivity and specificity for complete tears and 85% accuracy for partial tears and tendinitis.
MRI arthrography increases the accuracy, but requires a procedure.
Conventional (x-ray) arthrography may also be used.

What are the signs of a rotator cuff tear on MRI?

Increased signal intensity on T_2-weighted images or a gap in muscle (usually at a musculotendinous junction)

List 4 signs of a chronic rotator cuff tear on plain radiograph.

1. Narrow acromiohumeral space (i.e., < 6 mm)
2. Erosion of the inferior surface of the acromion
3. Atrophic changes of the greater tuberosity
4. Extravasation of contrast into the subacromial bursa

Adhesive capsulitis

What are the symptoms of adhesive capsulitis ("frozen shoulder")?

Pain, stiffness, decreased range of motion

What is the best imaging modality for diagnosing adhesive capsulitis?

Shoulder arthrogram

What are the radiographic features?

Decreased capacity of the joint capsule, loss of subscapular and axillary recesses, and possibly disuse osteoporosis

HUMERUS TRAUMA

What is the most common injury to the humerus?	Nondisplaced fractures (85% of humerus injuries)
How are proximal humerus fractures classified?	Neer's classification of proximal humerus fractures is based on the anatomic site and displacement of fracture fragments.
How is displacement defined?	Separation of fracture fragments by more than 1 cm or angulation between fragments of more than 45°

ELBOW TRAUMA

What is "tennis elbow?"	Inflammation of the extensor tendon where it originates on the lateral epicondyle
What is "golfer's elbow?"	Inflammation of the flexor tendon where it inserts on the medial epicondyle

Elbow fractures

What are the posterior fat pad and sail signs?	The posterior fat pad and sail signs indicate an elbow fracture. Ordinarily, the posterior fat pad is not visible on a lateral view and the anterior fat pad is seen as a small triangle adjacent to the anterior surface of the supracondylar humerus. With fractures of the elbow, the subsequent hemarthrosis distends the joint capsule, making the posterior fat pad visible and lifting the anterior fat pad away from the bone, causing it to look like a sail.

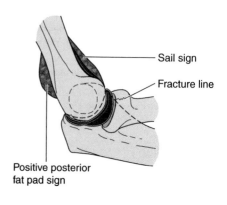

Sail sign

Fracture line

Positive posterior
fat pad sign

In adults, which two sites in the elbow are most commonly injured?

The radial head and the medial epicondyle

How are distal humerus fractures classified?

According to the anatomic location and fracture pattern:
Extra-articular
  Epicondylar: Fracture of the medial or lateral epicondyle
  Supracondylar: Fracture line is above the epicondyles
Intra-articular
  Transcondylar: The fracture plane is within the joint capsule, and either the lateral or medial condyle is fractured.
  Intercondylar (bicondylar): An intra-articular fracture line splits the medial and lateral condyles.

What is the mechanism of injury associated with radial head fractures?

Falling on an outstretched arm is the most common cause of radial head fracture.

Are radial head fractures easily missed on plain films?

Yes, especially if the fracture is non-displaced. Look for the fat pad sign.

What additional view should be ordered when there is strong clinical suspicion for radial head fracture but no visible fracture on a standard projection?

A radial head view; CT may also be helpful

What is an Essex-Lopresti injury?

A comminuted fracture of the radial head with disruption of the interosseous membrane and distal radioulnar joint dislocation

Elbow dislocations

How are elbow dislocations classified?

According to the direction of displacement of the radius, ulna, or both, relative to the distal humerus

What is the most common elbow dislocation?

Posterior or posterolateral dislocation of the ulna accounts for approximately 90% of all elbow dislocations.

What associated injuries should always be looked for?

Fracture of the olecranon, radial head, or distal humerus

FOREARM TRAUMA

What are the major types and frequency of forearm fractures?	Fracture of both the radius and ulna (60%) Ulna fracture only (25%) Radius fracture only (15%)

Describe the following fractures:

Monteggia fracture	Fracture of the ulna with accompanying radial head dislocation
Galeazzi ("reverse Monteggia") fracture	Fracture of the proximal radius with an associated distal radioulnar joint dislocation
Nightstick fracture	Isolated transverse fracture of the ulnar diaphysis (called a "nightstick fracture" because a person being subdued by a police officer wielding a nightstick instinctively raises his arm for protection, causing the baton to fall on the ulna)

WRIST TRAUMA

What is a Colles' fracture pattern?	Distal radius fracture with volar apex angulation and dorsal displacement of the fracture fragment (dinner fork deformity), often with impaction; associated with ulnar styloid fracture in 50% of cases
What is the mechanism of injury?	Usually caused by falling on an outstretched hand with the wrist extended and the forearm pronated
Among what group are Colles' fractures most common?	Elderly women
How are Colles' fractures classified?	The Frykman classification system distinguishes between intra- and extra-articular fractures and the presence or absence of an associated ulnar styloid fracture. More complex fractures are graded higher.

Describe the following types of fractures:

Smith's fracture	Distal radius fracture with volar displacement and dorsal apex angulation (opposite of a Colles' fracture); caused by falling on an outstretched arm with the wrist in flexion
Barton's fracture	Intra-articular fracture of the dorsal aspect of the distal radius
Reverse Barton's fracture	Intra-articular fracture of the volar aspect of the distal radius (same as a type III Smith's fracture)
Chauffeur's fracture	Fracture of the radial styloid (named in the early 1900s when the injury was commonly caused by a car backfiring while being crank-started)

What is the most commonly fractured carpal bone?

Scaphoid bone (90% of cases)

What is the frequency of scaphoid fracture (by type)?

Comminuted (70%), proximal (20%), distal (10%)

Why is osteonecrosis of the scaphoid bone a common complication of scaphoid fracture?

Blood supply to the proximal pole of the scaphoid flows from distal to proximal.

What is the "snuff box" and what is its significance?

The space on the dorsum of the proximal hand between the extensor indices tendon and the extensor pollicis tendon; this space lies over the scaphoid

What is the treatment of a patient with snuff box tenderness and no radiographic evidence of a scaphoid fracture?

Assume that the scaphoid is fractured—immobilize and follow up.

Name 3 common types of carpal dislocation.

1. Rotary subluxation of the scaphoid with scapholunate dissociation
2. Perilunate dislocation (i.e., the lunate is aligned with the radius and the carpals are dorsally displaced)

3. Lunate dislocation (i.e., the lunate is dislocated in the volar direction)

What are the radiographic features of:

Scapholunate dissociation?

Triangular or pie-shaped lunate on AP view of the wrist
Terry Thomas sign

Perilunate dislocation?

The capitate is not seated in the cup of the lunate on lateral view
Transcaphoid fracture common, as is fracture of the triquetrum and capitate
Radial styloid fracture often seen as well

Describe the following signs:

Signet ring sign

The scaphoid has the appearance of a signet ring when seen on an AP view of the wrist; seen with rotary subluxation

Terry Thomas sign

Scapholunate diastasis of more than 3 mm on an AP view of the wrist; pathognomonic for scapholunate dissociation (named for Terry Thomas, a famous comedian of the 20s and 30s known for the gap between his teeth—David Letterman would be a more easily recognized namesake today)

What are 2 types of carpal instability?

Volar intercalary segment instability (VISI)
Dorsal intercalary segment instability (DISI)

Which is the most common form of carpal instability?

DISI

Injury to which ligament is associated with DISI?

Scapholunate ligament

What are the radiographic signs of DISI?

On a lateral radiograph of the wrist, the lunate tilts dorsally and the scapholunate angle increases. The Terry Thomas sign may be seen on an AP view.

What is VISI?

Tilt of the lunate in a volar direction

Injury to which ligament is associated with VISI?   Lunotriquetral ligament

What are the radiographic signs of VISI?   A decreased scapholunate angle is noted on a lateral radiograph of the wrist.

HAND TRAUMA

Describe the following hand injuries:

    Bennett's fracture   Intra-articular fracture-dislocation of the base of the thumb metacarpal

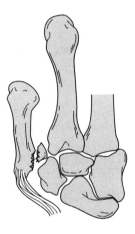

    Rolando's fracture   Comminuted Bennett's fracture

    Boxer's fracture   Fracture of the fifth metacarpal neck with dorsal apex angulation of the distal fragment (usually occurs secondary to striking a hard object with a closed fist)

    Gamekeeper's thumb   Disruption of the ulnar collateral ligament of the metacarpophalangeal joint of the thumb, often associated with an avulsion fracture of the base of the proximal phalanx [named for injury caused by breaking rabbit necks between the thumb and forefinger; now more commonly associated with skiing (falling with the thumb tangled in a ski pole) or kayaking]

Mallet (baseball) finger	Avulsion injury at the base of the distal phalanx at the insertion of the extensor digitorum tendon

PELVIC AND HIP TRAUMA

Pelvic fractures

What is the leading cause of pelvic fracture:

In patients younger than 60 years?	MVC
In patients older than 60 years?	Falling at home
What plain radiographs are required for patients with pelvic or hip trauma?	AP view of the pelvis, including the iliac crest, the inferior spine and sacrum, and both hips Cross-table lateral view Inlet and outlet views and Judet (oblique) views of the pelvis (used to define fractures)
What is the best imaging modality for pelvic fractures?	CT of the pelvis is the technique of choice for evaluating complex fracture patterns and the degree of displacement and soft tissue injury.
What makes a pelvic fracture stable or unstable?	The pelvic ring must remain intact in stable pelvic fractures. Unstable pelvic fractures are characterized by disruption of the bony or ligamentous structures of the pelvic ring.
List 4 stable fractures of the pelvis.	1. Avulsion fracture 2. Duverney's fracture (fracture of the iliac wing) 3. Isolated sacral fracture 4. Ischiopubic rami fracture
What is the most common cause of avulsion fractures?	Avulsion fractures occur most commonly in young athletes as a result of abnormal stress on the tendinous attachments of the muscles, prior to fusion of the ossification centers.
List 4 common locations for pelvic avulsion fracture.	1. Anterosuperior iliac spine: sartorius avulsion

2. Anteroinferior iliac spine: rectus femoris avulsion
3. Ischial tuberosity: hamstring avulsion
4. Lesser trochanter of the femur: iliopsoas avulsion

Name 4 unstable pelvic fractures.

1. Malgaigne fracture

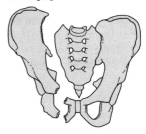

2. Straddle fracture

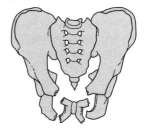

3. Bucket-handle fracture

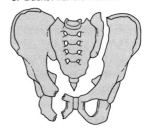

4. Sacroiliac joint dislocation

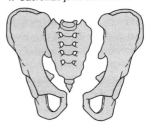

What is a Malgaigne fracture?	Articular or para-articular fracture of the sacroiliac joint and ipsilateral ischiopubic rami
What is a straddle fracture?	Bilateral fracture of the obturator rings
What is a bucket-handle fracture?	Fracture of an obturator ring and fracture or disruption of the contralateral sacro-iliac joint

Acetabular fractures

What plain film radiographs are usually obtained for evaluation of an acetabular fracture?	AP views (of both hips, not just the affected side) and Judet views (45° oblique views) of the pelvis
What other imaging modality should be considered?	CT should be considered for all patients with acetabular fractures. New techniques allow three-dimensional reconstruction and computer-guided surgical navigation to assist planning for repair of pelvic and acetabular fractures.

Describe the following acetabular fractures:

Anterior column fracture	Fracture through the iliopubic column
Posterior column fracture	Fracture through the ilioischial column
Transverse acetabular fracture	Fracture that involves both the anterior and posterior columns, cleaving the bone into superior and inferior segments (the superior fragment contains the acetabular roof and ilium, and the inferior fragment contains the ischiopubic bone)

Hip dislocation

What is a hip dislocation?	Displacement of the femoral head from the acetabulum
How can hip dislocations be classified?	As anterior, posterior, or central (fracture dislocation resulting in protrusio acetabuli)

What 5 radiographs are required for a patient with a dislocated hip?

1. AP film of the pelvis that includes both hips
2. AP film of the affected hip
3. Lateral film of the affected hip
4. Post-reduction AP film of the affected hip
5. Post-reduction lateral film of the affected hip

What is the most common type of hip dislocation?

Posterior (account for as many as 90% of all cases)

What is the most common mechanism of injury in posterior hip dislocations?

High-energy trauma, such as that seen with knee-to-dashboard injuries

What complication may be seen with a posterior hip dislocation?

Injury to the sciatic nerve (10% of patients)

List 4 radiographic features of posterior hip dislocation.

1. Femoral head lateral and superior to the acetabulum
2. Fracture of the posterior rim of the acetabulum in most cases
3. Femur in internal rotation and adduction
4. Affected femoral head may appear smaller secondary to magnification

What is protrusio acetabuli?

Femoral head protrudes into the pelvic cavity; associated with acetabular fracture

Name 4 causes of protrusio acetabuli.

PROTrusio
Paget's disease
Rheumatoid arthritis
Osteomalacia
Trauma

m

Why is hip dislocation an emergency?

It may result in osteonecrosis and osteoarthritis.

Femoral fractures

Which demographic group is most prone to femur fractures?

Elderly women with osteoporosis

Which 2 plain films should be obtained first?

AP view of the pelvis and cross-table lateral view of the affected hip

In a patient with a suspected hip fracture and negative plain films, what imaging study, if any, should be ordered next?

MRI may identify a nondisplaced femoral neck fracture that is not visible on plain radiographs. CT may miss these fractures because the fracture may be in the plane of the image.

How are proximal femur fractures classified?

By the anatomic location and pattern of the fracture

What is the anatomic classification of proximal femur fractures?

Intracapsular fractures involve the head or neck of the femur:

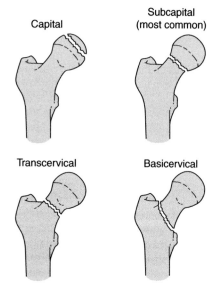

Extracapsular fractures involve the trochanters:

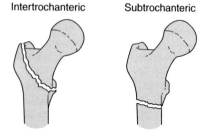

What is Garden's classification system for subcapital femoral fractures?

Garden's classification system for subcapital femoral fractures is based on displacement of the femoral head and is useful for estimating the patient's risk of osteonecrosis.

Stage I: Incomplete subcapital fracture (impacted or abducted); all patients achieve union

Stage II: Complete subcapital fracture without displacement; all patients achieve union

Stage III: Complete subcapital fracture with partial displacement; 95% of patients achieve union

Stage IV: Complete subcapital fracture with total displacement; only 55% of patients achieve union

KNEE TRAUMA

What views are standard when evaluating the knee?

AP and lateral views of the knee allow visualization of both the tibial and femoral metaphyses. In trauma, four views (i.e., an AP view, a lateral view, and two oblique views) are mandatory.

What does the tunnel view show and when is it useful?

A tunnel view shows the intercondylar notch and is useful for detecting loose bodies that may be hidden on AP films, and for evaluating patients with OCD.

What does a sunrise view show and when is it useful?

A sunrise view (taken from below at a 15° angle with the knee flexed at 115°) provides a tangential view of the patella and intercondylar fossa of the femur, demonstrating the patellofemoral joint. A sunrise view is good for showing subluxation of the patella from the trochlear groove.

What is a Merchant's view?

A Merchant's view is similar to a sunrise view, except that it is taken from above. This view provides a better image of the articular surface of the patella.

What is a knee dislocation?

Displacement of the tibia relative to the femur; often associated with femoral or tibial fractures and neurovascular compromise

Which type of knee disloca-tion is most common?	Posterior dislocation
What additional radio-graphic study is usually required for patients with knee dislocations?	Angiography to rule out vascular injury to the popliteal artery and vein

Patellar fractures and dislocations

What normal variant may mimic patella fracture?	Bipartite or multipartite patella
How is a multipartite patella differentiated from a fractured patella on radiographs?	Bony nonfusion (associated with bi- or multipartite patella) is most often seen along the superolateral margin. Patella fracture fragments fit together like puzzle pieces; bones of a bi- or multi-partite patella have more rounded margins and do not fit together.
What is the most common direction of patellar dis-location?	Lateral
What are the best plain film views for evaluating patellar dislocation?	Sunrise or Merchant's views of the knee
Patellar dislocation can be radiographically occult. What other imaging modal-ity may be useful?	MRI can demonstrate bone contusions and prove the diagnosis.
What are the plain film radiographic features of patellar dislocation?	Joint effusion Shallow, hypoplastic femoral groove Osteochondral fracture of the patella Lateral displacement of the patella (if not relocated by the time radiographic examination takes place)
What are the MRI findings?	Bony contusion of the femoral condyle and patella Disruption of the patellar retinaculum

Meniscal injury

Which meniscus is most commonly injured?	The medial meniscus sustains a higher rate of injury because it is less mobile

than the lateral meniscus. The most common injury is a longitudinal tear of the posterior horn of the medial meniscus.

What are the 3 patterns of meniscal injuries?

Longitudinal (vertical) tears (most common, occur secondary to acute trauma)

Horizontal (cleavage) tears (more common in older patients, occur secondary to degenerative changes)

Radial (oblique) tears

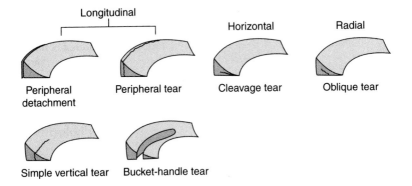

Longitudinal

Peripheral detachment   Peripheral tear

Horizontal

Cleavage tear

Radial

Oblique tear

Simple vertical tear   Bucket-handle tear

What is the best imaging modality for evaluating meniscal tears?

MRI

What is the normal appearance of the menisci on MRI?

Size: The medial and lateral menisci normally appear as two "bow ties" on sagittal images. The "bow tie" is the anterior and posterior horn of the meniscus joined by the body. The body is normally only seen on the most peripheral two images, both medially and laterally.

Shape: The anterior and posterior horns of the lateral meniscus are symmetric. The anterior horn of the medial meniscus is smaller than the posterior horn.

What is the appearance of a meniscal tear on MRI?

Linear or stellate area of signal abnormality in the meniscus; low signal on T_1-weighted images and high signal on T_2-weighted images

Describe 4 pitfalls associated with MRI diagnosis of meniscal injury.

1. Volume-averaging effects obscure fibrillatory degeneration of the free concave edge of the meniscal surface.
2. The transverse ligament, which courses through Hoffa's fat pad to connect the anterior horns of the medial and lateral meniscus, may mimic a meniscal tear or fragment.
3. Normal variant ligaments of Humphrey or Wrisberg (anterior and posterior to the posterior cruciate ligament, respectively) may mimic a meniscal tear.
4. Fibrous changes postmeniscectomy may have intermediate signal intensity.

What is a discoid meniscus?

A plate-shaped meniscus with a sagittal body dimension of more than 10 mm (i.e., it does not taper centrally); more common laterally; predisposes to injury

How does a discoid meniscus present clinically?

It may present as snapping of the knee during flexion and extension.

How does a discoid meniscus appear on MRI?

"Bow tie" meniscus seen on 3 or more MRI images (more than 10 mm total)

What is a meniscal cyst?

A cystic collection in continuity with a meniscal tear; usually related to the medial meniscus at the capsular margin; may occur following meniscectomy or trauma

What is the terrible triad of O'Donoghue?

The terrible triad of O'Donoghue is concomitant injury to the medial collateral ligament, anterior cruciate ligament, and medial meniscus, caused when a valgus load is applied to the externally rotated knee with the foot planted. This is the classic football clipping injury.

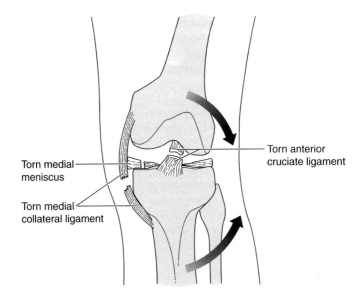

Torn anterior
cruciate ligament

Torn medial
meniscus

Torn medial
collateral ligament

(Note that lateral meniscal tears, as
opposed to medial meniscal tears, are
actually more commonly associated with
anterior cruciate ligament tears.)

Ligament tears

**What is the best imaging
modality for diagnosing
cruciate ligament tears?**

MRI

**What is the appearance of
a tear on plain film?**

Joint effusion is seen acutely.
Avulsion fracture of the tibial spine may
    be noted.
Segond fracture of the tibia is often
    associated with anterior cruciate
    ligament injury and may be visible on
    an AP view.

**What is the MRI appear-
ance of an anterior cruciate
ligament tear?**

Edematous pseudomass (may be visible
    with acute injury)
Wavy ligament
Ligament may end abruptly or lie on the
    tibial plateau
Associated bone contusion of
    posterolateral tibial plateau or lateral
    femoral condyle

Which collateral ligament is most commonly injured?

Medial collateral ligament

What are the radiographic features of a medial collateral ligament tear on plain film?

Widening of the tibiofemoral joint compartment on the side of the injury (seen on stress films)

Pelligrini-Stieda lesion (i.e., ossification at the site where the medial collateral ligament attaches to the femur)

What is the imaging modality of choice for patients with suspected medial collateral ligament tears?

MRI (best seen on coronal images)

List 5 MRI features.

1. Hyperintensity on T_2-weighted images in the ligament, which normally has low intensity (seen with sprain and tear)
2. Enlargement of the ligament
3. Avulsion from the attachment site
4. Wavy ligament
5. Disrupting ligament fibers

Tibial fractures

Describe 2 common mechanisms of injury in a tibial plateau fracture.

1. Fall from height onto the extended lower extremity
2. Fender or bumper fracture when the knee is struck by moving vehicle

How are tibial plateau fractures best described?

By location (i.e., medial, lateral, bicondylar), displacement of fragments, and the degree of depression

Which type of tibial plateau fracture is most common?

Lateral (75%), medial (10%), bicondylar (15%)

What injury may be seen in conjunction with a tibial plateau fracture?

Tibial spine avulsion and associated cruciate ligament injury

What imaging approach should be taken if a tibial plateau fracture is suspected?

Tibial plateau fractures are not always obvious on plain film. Often the extent of the fracture is underestimated and CT is necessary for evaluation.

What are the radiologic features of a tibial plateau fracture?	Knee effusion and the fat (marrow)/fluid (blood) interface sign (i.e., hemarthrosis) on a cross-table lateral view
What imaging modality can be helpful in further characterizing a tibial plateau fracture?	Spiral CT with coronal and sagittal reconstructions
What is a Segond fracture?	Avulsion of the lateral tibia at the attachment of the lateral capsule; commonly associated with an anterior cruciate ligament tear

ANKLE TRAUMA

Which radiographs are required for any patient with a suspected ankle injury?	AP, lateral, and mortise views of the ankle are required. Stress views of the ankle may be considered for patients with suspected joint instability.
What is a mortise view?	A mortise view is an oblique view at 20°–30° internal rotation. At this angle, the medial and lateral malleoli are on the same plane; therefore, congruity of the talus in relation to the medial and lateral malleolus and tibial plafond can be evaluated.
How are distal tibial and fibular fractures classified?	According to the mechanism of injury and the level of the fracture to the fibula
For each mechanism of injury, describe the resultant fracture pattern or patterns:	
Supination adduction	Transverse fracture of the lateral malleolus inferior to the tibial plafond Oblique fracture of the medial malleolus
Supination external rotation	Spiral fracture of the distal fibula Oblique fracture of the medial malleolus or deltoid ligament tear
Pronation abduction	Rupture of the medial collateral ligaments (deltoid ligament)

Transverse fracture of the medial
malleolus
Oblique fracture of the lateral malleolus
above the tibial plafond

**Pronation external
rotation**

Transverse medial malleolar fracture or
deltoid ligament tear
Anterior tibiofibular ligament disruption
Oblique fibula fracture above the level of
the tibial plafond

Pronation dorsiflexion

Medial malleolus fracture

**What are 3 critical clinical
factors to be considered in
an ankle fracture?**

1. **Malleolar involvement:** Medial,
   lateral, posterior, or a combination of
   the three?
2. **Stability of the fracture:** Widening
   of the ankle mortise or lateral clear
   space?
3. **Associated fibular fractures:** High
   or low?

Tibial and fibular fractures

What is a:

**Tibial plafond (pilon)
fracture?**

An intra-articular fracture of the distal
tibia caused by impaction of the talus;
often comminuted

Tillaux fracture?

Lateral margin avulsion of the distal tibia
(See figure next page)

A. Coronal section

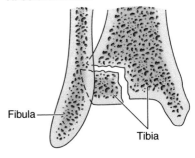

Fibula

Tibia

B. Axial section

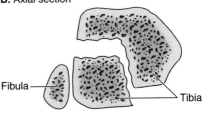

Fibula

Tibia

Wagstaffe-LeFort fracture?

Medial margin avulsion of the distal tibia with anterior disruption of the tibiofibular ligament from its fibular attachment

Triplane fracture?

Fracture in three planes

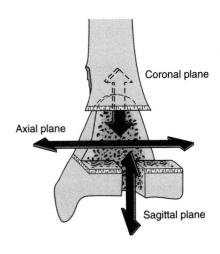

Coronal plane

Axial plane

Sagittal plane

Pott's fracture?

Fracture of the fibula above the tibiofibular syndesmosis with disruption of the deltoid ligament

Dupuytren's fracture?

Unstable distal fibula fracture characterized by disruption of the structural ring; two variants in fracture pattern are possible:

High variant: Fracture 2–7 cm above the distal end of the fibula with disruption of the tibiofibular syndesmosis and deltoid ligaments

Low variant: Fracture occurs distal to an intact tibiofibular ligament, but the deltoid ligament is disrupted

High variant

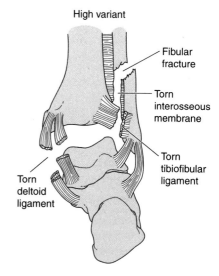

Low variant

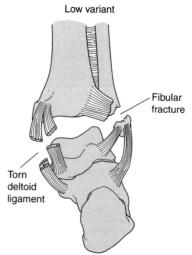

Maisonneuve fracture?   Fracture of the proximal half of the fibula with disruption of the interosseous membrane

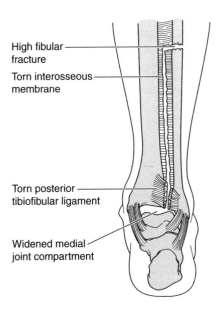

High fibular fracture

Torn interosseous membrane

Torn posterior tibiofibular ligament

Widened medial joint compartment

Ligamentous injury of the ankle

List 4 plain film radiographic findings associated with a deltoid ligament tear.

1. Soft tissue swelling
2. Lateral subluxation of the talus
3. Widening (more than 4 mm) of the clear space between the medial malleolus and the talus on a mortise view
4. A talar tilt angle of more than 10° between the tibial plafond and talar dome on an eversion stress AP view

List 3 plain film radiographic findings associated with a lateral collateral ligament tear.

1. Soft tissue swelling
2. Medial subluxation of the talus
3. A talar tilt angle of more than 10° on an inversion stress AP view

Which ligament in the ankle is most commonly injured?   Anterior tibiofibular ligament

FOOT TRAUMA

What is the site of most talus fractures?   The neck of the talus

What is the most common serious complication of talus fracture?

Osteonecrosis. The talus, like the scaphoid in the wrist, has distal to proximal blood perfusion.

What is the mechanism of injury in calcaneal fracture?

Calcaneal fractures (also known as "lover's fractures") are usually caused by a fall from height (e.g., by leaping out of a bedroom window).

What are the radiographic features of a calcaneal fracture?

Decreased Boehler's angle (i.e., < 20°); however, a normal Boehler's angle does not exclude a compression fracture

It is important to determine whether a calcaneal fracture involves which joint?

The subtalar joint (calcaneal fractures are intra-articular in 75% of patients)

What other injuries are associated with calcaneal fractures?

Fractures of the vertebrae and femoral neck

What other imaging modalities may be necessary in the evaluation of a patient with a calcaneal fracture?

1. CT is often required to evaluate the full extent of trauma in patients with complicated calcaneal fractures.
2. Thoracic and lumbar spine films are helpful to rule out possible associated spinal injury.
3. Films of the tibial plateau or femoral neck may be necessary to rule out fractures in these areas.

What is a Jones fracture?

Fracture of the base of the fifth metatarsal

What complication can occur if a Jones fracture is not immobilized?

Nonunion

With which normal variant is a Jones fractures sometimes confused?

An unfused apophysis of the fifth metatarsal

What is a march fracture?

A stress fracture of a metatarsal (usually the second); often seen in soldiers (hence the name) and runners

What is a Lisfranc injury?

A fracture-dislocation at the tarsometatarsal joint

What is the mechanism of injury in a Lisfranc injury?	These injuries are named after the surgeon in Napoleon's cavalry who originally described them. At that time, the most common mechanism of injury was getting a foot caught in a stirrup. Now, Lisfranc injuries are most often seen in patients with high-energy trauma as a result of a MVC. They are also seen in mountain bikers who get their feet caught in the pedal clips.
What are the radiographic features of a Lisfranc injury?	The medial border of the second metatarsal is not aligned with the medial border of the second cuneiform

RHEUMATOLOGIC DISORDERS

ARTHRITIS

What is the radiographic approach to arthritis?	**ABCDEs** **A**lignment—subluxations **B**one proliferation—periosteal reaction, soft tissue calcification **C**artilage—joint space narrowing **D**ensity—bone mineral **E**rosions **s**oft tissues

m

Osteoarthritis

What is osteoarthritis?	Degenerative arthritis characterized by deterioration of the articular cartilage and formation of new bone (osteophytes) at the joint surfaces and edges
What causes osteoarthritis?	Osteoarthritis may be primary or secondary to trauma, neurologic disease, or metabolic disorders
What is an osteophyte?	Outgrowth of ossified cartilage from the free articular surface of a joint
Name 8 joints that are commonly affected by osteoarthritis.	1. Distal interphalangeal joint 2. Proximal interphalangeal joint 3. Carpometacarpal joint 4. Metatarsophalangeal joint 5. Knee joint 6. Hip joint

7. Spinal joints
8. Ankle joint

What are Heberden's nodes and Bouchard's nodes?

Heberden's nodes: Osteophytes on the dorsal aspect of the distal interphalangeal joints of the hands
Bouchard's nodes: Osteophytes at the proximal interphalangeal joints of the hands

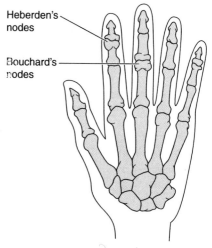

Heberden's nodes

Bouchard's nodes

Describe 4 classic radiographic findings in osteoarthritis.

1. Narrowing of the joint space and bone eburnation (caused by erosion of the cartilage)
2. Subchondral sclerosis
3. Osteophyte formation
4. Subchondral cysts

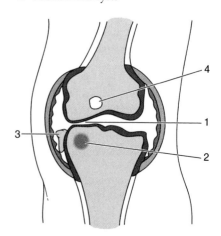

List 4 other radiographic findings that may be seen.

1. Heberden's and Bouchard's nodes in the hands
2. Deformity and malalignment secondary to joint space collapse and injury to the capsular ligaments (e.g., varus or valgus deformity of the knees)
3. Subchondral collapse
4. Vacuum disk sign (i.e., gas in the spinal apophyseal joints and intervertebral disks)

What does a bone scan reveal in a patient with osteoarthritis?

Increased uptake around the affected joints

What is the finding on MRI?

Degenerative changes—loss of cartilage, osteophytes, and subchondral cysts

What is erosive osteo-arthritis?

Inflammatory arthritis with distinct episodes that affects the interphalangeal joints and the first metacarpophalangeal joint and is often seen in perimenopausal women

What radiographic findings are associated with erosive osteoarthritis?

"Gull wing deformity" (i.e., severe central bony erosion with osteophytes laterally)

Neuropathic arthritis (Charcot's disease)

What is neuropathic arthritis?

A severe, destructive, degenerative arthritis resulting from the loss of sensation in a joint

List 6 causes of neuropathic arthritis.

1. Diabetes
2. Syringomyelia
3. Tabes dorsalis
4. Meningomyelocele
5. Spinal cord tumor
6. Congenital insensitivity to pain

What is the most likely cause if the neuropathic arthritis is in the:

Feet?

Diabetes

Knee?

Tabes dorsalis or meningomyelocele

Spine?

Tabes dorsalis

Shoulder?

Syringomyelia

List 5 radiographic hallmarks of neuropathic arthritis.

5 Ds
1. **D**estruction of the joint
2. **D**ebris
3. **D**islocation
4. **D**istention (effusion)
5. **D**ense bones

m

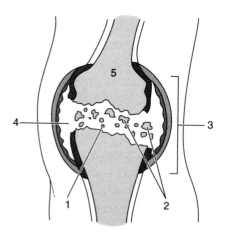

Rheumatoid arthritis

What is rheumatoid arthritis?

Inflammatory arthritis that originates in the synovium and can involve both small and large joints.

What are the clinical features of rheumatoid arthritis?

Usually symmetric and polyarticular, characterized by morning stiffness in the wrists and hands, may present as an acute or subacute process

Which joints are most often affected?

Early changes are typically found in the second and third metacarpophalangeal joints of the hands and the fourth and fifth metatarsophalangeal joints of the feet. The carpal joints, proximal interphalangeal joints, ankle, knee, shoulder, hip, or elbow may also be affected.

How can rheumatoid arthritis be distinguished from other arthritides clinically?

Usually, the distal interphalangeal joints are not affected in rheumatoid arthritis.

What are the best views for evaluating a patient with rheumatoid arthritis?

AP and "ballcatcher" views of the hands showing the carpal and phalangeal joints should be obtained.

Why is a "ballcatcher" view useful?

It may show early erosive changes at the metacarpophalangeal joints that were missed on a standard AP film.

List 3 early radiographic findings in a patient with rheumatoid arthritis.

1. Periarticular soft tissue swelling
2. Symmetric periarticular osteoporosis
3. Marginal erosions

List 5 late radiographic findings.
(See figure next page)

4. Boutonnière deformity
5. Swan-neck deformity
6. Subluxation of the affected joints (ulnar deviation)
7. Diffuse uniform joint space narrowing secondary to erosion of cartilage by pannus and granulation tissue
8. Ulnar and radial styloid erosion

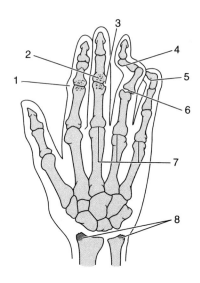

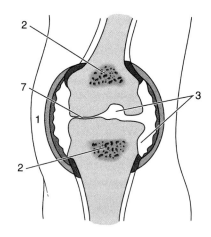

How can rheumatoid arthritis be differentiated from other types of arthritis radiographically?	Absent or minimal subchondral sclerosis, lack of osteophytes

Septic arthritis

What is the definition of septic arthritis?	Infection of the joint space and synovium

What is a potential complication if septic arthritis is not treated?	Uniform joint destruction caused by the release of proteolytic enzymes

Which joints are most susceptible to septic arthritis in:

Otherwise healthy patients?	Knee, hip, and elbow joints
Intravenous drug abusers?	Sacroiliac, sternal, and pubic joints
Patients with tuberculosis?	Hip, knee, intertarsal joints, and spine

Which organisms are most often cultured?

Staphylococcus aureus, Streptococcus, Gram-negative rods (especially in patients with diabetes), *Neisseria gonorrhoeae* (most common cause in sexually active young adults), *Salmonella* (in patients with sickle cell disease), *Mycobacterium tuberculosis*

How is septic arthritis diagnosed?

Joint aspiration

What are the characteristics of septic arthritis on plain film radiography?

Early films may reveal few if any bony changes, although soft tissue swelling and joint effusions may be present. Subsequent films may show juxta-articular osteomyelitis or osteopenia and secondary degenerative changes.

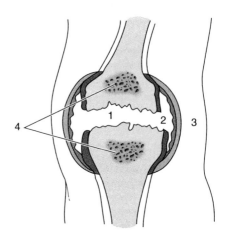

1. Joint space destruction
2. Joint effusion
3. Soft tissue swelling
4. Osteoporosis

How does septic arthritis appear on bone scanning?	Tc-99m diphosphate scanning shows uptake in the vascular phase, but not in the delayed phase.
Describe the radiographic appearance of tuberculous arthritis.	1. Phemister triad (osteoporosis, erosion at the joint margins, and cartilage destruction) 2. Gibbous deformity of the spine (secondary to vertebral body collapse) 3. Pott's disease (tuberculous disk space infection), a destructive process that spreads from the vertebral endplates to cross the intervertebral disk space, often affecting multiple levels 4. Paravertebral abscesses

Crystalline arthropathies

List the 3 major crystalline arthritides.	1. Gout (onosodium urate arthropathy) 2. Calcium pyrophosphate deposition disease (CPPD) 3. Calcium hydroxyapatite disease
Describe the pathogenesis of the crystalline arthropathies.	Crystals in the joint fluid act as abrasive agents on the articular surfaces. In addition, the accumulation of crystals in the cartilage matrix changes its mechanical properties, leading to hardening and microfracture. Crystals in the synovial fluid and soft tissues may also elicit an inflammatory response.
How do crystalline arthropathies present clinically?	With the abrupt onset of a painful, swollen, warm, erythematous and exquisitely tender joint
Which joint is most often involved in acute gout?	The first metatarsophalangeal joint is usually involved, but acute gout may also appear in any of the distal extremity joints, including the ankles, knees, wrists, fingers, and elbows. Acute gout is usually monoarticular.
How does gout appear radiographically?	Erosions away from the joint with overhanging margins and sclerotic borders, swelling, preservation of the joint space and bone density

What is pseudogout?

CPPD, which presents with an acute clinical picture similar to that of gout in 10%-20% of CPPD patients

What is the typical radiographic appearance of CPPD?

Osteoarthritis, but with prominent geodes and less prominent osteophytes, and chondrocalcinosis

What is chondrocalcinosis?

Calcification of cartilage, including hyaline and fibrocartilaginous tissues; lesions are linear and run parallel to subchondral bone

Which joints are most commonly involved in CPPD?

The larger joints are involved most often. Approximately 50% of cases involve the knees, but the shoulders, hips, elbows, wrists, or ankles may also be involved.

When CPPD affects the knee, what is the typical radiographic appearance?

Degenerative arthritis that affects the patellofemoral joint compartment more than the tibiofemoral joint compartments

SERONEGATIVE SPONDYLOARTHROPATHIES

List 5 common seronegative spondyloarthropathies.

1. Ankylosing spondylitis (AS)
2. Juvenile AS
3. Psoriatic arthritis
4. Reiter's syndrome (reactive arthritis)
5. Enteric arthropathies

What are the clinical features of seronegative spondyloarthropathies?

Axial skeleton involvement
Extra-articular involvement
Patients are usually young and male
Negative rheumatoid factor and associated with HLA-B27
Sacroiliitis or spondylitis, oligoarticular peripheral arthritis, and enthesopathy

What is enthesopathy?

Inflammation of the enthesis (i.e., the attachment of the ligament or tendon to the bone)

How does enthesopathy appear radiographically?

Often seen as calcification adjacent to the bone in the expected location of the tendon insertion

Ankylosing spondylitis (AS)

What are the clinical features of AS?

Slow onset of low back pain before the age of 40 years

As many as one third of patients have an acute, usually unilateral, uveitis

List 6 radiographic findings associated with AS.

1. Sacroiliitis (i.e., blurred and sclerotic sacroiliac joints), usually bilateral and symmetric
2. Enthesopathy
3. Peripheral arthritis (30% of patients)
4. Anderson lesion (pseudoarthrosis of the spine)
5. "Bamboo" spine [i.e., multilevel spinal fusion with syndesmophytes (calcification of the outer rim of the annulus fibrosis) and resorption of vertebral endplates]
6. Uniform joint space narrowing of the hips

What is osteitis condensans ilii (OCI)?

OCI is typically asymptomatic and found incidentally in young, multiparous women. It is demonstrated radiographically by a triangular area of radiodense sclerotic iliac bone that borders the inferior half of normal sacroiliac joints, and is easily confused by the unwary with AS.

Psoriatic arthritis

What are the clinical features of psoriatic arthritis?

Psoriatic skin lesions and asymmetric peripheral oligoarticular polyarthritis

What radiographic changes are associated with psoriatic arthritis:

Pertinent positive findings? (List 7)

1. Pencil-in-cup deformity of the distal interphalangeal or proximal interphalangeal joints (pathognomonic)
2. Fluffy periostitis
3. Ankylosis
4. Resorption of terminal tufts (acroosteolysis)
5. Severe joint space narrowing or fusion (arthritis mutilans)
6. "Sausage" digits

7. "Mouse ears" (bone proliferation adjacent to intra-articular bare areas)

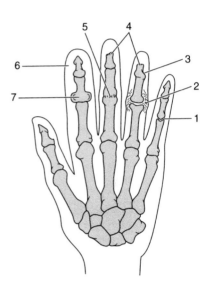

Pertinent negative findings? (List 3)	1. Lack of periarticular osteopenia (such as that seen with rheumatoid arthritis) 2. Lack of soft tissue calcifications 3. Little or no subluxation or dislocation

Reiter's syndrome (reactive arthritis)

What is reactive arthritis?	An idiopathic (probably infectious or autoimmune) disorder characterized by urethritis, conjunctivitis, and arthritis
Which sites are most often affected?	Foot, sacroiliac joint, and spine
List 5 radiographic characteristics of Reiter's syndrome.	1. Bilateral, symmetric sacroiliitis 2. Asymmetric syndesmophytes 3. Calcaneal enthesopathy and periostitis 4. "Sausage" digits (fingers) 5. Pencil-in-cup deformity of the fingers
What other imaging modality should be considered?	CT is the gold standard for examination of the sacroiliac joints.

Enteropathic arthropathies

What is the most common extraintestinal manifestation of ulcerative colitis and Crohn's disease?

Approximately 20% of patients have arthritis, either symmetric sacroiliitis and spondylitis such as that seen in AS or an oligoarticular peripheral arthritis of the lower limbs. Typically, the arthritis is nondeforming and parallels the activity of the inflammatory bowel disease in exacerbation and remission.

What other gastrointestinal conditions can be associated with arthropathy?

Whipple's disease, pancreatic disease, infection (e.g., *Salmonella, Shigella*), cirrhosis

What are the radiographic characteristics of enteric arthropathies?

The radiographic picture is similar to that of AS:
Symmetric sacroiliitis, spondylitis, or both
Swelling of the peripheral joints
Osteoporosis

SYNOVIAL OSTEOCHONDROMATOSIS AND PIGMENTED VILLONODULAR SYNOVITIS (PVNS)

What is synovial osteochondromatosis?

Synovial osteochondromatosis (idiopathic monoarticular synovial metaplasia) is a benign, self-limited condition in which cartilaginous nodules detach from the synovium and migrate into the joint space.

What are the typical locations?

The knee, hip, and elbow joints are most commonly affected.

What are the radiographic features of synovial osteochondrosis?

"Joint mice" are classic. Joint effusion and erosion may be the only evidence in the 30% of patients who do not have calcified loose bodies.

What is PVNS?

A monoarticular benign proliferation of the synovium characterized by a tendency toward hemorrhage. Pigmentation is caused by hemosiderin deposition.

What are the typical locations?

The knee (80% of cases), as well as the hip and ankle joints

What are the plain film radiographic features?

PVNS is indistinguishable from noncalcified synovial osteochondromatosis.

Findings include joint effusion and cystic erosions of periarticular bone.

What are the features of PVNS on MRI?

A decreased signal on T_2-weighted images (as a result of hemosiderin deposition) that increases in size ("blooms") on gradient-recalled echo (GRE) sequences.

SYSTEMIC LUPUS ERYTHEMATOSUS (SLE), SCLERODERMA, AND DERMATOMYOSITIS

What is the incidence of inflammatory arthritis in SLE?

As many as 90% of patients with SLE have polyarthritis similar to rheumatoid arthritis

What is the classic radiographic finding associated with SLE?

Joint subluxation in isolation

What is scleroderma?

Disease of systemic sclerosis featuring gastrointestinal, dermatologic, and renal abnormalities

Describe 3 radiographic hallmarks of scleroderma.

1. Acroosteolysis (i.e., bony damage with phalangeal tuft resorption secondary to pressure from overlying sclerotic skin)
2. Soft tissue calcification
3. Atrophy of soft tissues

What is the differential diagnosis of acroosteolysis?

Scleroderma (tips of fingers appear "bitten off" on radiographs)
Psoriasis (usually accompanied by nail pitting and ridging)
Hyperparathyroidism (usually accompanied by other resorptive changes)
Diabetes
Frostbite
Raynaud's phenomenon
Polyvinyl chloride poisoning

What are the radiographic findings in dermatomyositis?

Diffuse soft tissue calcification

BONE INFECTION (OSTEOMYELITIS)

How is osteomyelitis defined? Bacterial infection of the bone

Which organisms are commonly isolated in:

Otherwise healthy patients? *Staphylococcus aureus, Streptococcus,* Gram-negative bacilli, *Staphylococcus epidermidis*

Patients with sickle cell disease? *Salmonella* (although *Staphylococcus* is still most common)

Intravenous drug abusers? Uncommon organisms (e.g., *Pseudomonas, Klebsiella,* or *Enterobacter*) are more likely to cause infection.

Define the following pathologic findings:

Cloaca A canal formed in the cortex of a bone resulting from the formation of a draining sinus tract

Sequestrum Death of cortical bone secondary to occlusion of nutrient arteries leads to a fragment of necrotic bone embedded in pus

Involucrum Lesion in which new bone is laid down around a sequestrum

Brodie's abscess Reactive bone from the periosteum and endosteum surrounding and containing an infection

What is the approach to the patient with osteomyelitis? A plain radiograph of the affected extremity is obtained. If the film is positive, treatment is initiated. If the plain film is negative for osteomyelitis, an MRI or bone scan can be performed. A positive MRI or bone scan indicates a need for treatment.

How long does it take before bony changes are evident on a plain film radiograph? 7–10 days

What changes are seen on plain film and CT?	Acute changes include loss of the white cortical line and periosteal reaction. Subacute and chronic changes include mixed bone lysis and sclerosis.
What MRI changes are seen?	Bone marrow edema (high signal on T_2-weighted images and destruction of the cortex)
Which is more specific for osteomyelitis—MRI or bone scan?	MRI
How is cellulitis distinguished from osteomyelitis on bone scan?	Cellulitis is characterized by increased blood flow and blood pool images with a normal late phase. Osteomyelitis is characterized by increased activity in all three phases.
What conditions may complicate bone scan evaluation for infection?	Recent fractures typically demonstrate increased uptake on all three phases. A gallium scan or tagged white blood cell (WBC) scan may be necessary to differentiate a recent fracture from infection.

METABOLIC AND ENDOCRINE BONE DISORDERS

HYPERPARATHYROIDISM

What is the pathogenesis of hyperparathyroidism?	Parathyroid hormone (PTH) stimulates osteoclast activity, inducing bone resorption
What causes hyperparathyroidism?	Primary causes: Parathyroid adenoma, parathyroid hyperplasia, parathyroid carcinoma Secondary causes: Renal failure, ectopic PTH production Tertiary causes: Autonomous parathyroid hyperactivity seen in patients with chronic renal failure
List 4 radiographic signs of hyperparathyroidism.	1. Bone resorption (pathognomonic) 2. Osteopenia 3. Lytic bone lesions (brown tumors) 4. Soft tissue calcification and chondrocalcinosis
List 4 classic sites of bone resorption.	1. Radial aspect of the middle phalanges of the second and third digits

2. Distal clavicle
3. Medial tibia
4. Skull ("salt and pepper" skull)

What are brown tumors?

Radiolucent lytic or cystic lesions that replace bone

Are brown tumors seen more often in primary or secondary hyperparathyroidism?

Brown tumors are seen in a higher percentage of patients with primary hyperparathyroidism, but secondary hyperparathyroidism is much more common. Therefore, most brown tumors are seen in patients with secondary hyperparathyroidism.

What is the differential diagnosis for distal clavicle osteolysis?

Hyperparathyroidism, rheumatoid arthritis, myeloma, rickets, cleidocranial dysostosis, eosinophilic granuloma, post-traumatic or stress osteolysis

ACROMEGALY

What is the pathogenesis of acromegaly?

Excess pituitary growth hormone (GH) causes changes in the bones and soft tissues. In children, excess GH increases the linear growth of the long bones, leading to gigantism. In adults, gigantism cannot occur because the epiphyses have closed, but the excess GH leads to bone enlargement and soft tissue growth.

In adults, what is the clinical presentation of acromegaly?

Gradual enlargement of the hands and feet and coarsening of facial features

List 7 radiographic features of acromegaly.

1. Premature degenerative change
2. Ossicles at the tendonous insertions and exaggeration of ~ ~ ~
   ~~~~~~~~
   . Thickened, radi~
4. Prognathism
5. Large orbital ridges (frontal bossing)
6. Reduced frontal sinuses
7. Increased heel pad thickness (> 25 mm)

PAGET'S DISEASE

What is Paget's disease?	A disorder seen in patients older than 40 years and characterized by an increased rate of bone turnover, which can lead to polyostotic osteitis deformans
What is osteitis deformans?	Deformation of a bony structure
What are the main clinical features of Paget's disease?	Bowing of the weight-bearing long bones Neurologic disorders secondary to spinal compression Warmth and tenderness of the extremities High-output congestive heart failure (CHF) resulting from increased bone perfusion Enlarged hat size (resulting from growth of the skull)
Describe the 3 stages of Paget's disease.	**Hot stage:** Active (lytic) phase, characterized by aggressive bone resorption **Cold stage:** Inactive (quiescent) phase, marked by excess new bone formation **Mixed stage:** Both lytic and sclerotic changes occur concurrently
What bones are commonly involved?	More than 75% of patients have involvement of the pelvis. The femur, skull, tibia, vertebrae, clavicle, humerus, and ribs can also be affected.
What are the conventional radiographic findings?	**Hot stage:** "Candle flame"- or "V"-shaped lytic lesion involving the epiphysis and progressing toward the diaphysis **Cold stage:** Expansion of bone with thickening of the cortex and sclerosis **Mixed stage:** Bowing of the tibia and femur as a result of chronic stress insufficiency **Other findings:** Banana fractures (i.e., small pathologic cortical fractures along the convex border of bowed long bones), osteoarthritic changes, early thickening of the iliopubic and ilioischial lines, coarsened trabeculations of the sacrum and

ilium, acetabular protrusio, vertebral
body enlargement and ivory vertebrae

**How do changes in skull
vary during each stage?**

Hot stage: Osteoporosis circumscripta
Cold stage: Diploic widening of the
  inner and outer tables
Mixed stage: "Cotton wool" appearance
  of mixed lytic and sclerotic lesions

**What are the characteristics
of Paget's disease on bone
scan?**

Hot stage: "Hot" bone scans with
  increased radiotracer uptake adjacent
  to and extending away from the joints
Cold stage: "Cold" lesions in sclerotic
  bone

**What are the characteristics
of Paget's disease on CT?**

Dense enhancement of vascular lesions is
found during the hot stage.

**What is a complication of
Paget's disease?**

Malignant degeneration in as many as 5%
of patients (usually osteosarcoma, but any
sarcoma can develop)

GAUCHER'S DISEASE

What is Gaucher's disease?

A lysosomal storage disease—a defect in
glucocerebrosidase causes accumulation
of ceramide in the macrophages of the
reticuloendothelial system, resulting in
hepatosplenomegaly and, in many
patients, bone marrow involvement

**What radiographic changes
are seen in Gaucher's
disease?**

A generalized decrease in bone density,
the "Erlenmeyer flask" deformity of the
long bones, and osteonecrosis

HEMATOLOGIC DISORDERS WITH MUSCULOSKELETAL SEQUELAE

SICKLE CELL DISEASE

What is sickle cell disease?

A hemoglobinopathy in which polymeri-
zation of the affected hemoglobin (HbS)
causes deoxygenated erythrocytes to lose
their normal biconcave shape and
become sickle shaped

**What are the clinical fea-
tures of sickle cell disease?**

Hemolytic anemia, skeletal pain (as a
result of infarcts and osteomyelitis), chest
and abdominal pain and infections

List 6 radiographic findings in sickle cell disease.

1. Osteopenia
2. Osteonecrosis, especially of the hips and shoulders
3. "H"-shaped vertebrae
4. Bone infarcts
5. Osteomyelitis
6. Dactylitis

What is dactylitis?

Painful enlargement of a digit (seen in sickle cell disease, juvenile rheumatoid arthritis, and tuberculosis)

What organisms cause infection in patients with sickle cell disease?

Salmonella is classic, but *Staphylococcus* is more common.

THALASSEMIA

What are the thalassemias?

Hereditary disorders resulting in decreased production of either α or β globin chains

List 7 radiographic features of the thalassemias.

1. Expanded marrow space (sign of marrow hyperplasia)
2. "Hair-on-end" skull
3. "Erlenmeyer flask" modeling deformities of the long bones
4. Paravertebral masses (a sign of extramedullary hematopoiesis)
5. Premature growth plate closure
6. Diffuse bone sclerosis
7. "H"-shaped vertebrae

HEMOPHILIA

What are the musculo-skeletal sequelae of hemo-philia?

90% of patients with hemophilia suffer from spontaneous hemarthroses, many recurrently. Typically, the hemarthroses are monoarticular and occur most commonly in the knee, elbow, and ankle.

What are the radiographic findings?

Acute findings include joint effusion and periarticular osteopenia. Chronic findings include epiphyseal overgrowth, pseudo-tumor formation (i.e., a hematoma with a thick fibrous capsule), and possibly, osteoarthritic changes.

What condition can mimic the epiphyseal overgrowth of hemophilia?	Juvenile rheumatoid arthritis

BONE TUMORS

GENERAL CONSIDERATIONS

What is the most common malignant bone tumor?	Metastatic disease from a non-bone source
What is the most common primary malignant bone tumor?	Multiple myeloma
What features of bone tumors are important in terms of making a diagnosis?	Patient age, aggressiveness of the lesion, location of the lesion
How is lesion aggressiveness assessed?	By plain film radiography! Aggressiveness can be over- or underestimated by other modalities.
What 8 characteristics are used to judge lesion aggressiveness?	1. Pattern of bone destruction 2. Definition of the lesion 3. Periosteal reaction 4. Presence or absence of soft tissue expansion 5. Presence of tumor matrix 6. Site in skeleton 7. Location in bone 8. Patient's age

Patterns of bone destruction and lesion definition

Describe the 3 basic patterns of bone destruction.	**Geographic pattern:** The lesion is circumscribed. A sclerotic rim indicates relatively slow growth. Ill-defined borders or a wide transition zone indicates a moderately aggressive tumor. **Moth-eaten pattern:** The lesion is poorly circumscribed, with numerous defects of varying size in the cortical and trabecular bone. This pattern is indicative of aggressive behavior. **Permeative pattern:** This pattern is characterized by abundant elongated

perforations along the bone cortex and occasional decreases in cortical bone density and is indicative of aggressive behavior.

What does the term "sclerotic" refer to?

Bone proliferation (appears white on radiographs)

What does the term "lytic" refer to?

Bone loss (appears dark on radiographs)

Patterns of reactive bone formation

What are the 2 major patterns of reactive bone formation?

Periosteal pattern, endosteal pattern

Which periosteal responses suggest a more benign process?

Buttressing (i.e., a single thick layer of periosteal reaction) is nonspecific, but usually indicates slow growth.

Which periosteal findings are more suggestive of an aggressive process?

Uneven periosteal reactions that progress over weeks

Describe the following common periosteal reactions, which are suggestive of an aggressive lesion:

   Onion skin

Periosteum appears laminated

   Codman's triangle

Periosteal elevation from the bone at the margin of the tumor creates a triangular shape on the radiograph

   Sunburst pattern

Spiculations are directed toward the center of the lesion

   "Hair-on-end" (velvet) pattern

Spiculations are directed toward the marrow cavity

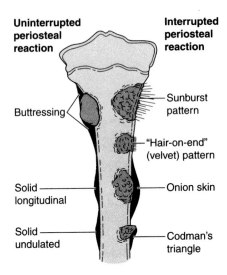

Uninterrupted periosteal reaction

Interrupted periosteal reaction

Buttressing

Sunburst pattern

"Hair-on-end" (velvet) pattern

Solid longitudinal

Onion skin

Solid undulated

Codman's triangle

What do the 3 types of endosteal responses indicate?	1. A thick rim of new bone suggests benign, slow growth. 2. A thin rim (or no rim) suggests a more active lesion. 3. A mottled appearance, caused by the mingling of new bone and a permeative or moth-eaten pattern of destruction, suggests an invasive process, either malignant or nonmalignant.
In general, what does a malignant tumor look like?	Poorly circumscribed lesion without sclerotic margins Soft tissue expansion Uneven or irregular progressive bone repair
What other process can mimic a malignant tumor?	Infection
In general, what does a benign tumor look like?	Well-circumscribed lesion with sclerotic margins and preserved cortical margins No soft tissue expansion Uninterrupted bone repair

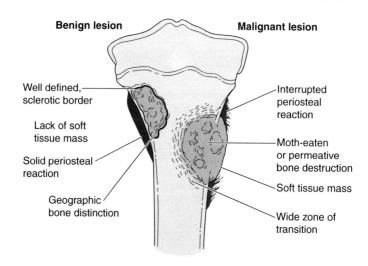

Benign lesion — Malignant lesion

Well defined, sclerotic border

Lack of soft tissue mass

Solid periosteal reaction

Geographic bone distinction

Interrupted periosteal reaction

Moth-eaten or permeative bone destruction

Soft tissue mass

Wide zone of transition

Tumor matrix

What is tumor matrix?

The intercellular substance produced by tumor cells

What are the 3 types of tumor matrix?

Osteoid, chondroid, and fibrinoid

What imaging modality is useful for evaluating the tumor matrix?

CT, because increased density on plain films may be attributable either to an osteoid tumor matrix or a periosteal or endosteal response

Describe the radiographic appearance of each of the following types of tumors:

Osteogenic tumor

Fluffy, cloud- or cotton-like densities within the lesion

Chondrogenic tumor

Annular, "popcorn" or comma-shaped calcifications (sometimes described as "rings and arcs" or "O's and C's")

List 5 osteogenic tumors.

Benign
1. Osteoid osteoma
2. Osteoblastoma
3. Osteoma
4. Enostosis (bone island)

Malignant
5. Osteosarcoma

List 5 chondrogenic tumors.

Benign
1. Enchondroma
2. Osteochondroma
3. Chondroblastoma
4. Chondromyxoid fibroma
Malignant
5. Chondrosarcoma

List 7 common fibrous tumors.

Benign
1. Fibrous cortical defects
2. Nonossifying fibroma
3. Fibrous dysplasia
4. Ossifying fibroma
Malignant
5. Malignant fibrous histiocytoma
6. Fibrosarcoma
7. Adamantinoma

Tumor site

Where do primary bone tumors usually arise?

Most primary tumors appear in areas of rapid growth (e.g., the distal femur, proximal tibia, and humerus).

Where do metastases usually occur?

Bone metastases tend to be located in the hypervascular red bone marrow in the spine and iliac wings, but can occur in any bone.

List 7 bone marrow tumors.

Benign
1. Giant cell tumor
2. Eosinophilic granuloma
3. Lymphangioma
Malignant
4. Multiple myeloma
5. Ewing's sarcoma
6. Lymphoma
7. Leukemia

List 4 epiphyseal tumors.

Benign
1. Chondroblastoma
2. Giant cell tumor
3. Intraosseous lipoma
Malignant
4. Clear cell chondrosarcoma

List 7 metaphyseal tumors.	**Benign**
	1. Osteoblastoma
	2. Osteochondroma
	3. Nonossifying fibroma
	4. Osteoid osteoma
	5. Chondromyxoid fibroma
	6. Giant cell tumor
	Malignant
	7. Osteosarcoma.
List 4 diaphyseal tumors.	**Benign**
	1. Enchondroma
	2. Fibrous dysplasia
	Malignant
	3. Ewing's sarcoma
	4. Chondrosarcoma

Tumor location

What is an "endosteal" lesion?	Endosteal lesions arise just deep to the inner layer of the cortex of the bone.
What is a "periosteal" lesion?	Periosteal lesions arise just superficial to the outer cortex of the bone.
What does the term "axial location" refer to?	The position of the lesion with respect of the long axis of the bone
Which lesions tend to be central (medullary)?	Enchondroma, unicameral bone cysts, and eosinophilic granuloma
Which lesions tend to be eccentric (i.e., non-central)?	Aneurysmal bone cysts, nonossifying fibroma, giant cell tumor, osteosarcoma
List 4 common benign cortical lesions.	Cortical defect, cortical desmoid, osteoid osteoma, periosteal chondroma
Which lesions tend to be juxtacortical (i.e., located adjacent to the cortex)?	All osseous, cartilaginous, and fibrous malignancies may be juxtacortical. In addition, chondroma and myositis ossificans may be juxtacortical.

Patient age

For each decade of life, name the most common malignant bone tumor or tumors:	
0–10 years (List 1)	Ewing's sarcoma

10–20 years (List 1)	Osteosarcoma
30–40 years (List 4)	Malignant fibrous histiocytoma, parosteal osteosarcoma, fibrosarcoma, lymphoma
40+ years (List 3)	Metastases, multiple myeloma, chondro-sarcoma

OSTEOGENIC TUMORS

Osteoid osteoma

What are the clinical features of osteoid osteoma?

The hallmark is pain (thought to be caused by increased prostaglandins) that increases at night and is improved with aspirin. Patients are typically younger than 25 years.

What is the typical site in the skeleton?

More than 50% occur in the femur and tibia. The feet and hands are the next most common location (20% of cases).

What are the classic plain film imaging features of osteoid osteoma?

Cortical sclerotic lesion with an oval or round radiolucent nidus that is larger than 2 centimeters in diameter
Lack of a soft tissue mass

Why might CT imaging be indicated?

The sclerosis may obscure detection of the nidus on plain films; CT can help to define the exact location of the nidus.

What are the features of osteoid osteoma on:

Bone scan imaging?

Hot focus

Angiography?

Dense nidus

MRI imaging?

Extensive reactive marrow edema

How is osteoid osteoma treated?

With surgical excision or percutaneous ablation

Osteoblastoma

What is an osteoblastoma?

Also called giant osteoid osteoma, osteoblastomas are larger than (but histologically comparable to) osteoid osteoma. In addition to size differences, however, osteoblastomas are more vascular, have higher numbers of osteoblasts, and are less organized than osteoid osteoma. Patients are typically younger than 30 years. Osteoblastomas are rare.

What is the typical site in the skeleton?

Osteoblastomas are most often seen in the posterior elements of the spine and the long bones of the appendicular skeleton. They also tend to occur in the hands and feet or skull and face.

List 4 radiographic features of osteoblastoma.

1. Dense sclerotic bone reaction around lesion
2. Lesion greater than 2 centimeters in size
3. Expansile, well circumscribed or calcified soft tissue mass
4. Speckled central calcification

Osteoma

What is the radiographic appearance of an osteoma?

Endosteal or periosteal localized masses of mature-appearing bone

Where are osteomas usually found?

The skull

With which condition is osteoma associated?

Gardner's syndrome (gastrointestinal polyps, desmoid tumors, and osteomas)

Enostosis (bone island)

What are the plain film radiographic features of enostosis?

Small (i.e., 1–4 cm) focus of cortical-like bone within cancellous bone

Lesion appears dense, homogenous, and well marginated

Bony trabeculae extend into the normal bone

Lesion is usually oblong and oriented along the long axis of the bone

What are the bone scan radiographic features of enostosis?

Little or no uptake

Osteosarcoma

How common is osteosarcoma?

Like all primary bone tumors, osteosarcoma is relatively rare (fewer than 1000 new cases are diagnosed per year in the United States). However, osteosarcoma is second only to multiple myeloma as the most common primary malignant bone tumor.

What is the age distribution in osteosarcoma?

There is a bimodal age distribution. The younger patients tend to be between 10 and 25 years of age, with a mean age of 17 years). The mean age for older patients tends to be 70 years.

What are the clinical features of osteosarcoma?

The affected area is painful, swollen, and warm, and the patient usually has a fever.

What is the typical location of osteosarcoma in the bone?

Osteosarcoma typically is located toward the ends of the bones, usually in the metaphyses of the long bones. The most common location is the femur, mostly around the knee (40% of cases). Approximately 30% of cases arise in either the tibia or humerus.

List 6 types of osteosarcoma.

1. Primary (conventional or central) osteosarcoma
2. Telangiectatic osteosarcoma
3. Post-radiation osteosarcoma (develops 3–50 years after radiation therapy)
4. Osteosarcoma secondary to Paget's disease
5. Dedifferentiated chondrosarcoma (lesions starts as chondrosarcoma and dedifferentiates to a more primitive tumor with multiple cell types)
6. Juxtacortical osteosarcoma

What is juxtacortical osteosarcoma?

Approximately 5% of osteosarcomas arise outside the bone, per se, and are termed juxtacortical. There are three main types of juxtacortical osteosarcoma: parosteal, periosteal, and surface.

Describe parosteal osteosarcoma.

Parosteal osteosarcoma originates from the outer periosteum and is most often located in the posterior distal femoral shaft. Parosteal osteosarcoma accounts for fewer than 5% of osteosarcomas and is usually seen in older patients (peak age = 40 years). Typically, it has central high density with surrounding lower density. Parosteal osteosarcoma is considered less aggressive than periosteal or central osteosarcoma.

Describe periosteal osteosarcoma.

Periosteal osteosarcoma, which arises from the deep periosteum, accounts for only 2% of all osteosarcomas and is usually seen in younger patients (peak age = 10–20 years). Periosteal osteosarcoma tends to appear as a sessile, elliptical, or saucer-shaped cortical depression with no involvement of the medullary space. An extensive chondroblastic matrix may be seen.

Describe surface osteosarcoma.

The lesion is histologically identical to a conventional osteosarcoma but arises on the cortex or "surface" of the bone; these tumors are usually high-grade.

Describe telangiectatic osteosarcoma.

Telangiectatic osteosarcoma is a lytic-appearing osteosarcoma characterized by the rapid growth of large extraosseous masses and little bone reaction. Cystic cavities may be filled with blood or fluid. Telangiectactic osteosarcoma may mimic an aneurysmal bone cyst or aggressive hemangioma.

What is the diagnostic approach to the patient?

An initial presumptive diagnosis is made by plain film radiography. Cross-sectional imaging (i.e., CT, MRI) is used to determine the extent of tumor spread within the bone marrow and adjacent soft tissues and the vascularity of the lesion, and to detect skip lesions.

What are the strengths of CT and MRI, respectively, for this application?

CT is more useful for defining cortical penetration and the matrix, and for performing guided biopsy. CT of the chest is also used for detecting pulmonary metastasis.

MRI is better for staging and determining tumor margins, and for detecting skip lesions.

Name 1 other way of detecting metastasis.

Bone scan

What are the imaging features of osteosarcoma on plain film?

Poorly defined, mass lesion that extends through the cortex

Obvious sclerosis usually present from the tumor and reactive processes

Codman's triangle and sunburst pattern

What are the bone scan findings?

Increased uptake with activity extending beyond the tumor margin

CHONDROGENIC TUMORS

Enchondroma

What is an enchondroma?

A benign cartilaginous growth of the medullary cavity

What age group is most often affected?

Patients are typically 10–30 years of age.

What is the most common location for enchondromas?

Enchondromas are the most common benign cystic lesion of the phalanges, but they may appear anywhere.

What approach should be taken to the patient?

Pain at the site of an enchondroma is considered a fracture or malignancy until proved otherwise.

List 4 radiographic features of an enchondroma.

1. Oval lucency in the metaphysis
2. Chondroid calcification ("rings and arcs" pattern)—seen in all endochondromas except for those arising in the phalanges
3. No periostitis
4. No cortical breakthrough

What is Ollier's disease?

Nonhereditary multiple enchondromatosis. Patients are at increased risk for chondrosarcoma and often have hand and foot deformities.

What is Maffucci's syndrome?

Multiple enchondromatosis associated

with multiple soft tissue hemangiomas. Patients are at higher risk of malignant transformation than those with Ollier's disease. Unilateral involvement of the distal extremities is characteristic.

Osteochondroma

What is osteochondroma?

Osteochondroma, the most common benign bone lesion, is a painless, slow-growing osteocartilaginous exostosis (i.e., cartilage-capped bony projection). Boys are affected more often than girls (2:1). Growth of the lesion continues until the growth plate closes.

Name 2 complications that can be associated with osteochondroma.

Mass effect on nearby soft tissue and bone, malignant transformation

Where are the lesions typically located?

Tibia, femur, and humerus

What are 4 radiographic features?

1. The lesion arises from the metaphysis.
2. The cortex of the lesion is continuous with the adjacent bone.
3. The medullary bone is interrupted and continuous with the adjacent bone.
4. The lesion grows away from the joint.

List 3 situations when malignancy should be suspected.

1. Pain without nerve compression or fracture
2. Late tumor growth following growth plate closure
3. Large cartilaginous cap with diffuse calcifications

What is multiple osteocartilaginous exostoses?

A hereditary, autosomal dominant disease characterized by multiple, usually sessile, osteochondromas. The knee, ankle, and shoulder are often simultaneously affected. Patients may have severe growth abnormalities as a result of the multiple lesions, and as many as 20% of patients undergo malignant transformation to chondrosarcoma.

What is Trevor's disease (dysplasia epiphysealis hemimelica)?	Epiphyseal osteochondroma

Chondroblastoma (Codman's tumor)

What is a chondroblastoma?	An uncommon benign neoplasm of immature cartilage cells
How old are patients at the time of presentation?	Usually, 5–25 years
Where are chondroblastomas typically located in the bone?	The epiphysis. Approximately 50% extend across the physeal plate to the metaphysis.
Which joint is most often affected?	The knee (50% of cases)
How does a chondroblastoma appear radiographically?	As a lytic round or oval lesion in the epiphysis with a well-defined sclerotic margin
What is the differential diagnosis of an epiphyseal lesion?	Infection, eosinophilic granuloma, chondroblastoma

Chondromyxoid fibroma

What is a chondromyxoid fibroma?	An extremely uncommon benign neoplastic growth of the chondrogenic and myxoid tissue
What are the clinical features?	Patients may present with pain.
How does a chondromyxoid fibroma present radiographically?	The radiographic appearance is similar to that of a nonossifying fibroma (i.e., a "bite-like" lytic lesion with a well-defined sclerotic margin).

Chondrosarcoma

What is a chondrosarcoma?	A malignant cartilaginous tumor that may arise *de novo* or secondary to a benign cartilage tumor.
What is the typical age of patients?	Almost all occur in patients between the ages of 40 and 45 years.

How are the different forms of chondrosarcoma classified?

By tumor location (medullary, exostotic, juxtacortical) within the bone and by histology (well-differentiated or dedifferentiated)

Describe the following types of chondrosarcoma:

Medullary (central) chondrosarcomas

Arise within the cancellous bone or the medullary cavity; seen most often in the pelvis (25% of cases), femur (20%), ribs (10%), and humerus (10%)

Exostotic (peripheral) chondrosarcoma

Often occurs in the cartilage of a prior osteochondroma

Juxtacortical chondrosarcoma

Least common form; probably periosteal or parosteal origin, lies on the outer surface of the metaphysis

Define the following histologic classifications of chondrosarcoma:

Well-differentiated

Low-grade tumor; difficult to distinguish from a benign tumor

Dedifferentiated

High-grade tumor; large areas of noncalcified matrix

What are the common tumor sites?

Chondrosarcomas demonstrate a propensity for the long bones (45% of cases), especially the femur

What are the radiographic features of a chondrosarcoma?

Lytic destructive lesion (large, with endosteal scalloping)
Snowflake (punctate) stippling of amorphous calcification
May present as extraosseous mass with a chondroid matrix

FIBROUS LESIONS

Nonossifying fibroma

What is a nonossifying fibroma?

A common, benign, asymptomatic medullary bone lesion, occurring in as many as 20% of children, that typically

regresses spontaneously and is rarely
seen in patients older than 30 years

Where are nonossifying fibromas typically located?

Nonossifying fibromas are located
eccentrically in the metaphyseal region of
a long bone. The tibia and fibula are most
often affected (90% of cases).

What is a fibrous cortical defect?

A lesion that is histologically identical to a
nonossifying fibroma. The two differ only
in size (fibrous cortical defects are
smaller).

What are the radiographic features of nonossifying fibroma?

Radiolucent cortical lesion with a thin
sclerotic margin that may be scalloped
and expansile; frequently located on the
posteromedial metaphysis

Fibrous dysplasia

What is fibrous dysplasia?

A developmental disorder characterized
by the replacement of medullary bone
with fibrous tissue and abnormal bone

What are the clinical features of fibrous dysplasia?

Typically occurs in children between the
ages of 5 and 20 years and is associated
with endocrine disorders (e.g., hyperthyroidism, hyperparathyroidism)

What is the risk of malignant transformation?

Very low

Describe the 2 types of fibrous dysplasia.

Monostotic fibrous dysplasia occurs in
85% of patients and has a predilection
for the ribs, femur, and skull.

Polyostotic fibrous dysplasia occurs in
15% of patients, typically the younger
ones (mean age = 8 years). This form
is more likely to occur in the pelvis,
and when it does is nearly always also
present in the ipsilateral proximal
femur. It is also common to the
proximal femur without pelvic
involvement and the tibia.

What are the classic radiographic features?

The lesions are radiolucent, irregular,
marginated, and medullary, with a
"ground glass" or "soap bubble" appear-

ance and thick sclerotic borders. Bony expansion (i.e., cherubism, frontal bossing, leontiasis ossea) and bowing deformities (i.e., shepherd's crook deformity of the proximal femur) may also be seen.

What is cherubism?

Polyostotic symmetric involvement of the mandible and maxilla that results in an "angelic-looking" child with puffed-out cheeks (autosomal dominant condition)

What is leontiasis ossea?

Craniofacial fibrous dysplasia

List the 3 features of McCune-Albright syndrome.

1. Polyostotic unilateral fibrous dysplasia
2. Precocious puberty
3. Café au lait spots

What is the most common cause of an expansile lytic lesion in a rib in an adult?

Fibrous dysplasia

What is the differential diagnosis of an expansile rib lesion?

Fibrous dysplasia, metastasis, plasma-cytoma, enchondroma, eosinophilic granuloma, aneurysmal bone cyst, chondromyxoid fibroma

Ossifying fibroma (Sisson's disease)

What is ossifying fibroma?

Ossifying fibroma is similar to fibrous dysplasia. It is characterized by a highly vascularized fibrous stroma intermixed with trabeculae of new bone and is typically painless.

What is the typical location?

The tooth-bearing portion of the mandible or maxilla; rarely, lesions are isolated to the anterior tibial diaphysis and ipsilateral fibula

What are the imaging features?

Small (i.e., 1–5 cm in diameter), well-defined unilocular or multilocular areas of osteolysis

Malignant fibrous histiocytoma

What is malignant fibrous histiocytoma?

The most common soft tissue malignant mass in adults, malignant fibrous histiocytoma is a tumor of fibrous origin that arises from histiocytes. It rarely arises in bone. There is a high frequency of local recurrence.

What are the radiographic characteristics?

Aggressive-appearing lesion, usually without calcifications or a sclerotic border
Little or no periosteal reaction
Density of tumor is similar to that of muscle (10–60 HU)

Fibrosarcoma

What is fibrosarcoma?

A malignant tumor of pleomorphic fibroblasts that is similar (both clinically and radiographically) to malignant fibrous histiocytoma

What is the radiographic appearance?

Lesions are typically lytic and do not elicit reactive new bone formation; may form bony sequestrum

What is a desmoid tumor?

A mid-grade fibrosarcoma

What is the radiographic appearance of a desmoid tumor in soft tissue?

An infiltrating mass

What is the radiographic appearance of a desmoid tumor in bone?

Well-circumscribed, lytic lesion (often multilocular) with thick septa
Periostitis may appear benign or aggressive (Codman's triangle or thick spicules)
May form bony sequestrum

BONE MARROW TUMORS

Giant cell tumor

What is a giant cell tumor?

A locally aggressive and potentially malignant lesion of the skeletally mature thought to be derived from osteoclastic cells

What is the typical location?

50% arise around the knee; also common to the distal radius

List 4 radiographic features of giant cell tumors.

1. Expansile, lytic epiphyseal lesion abutting the articular surface

2. Thin overlying cortex with sclerotic outline
3. Usually eccentrically located in bone
4. Closed growth plate

Eosinophilic granuloma

What is eosinophilic granuloma?

An aberrant proliferation of histiocytes in the organs of the reticuloendothelial system

What is the typical age of patients?

Younger than 30 years

What are typical locations?

As many as 50% of cases involve the skull, and 25% of cases involve the vertebrae. Lesions may also be found in the epiphyses of the long bones.

What are the radiographic features of eosinophilic granuloma?

Lytic defects are common; the lesions may be ill-defined or have sclerotic borders and are often multifocal. A periosteal reaction may be present.
"Hole-within-a-hole" sign: The outer table of the skull is more damaged than the inner table, leading to the formation of button sequestrum.
Vertebra plana (i.e., complete collapse of the vertebral body) may be seen.

What is the differential diagnosis of vertebra plana?

Single: Gaucher's disease, eosinophilic granuloma, lymphoma, metastasis, myeloma, radiation
Universal: Leukemia, steroid therapy, osteogenesis imperfecta, mucopolysaccharidoses

What are some of the extra-skeletal manifestations of eosinophilic granuloma?

Pulmonary involvement (i.e., upper lobar interstitial disease), central nervous system (CNS) and meningeal manifestations are possible.

Multiple myeloma

What is multiple myeloma?

A multifocal bone marrow malignancy composed of monoclonal Ig (usually IgG)-producing plasmacytes

How common is multiple myeloma?

Multiple myeloma is the most common primary bone tumor in adults, accounting for more than 12,000 new cases in the United States each year.

What is the mean age at the time of diagnosis?

65 years

What is the typical location of the bone lesions?

The vertebral bodies (as opposed to the pedicle destruction seen more commonly with metastases), the ribs, the pelvis, the shoulder, the long bones, and the flat bones (e.g., skull, mandible)

List 4 plain film radiographic characteristics of multiple myeloma.

1. Well-defined lytic lesions with a "punched-out" appearance
2. Typically no reactive bone formation
3. Pathologic fracture common
4. Diffuse osteoporosis of the spine with multiple compression fractures may be seen

What are the atypical findings?

Sclerosing myeloma or myelomatosis (POEMS syndrome)
Osteolytic or mixed blastic and lytic lesions with reactive sclerosis

What is POEMS syndrome?

Polyneuropathy, **O**rganomegaly, **E**ndocrinopathy, **M**yeloma, **S**kin changes

What are the bone scan findings in multiple myeloma?

Bone scan is often **normal;** cold spots are common.

What are the MRI findings?

Normal marrow replaced with tumor

What is a plasmacytoma?

Myeloma presenting as a mass lesion

Ewing's sarcoma

What is Ewing's sarcoma?

Malignant, small, round cell bone tumor of uncertain origin (may arise from primitive marrow elements or immature mesenchymal cells)

Which age group is most often affected?

Patients between the ages of 5 and 30 years (mean age is 11 years)

What locations does the tumor favor?

The diaphysis of the femur, tibia, fibula, or humerus is the most common location, but the tumor can arise in any bone, including flat bones (25% of cases) and the vertebral bodies.

What are the radiographic features?

An aggressive permeative or moth-eaten osteolytic lesion with internal bony destruction is classic. Onion skin periostitis is common, but sunburst or amorphous reactive bone formation may be seen. Extraosseus soft tissue masses are fairly common. Metastases are common.

MISCELLANEOUS BONE TUMORS

Unicameral bone cyst (solitary or simple bone cyst)

What is a unicameral bone cyst?

An expansile lytic lesion of bone that tends to arise in patients between the ages of 10 and 20 years and resolves with maturity

Where are unicameral bone cysts typically located?

Proximal humerus or femur (two thirds of cases): 90% arise in the physeal plate and grow into the long bone shaft
Calcaneal lesions not uncommon

What are the radiographic characteristics?

Central (medullary) expansile lesion
Cystic cavity with air-fluid levels
"Fallen fragment" sign (pathognomonic): fragment from pathologic fracture sunken to the bottom of the fluid-filled lesion

Aneurysmal bone cyst

What is an aneurysmal bone cyst?

Named for its radiographic appearance, it is an expansile (or aneurysmal) nonneoplastic lesion of thin-walled, blood-filled cystic cavities.

Among what age group are aneurysmal bone cysts most common?

Patients between the ages of 10 and 20 years

What are the 2 types of aneurysmal bone cyst?

Primary (70% of cases) and secondary (i.e., those arising in preexisting bone lesions)

What are the common locations?

The posterior elements of the spine (30% of cases) and the long bones

What are the radiographic features?	Eccentric expansile lytic lesion that may have a sclerotic border No periosteal reaction unless fractured Thin residual cortex (best seen by CT) "Bubbly" (i.e., bone lucency gives the lesion a "soap bubble" appearance)
What is the differential diagnosis of "bubbly" bone lesions?	**FEGNOMASHIC** **F**ibrous dysplasia and **F**ibrous cortical defect **E**nchondroma and **E**osinophilic granuloma **G**iant cell tumor **N**onossifying fibroma **O**steoblastoma and **O**steoid osteoma **M**etastases and **M**ultiple myeloma **A**neurysmal bone cyst **S**olitary (unicameral) bone cyst **H**yperparathyroidism (brown tumor) and **H**emophilia **I**nfection **C**hondrosarcoma and **C**hondroblastoma

Adamantinoma

What is an adamantinoma?	A rare, locally aggressive malignant bone tumor consisting of epithelial-like cells in a dense fibrous stroma
Where do most adamantinomas arise?	The tibia
How does the lesion appear radiographically?	Well-defined mixed osteolytic and sclerotic lesion

Hemangioma

What is a hemangioma?	A tumor of vascular origin that is common in soft tissues and bone
What are the clinical features of a hemangioma?	Soft tissue mass, asymptomatic when in bone
What are the typical locations?	Most prevalent in the vertebral bodies; also seen in the craniofacial bones
What are the imaging features?	Corduroy pattern: Coarse, vertical, trabeculae among wide venous spaces (in the vertebrae)

Multiple, irregular, somewhat expansile lytic cortical lesions (in extraspinal sites)

Phleboliths

Chordoma

What is a chordoma?

A relatively uncommon, locally aggressive but slow-growing tumor that arises from the residual primitive notochord of the early fetal axial skeleton; although locally aggressive, chordoma is not considered malignant because it does not metastasize

What are the common locations?

Sacrococcygeal (50% of cases), naso-pharyngeal (i.e., the clivus; 35% of cases), vertebral bodies (15% of cases)

Mastocytosis

What is mastocytosis?

A rare disorder characterized by mast cell infiltration of the skin and bone marrow

What are the radiographic findings?

Mixed lytic-sclerotic process with thickened trabecula

Uniform increase in bone density

May see thickened small bowel folds with nodules on pelvic or abdominal films

Myeloid metaplasia (myelofibrosis)

What is myeloid metaplasia?

Fibrotic replacement of hematopoietic bone marrow that leads to hepa-tosplenomegaly as a result of extramed-ullary red blood cell (RBC) production

What are the radiographic features?

Transient osteolytic lesions, subsequent formation of radiodense bone, hepa-tosplenomegaly

METASTATIC BONE TUMORS

Which is more common, primary or metastatic bone tumors?

Metastatic bone tumors are much more common.

When should metastasis be considered on the differential diagnosis of radiographic bone lesions?

Metastasis should be considered whenever a lytic lesion (regardless of appearance) is seen in a patient older than 40 years or in a patient with a known primary malignancy.

Which tumors commonly metastasize to bone?

These **P**rimarily **L**ike **K**illing **B**one
Thyroid
Prostate
Lung
Kidney
Breast

m

What are the common metastatic origins by stage of life and gender?

Man: Prostate (60%), lung (15%), kidney (5%), other (20%)
Woman: Breast (70%), lung (5%), kidney (5%), other (20%)
Child: Neuroblastoma, leukemia or lymphoma, Wilms' tumor, medulloblastoma, sarcomas

How are metastases disseminated to the bones?

Hematogenous spread (either via arterial circulation to the vascular red marrow or via retrograde venous flow) is the most common means of dissemination. Direct extension is less common and lymphatic spread is rare.

What are the radiographic features of metastatic bone tumors?

The appearance usually reflects the aggressiveness of the primary tumor, although metastases may appear quite benign. The lesions may be lytic, sclerotic, or mixed. Involvement of the vertebrae, especially the posterior elements, may be seen. Pathologic fractures are common.

Which common metastases usually appear lytic?

Kidney, lung, thyroid, and melanoma

What is the differential diagnosis of multiple lytic bone lesions?

Metastases, myeloma, fibrous dysplasia, Gaucher's disease, brown tumors, infection, enchondromatosis, eosinophilic granuloma, hemangiomatosis, lymphangiomatosis

Which common metastases usually appear more sclerotic?

6 Bs Lick Pollen
Breast tumors
Bone tumors (osteosarcoma)
Bowel tumors (mucinous tumors)
Bronchogenic (carcinoid) tumors
Bladder tumors
Brain tumors (medulloblastoma)
Lymphoma
Prostate tumors

m

The first and last tumors of the mnemonic are by far the most common sources of metastasis to the bone.

What is the differential diagnosis of a solitary sclerotic area?

Osteoma
Osteoblastic metastasis
Osteoid osteoma
Sclerosing osteomyelitis
Healing benign lesion (fibrocystic dysplasia, nonossifying fibroma, bone cyst)
Callus
Enostosis (bone island)
Bone infarct
Avascular necrosis
Enchondroma
Paget's disease

What is the differential diagnosis of an ivory vertebral body?

Metastasis, osteomyelitis, myeloma, Paget's disease, osteosarcoma, lymphoma

What is the differential diagnosis for generalized dense bones?

Regular **S**ex **M**akes **O**rnery **P**eople **M**uch **M**ore **P**leasant **A**nd **F**riendly

m

Renal osteodystrophy
Sickle cell disease
Myelofibrosis
Osteopetrosis
Pyknodysostosis
Mastocytosis
Metastasis
Paget's disease
Athlete (stress reaction)
Fluorosis

7 Gastrointestinal Imaging

Eric J. Udoff
John J. Smith

ANATOMY

ESOPHAGUS

Which structures make impressions on the esophagus as the esophagus passes through the chest?

Aortic arch and left atrium

How many layers does the esophageal wall have?

Two—mucosa and submucosa (no serosa is present)

Why is the number of layers in the esophageal wall significant?

Lack of serosa makes spread of tumor to adjacent structures more likely

Identify the components of the esophagogastric junction:

A = Tubular esophagus
B = A line (i.e., demarcation of the beginning of the ampulla)
C = Phrenic ampulla
D = Submerged segment of the esophagus
E = B line (i.e., junction between the squamous esophageal mucosa and the columnar gastric mucosa)
F = Diaphragm
G = Gastric fundus

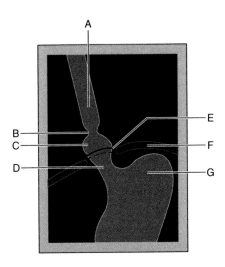

Describe the 3 types of muscle contractions seen in the esophagus.

1. Primary muscle contraction is coordinated, smooth contraction of the muscle that is initiated by swallowing.
2. Secondary muscle contraction clears material that is not cleared by the primary stripping wave.
3. Tertiary muscle contraction is irregular, uncoordinated, and nonpropulsive; the incidence of this type of muscle contraction increases with age.

STOMACH

Which part of the stomach is:

Posterior?

The fundus

Anterior?

The antrum and distal body

Where is air seen in the stomach on:

Upright abdominal radiographs?

The fundus, just under the left hemi-diaphragm

Supine abdominal radiographs?

Distal body

The following views depict various postoperative appearances of the stomach. For each view, identify the procedure that was performed and name the condition the procedure is most often used to treat.

A = Billroth I procedure (gastroduodenostomy), used to treat peptic ulcer disease

B = Roux-en-Y procedure (gastrojejunostomy), used to treat peptic ulcer disease

C = Billroth II procedure (gastrojejunostomy), used to treat peptic ulcer disease

D = Whipple procedure (pancreatectomy), often used to treat resectable pancreatic carcinoma

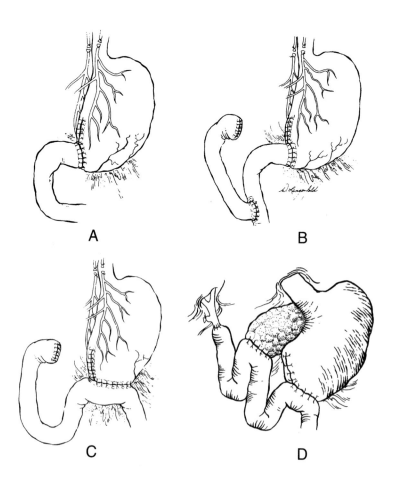

SMALL BOWEL (DUODENUM, JEJUNUM, AND ILEUM)

What is the normal position of the ligament of Treitz?	Left of the spine and as cephalad as the pylorus
Is the duodenum intra- or retroperitoneal?	The first and fourth portions are intraperitoneal, and the second and third portions are retroperitoneal.
What features are typical of the:	
Jejunum?	Feathery mucosal pattern, usually larger in caliber than the ileum, and generally located in the left abdomen
Ileum?	Fewer folds than the jejunum, smoother mucosal pattern, and generally located in the right abdomen
How can you find the terminal ileum?	Look for the cecum in the right lower quadrant (RLQ) and find a loop of bowel entering it from the medial aspect. Remember, the terminal ileum enters several centimeters cephalad to the cecal tip!

LARGE BOWEL (CECUM, COLON, RECTUM, ANAL CANAL)

Which parts of the colon are retroperitoneal?	The ascending and descending colon are retroperitoneal. The cecum may have a mesocolon or can be retroperitoneal. The rectum is extraperitoneal.
How can you locate the colon on a computed tomography (CT) scan?	Look for the bowel that is posterolateral in the retroperitoneum at the level of the mid-abdomen. This is the ascending colon (right side) and descending colon (left side). Then follow the ascending or descending colon to trace the colon from one end to the other.
How do you distinguish the large bowel from the small bowel?	The **large bowel** has **plicae semilunaris** (i.e., folds that extend part of the way across the lumen in between the haustra). The large bowel may contain stool and usually frames the abdomen.

The **small bowel** has **valvulae conniventes** (i.e., folds that extend all of the way across the lumen), except in the distal ileum. The small bowel is usually more centrally located than the large bowel.

What are the normal calibers of the small bowel, the transverse colon, and the cecum?

Remember the "3, 6, 9 rule:"
Small bowel < **3** cm
Transverse colon < **6** cm
Cecum < **9** cm

What is the "rule of 3s" for the small bowel?

The **bowel wall** should be **less than 3 mm thick.**
The **bowel folds** should be **less than 3 mm thick.**
The **bowel diameter** should be **less than 3 cm wide.**
No more than 3 air-fluid levels should be present.

LIVER

What criteria defines hepatomegaly?

Craniocaudal liver span of more than 15 cm

What is the blood supply to the normal liver?

Portal vein (75%) and hepatic artery (25%)

What are the 5 segments of the liver?

Right lobe (anterior segment and posterior segment)
Left lobe (lateral segment and medial segment)
Caudate lobe

What are the 9 liver subsegments according to Couinaud?

Couinaud divides the liver into superior and inferior portions at the porta, creating 9 liver subsegments.
1 = Caudate lobe
2 = Superior lateral segment (left lobe)
3 = Inferior lateral segment (left lobe)
4a = Superior medial segment (left lobe)
4b = Inferior medial segment (left lobe)
5 = Inferior anterior segment (right lobe)
6 = Inferior posterior segment (right lobe)
7 = Superior posterior segment (right lobe)

8 = Superior anterior segment (right lobe)

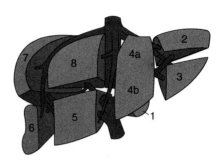

How can I reconstruct this arrangement at the view-box?

Make a table like the one below. Start numbering with the caudate lobe (*1*), then go directly to the superior lateral segment and number clockwise. Just remember that the medial segment of the left lobe is identified as *4a* and *4b*—if you remember where *4a* and *4b* are, the rest of the subsegments will fall into place.

	Right Lobe		**Left Lobe**		
	Posterior	**Anterior**	**Medial**	**Lateral**	**Caudate**
Superior	*7*	*8*	*4a*	*2*	*1*
Inferior	*6*	*5*	*4b*	*3*	

Why is it important to know the location of the sub-segments of the liver?

In order to perform segmental or subsegmental resection of the liver, the surgeon must know exactly which parts of the liver are diseased so that vascular supply and venous and biliary drainage can be preserved. Knowing the sub-segments helps the radiologist communicate with the surgeon.

Identify the structures on the following drawing:

A = Inferior vena cava (IVC)
B = Left hepatic vein
C = Left portal vein, lateral segment
D = Left portal vein, medial segment
E = Falciform ligament
F = Main portal vein
G = Left portal vein
H = Gallbladder
I = Right portal vein

J = Right portal vein, anterior segment
K = Right portal vein, posterior segment
L = Middle hepatic vein
M = Right hepatic vein

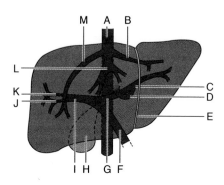

What are the landmarks that separate the lobes and segments?

The **hepatic veins** lie **between** segments; the **portal veins** lie **within** segments. (The left portal vein is the exception to this rule.) Therefore:

The posterior segment is separated from the anterior segment by the right hepatic vein cephalad in the liver. More caudally, the posterior and anterior segments are separated by a line that bisects the angle between the anterior and posterior right portal veins.

The right lobe is separated from the left lobe by the middle hepatic vein (cephalad) and the gallbladder (caudal).

The medial segment is separated from the lateral segment by the left hepatic vein (cephalad), the left portal vein (mid-level), and the ligamentum teres (caudal).

Identify the structures on the four axial sections below:

A = Right hepatic vein
B = Middle hepatic vein
C = Left hepatic vein
D = IVC
E = Main portal vein
F = Right portal vein
G = Right portal vein, anterior segment
H = Right portal vein, posterior segment

I = Left portal vein
J = Left portal vein, medial segment
K = Left portal vein, lateral segment
L = Ligamentum teres
M = Falciform ligament
N = Fissure for the ligamentum venosum
O = Gallbladder
P = Right hepatic duct
Q = Left hepatic duct
R = Common hepatic duct
S = Caudate lobe
T = Superior lateral segment, left lobe
U = Inferior lateral segment, left lobe
V_1 = Superior medial segment, left lobe
V_2 = Inferior medial segment, left lobe
W_1 = Superior anterior segment, right lobe
W_2 = Inferior anterior segment, right lobe
X_1 = Superior posterior segment, right lobe
X_2 = Inferior posterior segment, right lobe

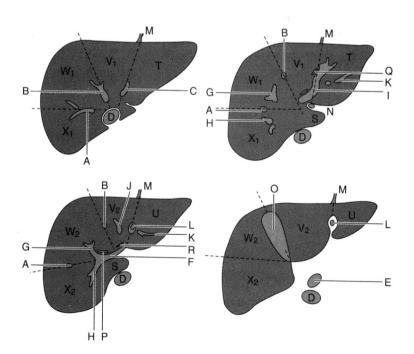

BILIARY SYSTEM, PANCREAS, AND SPLEEN

Identify the labeled struc-
tures on the following figure:

A = Right hepatic duct
B = Left hepatic duct
C = Common hepatic duct
D = Duct of Wirsung (major duct)
E = Tail of the pancreas
F = Body of the pancreas
G = Ligament of Treitz
H = Third part of the duodenum
I = Ampulla of Vater
J = Head of the pancreas
K = Duct of Santorini (lesser duct)
L = Common bile duct
M = Cystic duct

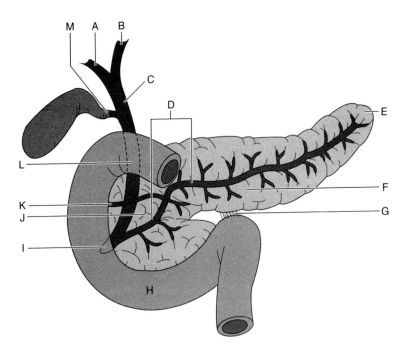

What is the caliber of the
normal common bile duct?

≤6 mm (in patients older than 60 years,
the rule is 1 mm for each decade of age)

What is the caliber of the
common bile duct in
patients who have under-
gone cholecystectomy?

8–10 mm

What is a useful landmark for locating the pancreas on a CT scan?

Find the third part of the duodenum [i.e., the most cephalad loop of small bowel passing immediately anterior to the aorta and posterior to the superior mesenteric artery (SMA) in the abdomen]. Then, move through the slices in a cephalad direction to identify the uncinate process, head, neck, body, and tail of the pancreas.

What is the best landmark for identifying the pancreas on ultrasound?

The body of the pancreas is usually anterior to the splenic vein. Scan up and down to visualize the entire gland (ability to visualize may be limited by bowel gas).

What is the normal short axis measurement of the pancreas?

The normal short axis measurement of the pancreas is less than 2.5 cm at the head and less than 1.5 cm at the tail. However, it is best not to rely on strict measurements. A better approach is to get a sense of the proportions of the patient's pancreas and then to look for a focal mass or atrophy.

In general, does the pancreas increase or decrease in size with age?

Decrease

What is pancreas divisum?

A congenital anomaly of failure of fusion of the dorsal and ventral pancreatic buds, resulting in two ducts. The major pancreatic duct (i.e., the duct of Wirsung) drains through the lesser papilla, and is seen to cross the common bile duct (rather than join it) on magnetic resonance cholangiopancreatography (MRCP) or endoscopic retrograde cholangiopancreatography (ERCP). The lesser duct (i.e., the duct of Santorini), rather than the major duct (i.e., the duct of Wirsung), drains most of the pancreas. The orifice of the duct may be too small, leading to pancreatitis.

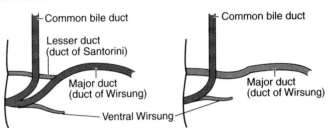

A. Normal

Common bile duct

Lesser duct
(duct of Santorini)

Major duct
(duct of Wirsung)

Ventral Wirsung

B. Pancreas divisum

Common bile duct

Major duct
(duct of Wirsung)

What is an accessory spleen?	A small portion of splenic tissue that is separated from the spleen but has the same enhancement characteristics. Accessory spleens may be seen after splenectomy or confused for pathology.
What percentage of patients have accessory spleens?	10%–25%
Where are accessory spleens located?	Splenic hilus (20% of cases), adjacent to the pancreatic tail, and rarely, elsewhere in the abdomen

PERITONEUM

Identify the peritoneal structures on the following anatomic view:	A = Right paracolic space (gutter) B = Hepatorenal recess (Morrison's pouch) C = Right subphrenic space D = Falciform ligament E = Left subphrenic space F = Perisplenic space G = Phrenicocolic ligament H = Left paracolic space (gutter) I = Root of the mesentery J = Cul de sac

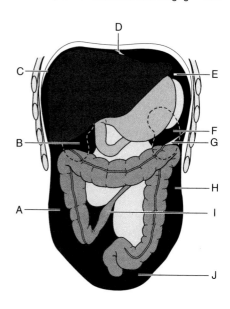

Identify the structures on the following CT scan:

A = Hepatorenal recess (Morrison's pouch)
B = Right subphrenic space
C = Gastrohepatic ligament
D = Falciform ligament
E = Lesser sac
F = Gastrocolic ligament
G = Splenic flexure of the left colon
H = Phrenicocolic ligament
I = Anterior pararenal space
J = Spleen
K = Pancreas
L = Perisplenic space

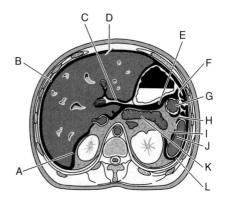

Where does peritoneal fluid accumulate in the supine position?	The hepatorenal recess (Morrison's pouch)
Where is the hepatorenal recess?	Between the anterior surface of the right kidney and the posterior surface of the right lobe of the liver
Where does peritoneal fluid accumulate in the upright position?	In the pouch of Douglas, which is located posterior to the uterus (in women) or the bladder (in men) and anterior to the rectum

GENERAL GASTROINTESTINAL ANATOMY

Identify the structures on the following CT slices:

A = Aorta
B = IVC
C = Azygos vein
D = Hemiazygos vein
E = Vertebral body
F = Spleen
G = Diaphragm
H = Rib
I = Lung
J = Splenic flexure
K = Stomach
L = Hepatic veins
M = Gastric fundus
N = Left portal vein
O = Falciform ligament
P = Left adrenal gland
Q = Left kidney
R = Pancreatic tail
S = Small bowel
T = Right portal vein
U = Right adrenal gland
V = Celiac axis
W = Splenic vein
X = Pancreatic body
Y = Gastric antrum
Z = Common bile duct
AA = Main portal vein
BB = Right kidney
CC = SMA
DD = Collecting system
EE = Transverse colon
FF = Duodenal bulb
GG = Head of the pancreas

HH = Gallbladder
II = Left renal vein
JJ = Descending colon
KK = Superior mesenteric vein (SMV)
LL = Uncinate process of the pancreas
MM = Crus of the diaphragm
NN = Right renal artery
OO = Third portion of the duodenum

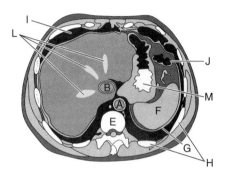

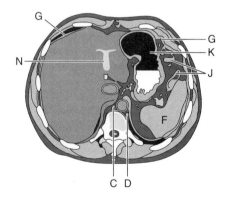

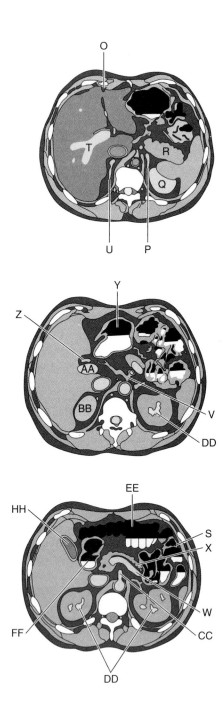

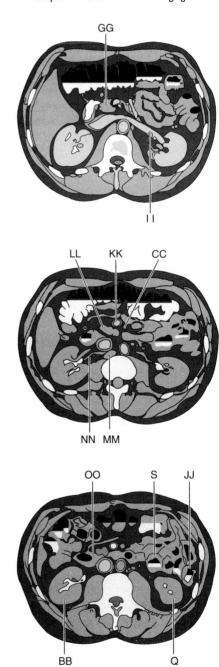

DEFINITIONS

TERMINOLOGY

Define the following terms:

Adynamic (paralytic) ileus	A condition characterized by hypomotility and distention of the bowel
Appendicolith	A calcified concretion in the appendix, seen in approximately 10%–20% of patients with appendicitis
Ascites	Fluid in the peritoneal cavity
Closed loop obstruction	A loop of bowel obstructed at two points, usually caused by adhesions or volvulus
Hematocrit effect	Layering of the components of a hematoma into serum and sediment
Hemoperitoneum	Blood in the peritoneal cavity
Intussusception	Invagination of the bowel wall into the lumen of the immediately contiguous segment of bowel; intussusception can be ileocolic, colocolonic, or enteroenteric
Pneumatosis intestinalis	Gas within the bowel wall
Pneumoperitoneum	Extraluminal gas in the peritoneal cavity
Sepsis	Infection resulting from bacteremia; the release of endotoxins may lead to unstable blood pressure and fever
Strangulation	Closed loop obstruction that leads to bowel ischemia
Thumbprinting	Thickening of the large bowel wall owing to infiltration by fluid (often blood); often demonstrated by thickening of the bowel wall folds
Volvulus	Twisting of the bowel about its mesentery

RADIOGRAPHIC SIGNS

Describe the following radiographic signs:

"Bird's beak" sign	1. The appearance, on barium enema, of the tapered end of the rectosigmoid colon in a patient with sigmoid volvulus
	2. The appearance of the esophagus in advanced achalasia (i.e., dilated proximal end and tapered distal end)
Border sign	On an air-contrast barium study, the outer border of the film of barium that coats the surface of a diverticulum or ulcer is often sharp, becoming less well defined centrally. In contrast, on a polyp, the inner border of the barium film is sharp, fading as it radiates.
Bull's-eye (target) sign	A filling defect in the wall of the bowel with a punctate collection of contrast centrally
"Coffee bean" sign	An air-filled closed loop obstruction (e.g., sigmoid volvulus) may look like a coffee bean on a plain film radiograph.
Colon cut-off sign	An abrupt termination of gas, usually at the distal transverse or proximal descending colon, results when inflammatory fluid spreads from the pancreas through the transverse mesocolon, narrowing the colon. Although this finding is classically associated with pancreatitis, it is only seen in a minority of cases.
Concave margin sign	Fluid in the peritoneum forms concave margins with loops of bowel. This extraluminal fluid should not be confused with fluid-filled loops of bowel or ovaries, which have round, convex margins on CT.
Diaphragm sign	Fluid posterior to the diaphragm on a CT scan is pleural fluid, not ascites. Fluid within the dome of the diaphragm (centrally) is ascites. Note that ascites cannot come between the liver and the

diaphragm posteriorly owing to the bare area of the liver.

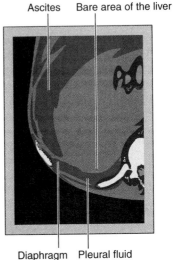

Ascites   Bare area of the liver

Diaphragm   Pleural fluid

"Dog ears" sign

Fluid in the peritoneum may accumulate in the peritoneal recesses superolateral to the bladder. These accumulations occasionally look like "ears" on the bladder, referred to as "dog ears."

Double duct sign

Enlargement of the pancreatic and biliary ducts caused by obstruction of the common bile duct

Double wall (Rigler's) sign

If you can see air outlining both the inside and outside walls of the bowel, the patient has a pneumoperitoneum.

Falciform ligament sign

Pneumoperitoneum outlines the falciform ligament in the supine position.

Flank stripe sign

The accumulation of peritoneal fluid displaces the colon away from the lateral peritoneum when the patient is supine. The properitoneal fat just outside the peritoneum laterally is also known as the flank stripe.

Ground glass sign

Large amounts of fluid in the peritoneum can cause a hazy appearance (described as "ground glass") on a plain abdominal film.

Inverted "3" sign

Enlargement of the pancreatic head as a result of pancreatitis or advanced pancreatic cancer can cause an impression on the barium-filled duodenum that resembles an inverted "3" (i.e., pancreatic tissue bulges above and below the duodenal insertion of the pancreatic duct).

"Mercedes-Benz" sign

Gas-containing gallstones occasionally have a central lucency that mimics the logo of the Mercedes-Benz automobile company.

"Mickey Mouse" sign

The portal vein, hepatic artery, and common bile duct form Mickey's head, left ear, and right ear, respectively, when seen on a transverse view of the porta on ultrasound.

Pseudocalculus sign

Transient spasm of the sphincter of Oddi can cause a defect in the column of contrast on a cholangiogram or endoscopic retrograde cholangio-pancreatogram.

Psoas sign

The margin of the psoas can usually be seen on plain films of the abdomen, because the margin is outlined by retroperitoneal fat. If fluid (e.g., as a result of pancreatitis) or blood infiltrates the retroperitoneum, the interface is lost and the psoas sign (i.e., loss of the psoas margin) is seen.

Sandwich sign

The sandwich sign is seen with soft-tissue infiltration of the mesentery by a process such as lymphoma. Lymphoma (the "bread") surrounds the mesenteric fat (the "mayo") and the mesenteric vessels (the "meat").

Sentinel clot sign

Clotted components of a hemoperitoneum, which have higher attenuation on CT, are likely to be found near the site of bleeding.

Shadow sign

Stones within a completely contracted gallbladder cast a shadow on ultrasound, but the gallbladder is not visualized.

Shotgun (parallel channel) sign

Dilated intrahepatic bile ducts and the normal portal vein branches give the appearance of a "double-barreled shotgun" on ultrasound. This sign is best seen in the left lobe.

"Stack of coins" sign

Thickening of parallel folds in the wall of the small bowel can resemble a stack of coins.

"String of pearls" sign

Small pockets of gas trapped between the small bowel valvulae conniventes form a chain of bubbles, or "string of pearls." This sign is seen in small bowel obstruction.

IMAGING STUDIES

RADIOGRAPHY

Plain film studies

What is the approach to evaluating a plain abdominal film?

Bones: Evaluate the integrity of the bones.

Stones: Check for calcifications or foreign bodies.

Gas: Check for extraluminal gas—for example, subdiaphragmatic (free air), between the bowel loops, or in the bowel wall (pneumatosis)—and intraluminal gas (note dilatation of the bowel, thickness of the wall, air-fluid levels, and displacement of loops). Check for peritoneal fluid between the flank stripe and the bowel.

Mass: Check the normal viscera (i.e., the liver, spleen, bladder, and flank) and note any abnormal masses.

You need to evaluate a film that is not labeled. How can you determine which position the patient was in when the film was taken?

There are two ways you may be able to tell which position the patient was in when the film was taken:

1. **Evaluate which structures contain air.** If ventral structures (e.g., the

antrum of the stomach) contain air, the patient was probably in the supine position when the film was taken. If the gas is in the fundus, the film was taken with the patient upright.

2. **Look for horizontal interfaces consisting of air above and fluid below (i.e., air-fluid levels).** These interfaces indicate that the film was taken with the patient either upright or in the decubitus position. Air-fluid levels can be key to diagnosing bowel obstruction.

Intraluminal contrast studies

What are the advantages of barium over water-soluble contrast agents, such as Gastrografin or Hypaque?

Barium provides better anatomic detail and easier visualization than water-soluble contrast agents.

What complication is associated with barium?

Free barium in the peritoneal cavity induces a granulomatous response that can lead to adhesions and obstruction.

When can barium be used?

Barium is acceptable for evaluating partial or complete small bowel obstructions.

When should a water-soluble contrast agent be used?

Immediately post-operatively (to assess anastomoses for leak or obstruction), or when perforation is suspected

What complication is associated with water-soluble contrast?

Massive aspiration can cause pulmonary edema.

What is a barium swallow?

The patient swallows barium and the radiologist observes the swallowing mechanism. Films of the cervical and thoracic esophagus are obtained.

What is an upper gastrointestinal study?

The patient swallows barium under fluoroscopic observation. Films of the thoracic esophagus, stomach, and duodenal bulb are obtained.

What is the difference between a small bowel follow-through (SBFT) study and enteroclysis?

SBFT study: The patient swallows barium (as for an upper gastro-intestinal study), and sequential abdominal films are obtained at 15- to 30-minute intervals. The abdomen is palpated until the terminal ileum is identified; the terminal ileum can then be examined with fluoroscopy and spot films.

Enteroclysis (small bowel enema): A tube is passed through the patient's nose or mouth into the duodenum. Barium is pumped through the tube into the gastrointestinal tract, distending it more fully and yielding a more complete exam. The sensitivity for subtle disease is better, but the radiation dose is six times that of an SBFT study.

List 3 absolute contraindi-cations to barium enema.

1. Toxic megacolon
2. Severe pseudomembranous colitis
3. Suspected perforation (suggested by free air or peritonitis)

List 4 relative contraindica-tions to barium enema.

1. Sigmoidoscopy within the past 24 hours
2. Colonic biopsy performed with a flexible scope within the past 48 hours
3. Colonic biopsy performed with a rigid scope within the past 6 days
4. Any acute colitis

Should the gastrointestinal tract be prepared prior to performing a barium enema?

Yes. A clean colon makes for a much more valuable study, because stool can mimic lesions.

How is a double-contrast barium enema different from a single-contrast barium enema?

A double-contrast barium enema is performed with thick barium and air (the barium coats the wall of the colon and the air distends the lumen). A single-contrast barium enema uses thin barium to fill the colon. In general, a single-contrast barium enema study is quicker and more comfortable than a double-contrast barium enema study.

What are the strengths of a double-contrast barium enema study?

Visualization of mucosal detail and diagnosis of mucosal lesions, such as polyps

When is a single-contrast barium enema used?

A single-contrast barium enema is used to rule out diverticulosis in patients who are too ill to roll over (a requirement for double-contrast barium enema studies, because air must be moved throughout the bowel). It can also be used for rapid assessment to obtain answers to relatively simple questions (e.g., "rule out obstruction").

Why would glucagon (1 mg) be administered intra-venously prior to performing a barium enema?

To reduce spasm of the bowel

How can mucosal, deep mucosal or submucosal, and extraluminal and subserosal lesions be differentiated from one another on a contrast study?

Mucosal, deep mucosal or submucosal, and extraluminal or subserosal lesions may be difficult to distinguish on a contrast study. The key is the angle (*arrows*) that the mass makes with the wall (i.e., acute versus obtuse).

Mucosal

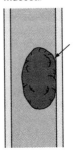

Deep mucosal
or submucosal

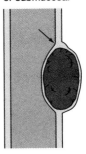

Extraluminal or
subserosal

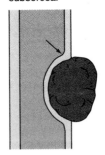

How do intraluminal masses appear on a contrast study?

The intraluminal mass is surrounded by barium.

What is the difference between ERCP and percutaneous transhepatic cholangiography (PTC)?

ERCP is performed, usually by a gastroenterologist in cooperation with a radiologist, via endoscopy with cannulation of the ampulla of Vater. PTC is done by cannulating a bile duct with a needle placed percutaneously by a radiologist. PTC is better for visualizing the proximal bile duct, whereas ERCP is better for visualizing the distal bile duct.

ULTRASOUND

What is the normal echo-genicity of the liver, kidney, and pancreas (in order of most to least)?

Pancreas, liver, kidney

What is the normal Doppler appearance of the:

Hepatic artery?

The hepatic artery shows flow toward the liver with a sharp upstroke (representing the systolic velocity) and a tail (representing the diastolic velocity).

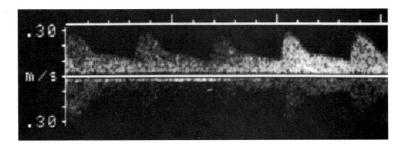

Hepatic veins?

The hepatic veins demonstrate flow toward the heart with pulsatility (caused by waves transmitted from the heart) and respiratory phasicity (i.e., flow increases with inspiration as blood is drawn into the thorax, and nearly ceases when a Valsalva maneuver is performed).

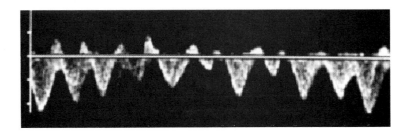

Portal vein?

The portal vein demonstrates flow toward the liver (i.e., hepatopetal flow) that is phasic. In patients with portal hypertension, the flow can reverse direction (i.e., it can become hepatofugal).

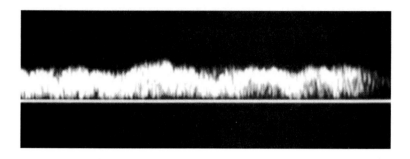

How can the following structures be best identified on color Doppler ultrasound?

The left portal vein?

Scan in the sagittal plane in the region of the falciform ligament. The left portal vein appears as a "shepherd's crook" with flow toward the transducer.

Right portal vein?

Scan in the right flank in the transverse plane midway through the liver at the level of the porta and look for the "Y" (i.e., the right portal vein bifurcating into the anterior and posterior segmental branches). Normal flow should be toward the transducer.

How do you find the common bile duct by ultrasound?

Find the "Mickey Mouse" sign on a transverse oblique view (A on the figure on the following page); the common bile duct forms the right "ear." In a longitudinal oblique section (B), the hepatic artery runs between the common bile duct and the right portal vein. Color Doppler ultrasound can be used to confirm flow through the artery.

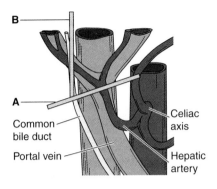

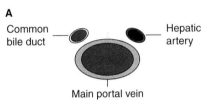

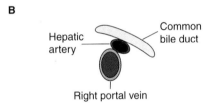

COMPUTED TOMOGRAPHY (CT)

What are the phases of hepatic enhancement on CT?

Arterial, portal venous, and equilibrium (see figure on next page)

What are the appropriate delay times for scanning in the arterial phase and portal venous phase for a 2 ml/sec injection?

Arterial phase: 25 seconds
Portal venous phase: 70 seconds

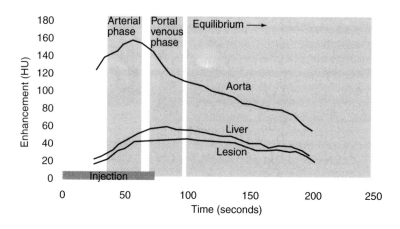

NUCLEAR MEDICINE (HEPATOBILIARY SCAN)

See also Chapter 2, "Imaging Techniques"

On a hepatobiliary scan, what are the causes of:

Poor liver uptake?	Hepatic insufficiency from any cause (e.g., hepatitis, cirrhosis)
Delayed liver clearance of tracer (i.e., cholestasis)?	Biliary obstruction, hepatitis, or hepatotoxicity
Nonvisualization of the gallbladder?	Acute cholecystitis Biliary tract obstruction Failure to maintain NPO status for 4 hours prior to the procedure, or failure to eat within the previous 24 hours Surgical removal of the gallbladder Hepatic insufficiency
A delayed biliary-to-bowel transmit time?	Biliary obstruction, poor hepatic function, or physiologic delay (i.e., delayed but visualized bowel activity)
What is the significance of visualizing the gallbladder and bowel activity within 1 hour on a hepatobiliary scan?	Acute cholecystitis, for practical purposes, has been excluded.

What is the implication if the gallbladder is not seen within 1 hour of injecting a Tc-99m-labeled iminodiacetic acid derivative (Tc-99m IDA), such as disopropyliminodiacetic acid (DISIDA) or hepatobiliary iminodiacetic acid (HIDA), but is seen within 30 minutes of morphine administration (or within 4 hours of injection on studies without morphine)?	Acute cholecystitis is excluded as a possible diagnosis; though this finding is nonspecific; diagnostic considerations include normal physiology and chronic cholecystitis.
What are the diagnostic considerations if there is no activity seen in the bile ducts? What conclusions can be drawn about the likelihood of acute cholecystitis as a diagnosis?	If there is no activity in the bile ducts, diagnostic considerations include high-grade obstruction of the biliary tree and poor hepatic function (look for blood pool activity). It is not possible to draw any conclusions about the presence or absence of acute cholecystitis.
What are the causes of lack of bowel activity at 1 hour?	Low biliary tract obstruction Physiologic delay (i.e., bowel activity will be seen promptly after offering a fatty challenge, such as a candy bar or ice cream)
What are the diagnostic considerations if there is no gallbladder activity after a morphine challenge or after 4 hours in a patient with normal hepatic function and a normal biliary-to-bowel transit time?	Acute cholecystitis (in the appropriate clinical setting) Post-cholecystectomy Obstructing lesion of the cystic duct
When should a hepatobiliary scan be performed in a patient who has undergone cholecystectomy or liver transplantation?	When there are clinical signs of a biliary leak, such as ascites, increasing abdominal girth, or abdominal pain
How is the scan performed in these patients?	A normal scan is performed, although, naturally, one does not expect to opacify the gallbladder. If no abnormality is seen after 60 minutes, late images (typically at

2 and 4 hours post-injection) are obtained.

What are the nuclear medicine signs of a leak?

Activity outside the expected confines of the biliary system and bowel; may see activity increasing behind the liver

ESOPHAGUS

Describe 2 ways of assessing the esophagus radiographically, and the best applications for each modality.

An esophagogram (barium swallow) is optimal for evaluating mucosal disease, primary neoplasia, and symptoms of dysphagia. A CT scan (with or without contrast) evaluates the surrounding mediastinum for adenopathy as well as the esophagus and is best used when structures adjacent to the esophagus (e.g., the aorta) need to be evaluated for invasion.

List 5 causes of esophageal dilatation.

1. Postinflammatory distal stricture [e.g., as a result of gastroesophageal reflux disease (GERD)]
2. Carcinoma
3. Achalasia
4. Scleroderma
5. Diabetes (hypomotility)

What is achalasia?

Failure of the lower esophageal sphincter to relax and open; caused by degeneration of Auerbach's plexus

How does achalasia appear on barium swallow?

The distal esophagus has a "rat tail" appearance.

What is a potential complication of achalasia?

Tertiary contractions can lead to aspiration.

How is achalasia treated?

With balloon dilatation or a myotomy

What is scleroderma?

Scleroderma is a collagen vascular disease that can affect multiple parts of the gastrointestinal tract, including the esophagus, the stomach, and the small bowel. The process usually affects the lower two thirds of the esophagus, leaving the gastroesophageal junction wide open.

What is the radiographic appearance of the esophagus in scleroderma?

Esophageal dilatation with an open gastroesophageal junction

Absence of the primary stripping wave, indicating neuromuscular dysfunction

What are the characteristic findings of scleroderma in the small bowel?

Dilatation with malabsorption and tightly packed mucosal folds ("hide-bound" bowel)

What is a Zenker's diverticulum?

An outpouching of the lower hypopharynx through a weakness in the posterior wall just above the cricopharyngeus muscle (i.e., the upper esophageal sphincter)

What is the most common cause of Zenker's diverticulum?

Idiopathic dysfunction of the cricopharyngeus muscle

Name 4 causes of esophageal ulceration.

1. GERD
2. Infection [e.g., candidiasis, herpes simplex virus (HSV) infection, cytomegalovirus (CMV) infection]
3. Corrosive ingestion
4. Esophageal carcinoma (occasionally)

Name 3 causes of esophageal narrowing.

1. Esophageal carcinoma
2. Inflammatory strictures (e.g., as a result of GERD, surgical anastomosis, Barrett's esophagus, corrosive ingestion, nasogastric tube insertion, or *Candida* infection)
3. Extrinsic mass

What is the typical appearance of a reflux stricture?

Smooth area of narrowing in the mid- to distal esophagus

How does a reflux stricture differ in appearance from esophageal carcinoma?

A reflux stricture usually tapers, whereas an esophageal carcinoma often shows shouldering (*arrow*).

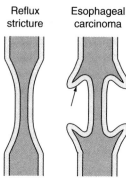

Reflux stricture   Esophageal carcinoma

List 4 radiographic features of GERD.	1. Evidence of reflux from the stomach into the esophagus on barium swallow 2. Ulceration 3. Strictures 4. Associated hiatal hernia (in some patients)
What is Barrett's esophagus?	A complication of GERD that changes the esophageal mucosa epithelium from squamous to columnar
What is the special concern associated with Barrett's esophagus?	Adenocarcinoma (risk is increased by approximately 10%)
Name 10 entities in the differential diagnosis of an esophageal filling defect.	**Intramural masses** 1. Esophageal carcinoma 2. Leiomyoma 3. Hematoma 4. Esophageal duplication **Intraluminal masses** 5. Foreign body or food **Extramural masses** 6. Mediastinal tumor or lymphadenopathy 7. Aortic aneurysm 8. Enlargement of the left atrium 9. Pancreatic pseudocyst 10. Anomalous subclavian artery
What are 3 causes of thick esophageal folds?	1. Esophagitis 2. Varicoid type of esophageal carcinoma (infiltrates submucosally) 3. Esophageal varices

What type of esophageal carcinoma is most common?

Squamous cell carcinoma (95% of cases)

What unique feature of the esophageal wall predisposes to mediastinal spread of tumor?

There is no serosal layer in the esophagus, so once the tumor spreads through the muscular wall, there is no barrier to prevent further spread.

What are the 4 radiologic types of esophageal carcinoma?

1. Polypoid (mass has a lobulated surface)
2. Varicoid (mass spreads superficially)
3. Ulcerating (mass with an ulcer)
4. Infiltrating (mass spreads rapidly deep in the wall, resulting in a diffuse narrowing, also known as "linitis plastica")

What are esophageal varices?

Dilated esophageal veins that serve as pathways for collateral flow

Trace the paths of flow that cause:

   Uphill varices

Portal vein, coronary vein, esophageal venous plexus, azygos/hemiazygos vein, superior vena cava (SVC), right atrium

   Downhill varices

SVC, azygos/hemiazygos vein, esophageal venous plexus, coronary vein, portal vein

List 4 causes of uphill varices.

Uphill varices result from portal venous hypertension or obstruction. Therefore, causes can include:
1. Alcoholic cirrhosis
2. Hepatic mass
3. Pancreatitis or pancreatic carcinoma
4. Portal vein thrombosis

List 3 causes of downhill varices.

Downhill varices are caused by SVC obstruction. Therefore, causes can include:
1. Mediastinal tumor (metastatic lung cancer most common)
2. Fibrosing mediastinitis
3. Thymoma

How are bleeding varices treated?

Short-term therapeutic measures include balloon tamponade with a Sengstaken-

Blakemore tube, endoscopic sclerotherapy, and endoscopic rubber banding. In order to achieve definitive treatment, however, the underlying cause must be addressed after bleeding has been controlled.

STOMACH

How is the stomach assessed radiographically, and what are the best applications for each modality?

An upper gastrointestinal study is the study of choice for evaluating malignancy and peptic ulcer disease. A gastric emptying study (a nuclear medicine examination) can be used to assess function.

What is a hiatal hernia?

A condition in which the proximal portion of the stomach slips through the esophageal hiatus into the thorax

What finding suggests a hiatal hernia?

Gastric folds more than 2 cm above the diaphragm

Describe the 2 types of hiatal hernia.

Sliding (axial) hiatal hernia: The gastroesophageal junction (B line) slides into the mediastinum above the diaphragm.

Rolling (paraesophageal) hiatal hernia: The gastroesophageal junction is in a normal location, but the gastric fundus "rolls" into the mediastinum. The potential for infarction makes this type of hiatal hernia a surgical emergency.

Which type of hiatal hernia is most common?

Nearly all hiatal hernias are of the sliding type.

List 6 causes of gastric outlet obstruction.

1. Benign stricture (e.g., as a result of acute or chronic peptic ulcer disease)
2. Crohn's disease of the stomach
3. Gastric neoplasm
4. Metastasis
5. Invasion of the stomach by pancreatic or colon cancer
6. Prior vagotomy or partial gastrectomy with anastomotic ulcer or bezoar

List 6 causes of nonobstructive gastric dilatation.

1. Neuromuscular disease (gastroparesis)
2. Diabetes (hypomotility)
3. Drug-induced dilatation
4. Vagotomy or other abdominal surgery
5. Swallowed air (anxious patients, patients in pain)
6. Recent endoscopy

Where do gastric ulcers usually occur?

On the lesser curvature near the antrum

Are most gastric ulcers benign or malignant?

Benign (95%)

Name 5 findings on an upper gastrointestinal study that indicate that a gastric ulcer is benign.

1. Extension of smooth gastric folds to the ulcer crater margin
2. Penetration of the crater beyond the normal margin of the lumen
3. Presence of Hampton's line (i.e., a thin mucosal line across the ulcer neck)
4. Presence of an ulcer collar (i.e., an edematous mucosal band across the ulcer neck)
5. Smooth transition from the surrounding edema mound to the normal stomach contour

List 3 findings that suggest that a gastric ulcer is malignant.

1. The ulcer crater is nodular and within the lumen of the stomach, suggesting ulceration of a mass projecting into the lumen.
2. A mass with irregular folds surrounds the ulcer.
3. The folds do not radiate to the ulcer.

How long should a gastric ulcer be followed?

Until complete healing is achieved

What are 11 causes of a gastric filling defect?

1. Gastric carcinoma
2. Lymphoma, especially non-Hodgkin's lymphoma
3. Metastatic disease, especially melanoma or breast tumors
4. Polyps (hyperplastic or adenomatous)
5. Leiomyoma
6. Leiomyosarcoma
7. Lipoma

8. Ectopic pancreas
9. Carcinoid
10. Hamartoma (Peutz-Jeghers syndrome, Cronkhite-Canada syndrome)
11. Kaposi's sarcoma

What is ectopic pancreas?

A pancreatic rest found in the greater curvature or the antrum of the stomach, or in the duodenum

How does ectopic pancreas appear radiographically?

As a solitary submucosal nodule with a central dimple (umbilication)

What is the most common histologic type of gastric malignancy?

Adenocarcinoma

Name 3 typical radiographic appearances of gastric carcinoma.

1. Polypoid (appears as a filling defect on barium study)
2. Ulcerative (a mass with an ulceration)
3. Infiltrating (results in a "linitis plastica" stomach)

What are the radiographic characteristics of each of the following types of gastric masses?

Gastric carcinoma

Irregular surface, may ulcerate

Metastatic disease

May ulcerate and have a "bull's-eye" appearance, usually multiple

Hyperplastic polyp

Smooth, approximately 1 cm in diameter, usually multiple

Adenomatous polyp

Irregular surface, solitary or few in number

Leiomyoma

Smooth, submucosal mass without mucosal irregularity

Leiomyosarcoma

Large, necrosis common, solitary

Carcinoid tumor

May ulcerate, solitary

Which type of gastric polyp is most common, adenomatous or hyperplastic?

Hyperplastic (75% of cases)

Which type of gastric polyp has malignant potential?	Adenomatous
Name the 4 most likely intraluminal gastric masses.	Food, bezoar, foreign body, blood clots
What is a linitis plastica stomach?	A narrowed stomach with a thickened wall and decreased motility; most often caused by malignancy or chronic inflammation and fibrosis

List 9 causes of a linitis plastica stomach.

1. Scirrhous carcinoma
2. Lymphoma
3. Metastatic disease, usually from the breast or lung
4. Neoplastic spread from an adjacent structure, such as the pancreas or transverse colon
5. Gastritis, especially that caused by peptic ulcer disease
6. Corrosive ingestion
7. Infection (e.g., tuberculosis or syphilis)
8. Sarcoidosis
9. Crohn's disease

List 6 causes of thickened gastric folds.

1. Gastritis (*Helicobacter pylori* gastritis, alcoholic gastritis, peptic ulcer disease, Zollinger-Ellison syndrome)
2. Gastric varices
3. Adjacent pancreatitis
4. Ménétrier's disease
5. Carcinoma
6. Lymphoma

What is the appearance of gastritis?	Gastritis is characterized by an area of focal thickening (usually in the gastric antrum) with punctate ulcerations
What is Ménétrier's disease?	A protein-losing enteropathy of unknown cause that results in gastric fold thickening, increased mucus production, and hyperchlorhydria
What is the appearance of Ménétrier's disease on an upper gastrointestinal study?	Diffuse gastric fold thickening

What is emphysematous gastritis?

Infection with a gas-forming organism results in gas in the gastric wall; can lead to infarction

Describe the 2 types of gastric volvulus.

1. Mesenteroaxial: Stomach twists perpendicular to the long axis on the mesentery
2. Organoaxial: Stomach twists around the long axis of the stomach

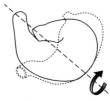

Mesenteroaxial

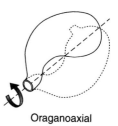

Oraganoaxial

Which type of volvulus is more serious?

Mesenteroaxial volvulus, because of the potential for ischemia

What is the treatment of volvulus?

Surgery

SMALL BOWEL

Describe a logical approach to evaluating the abnormal small bowel.

Dilatation (3 cm or more): Is the dilatation caused by mechanical obstruction or muscle dysfunction (e.g., adynamic ileus)?

Fold thickening (3 mm or more): Are the folds regular or irregular? Is the stomach involved?

Filling defects: Are the defects multiple or solitary? Is the "bull's-eye" sign present?

Loop separation: Are the loops separated from one another by more than 6 mm?

List 10 causes of duodenal obstruction.

1. Inflammation
2. Peptic ulcer disease
3. Pancreatitis
4. Congenital annular pancreas
5. Pancreatic neoplasia (e.g., pancreatic carcinoma)
6. Duodenal neoplasia (e.g., duodenal adenocarcinoma)
7. Metastasis
8. Intraluminal diverticulum (windsock deformity)
9. SMA syndrome
10. Hematoma

What is congenital annular pancreas?

The ventral pancreatic bud develops abnormally and encircles the duodenum.

What may congenital annular pancreas be confused with?

Duodenal carcinoma

What is the most common cause of hemorrhage in the duodenal wall?

Trauma (crushing of the duodenum against the vertebrae)

What is SMA syndrome?

Relative obstruction of the third portion of the duodenum owing to compression from the SMA; usually seen in cachectic patients

Name 4 causes of jejunal or ileal dilatation.

1. Mechanical obstruction
2. Adynamic ileus
3. Scleroderma
4. Malabsorption syndromes (e.g., sprue)

How are mechanical obstruction and adynamic ileus distinguished from one another?

In obstruction, there is a distinct transition point between the dilated segment and the normal segment, whereas in adynamic ileus, the entire bowel is dilated. In obstruction, dynamic air-fluid levels (i.e., air-fluid levels at different levels within the same loop of bowel) are present, which indicates peristalsis.

Name 10 causes of mechanical small bowel obstruction.

Extrinsic causes
1. Adhesions (75% of cases)
2. Hernia (20% of cases)
3. Extrinsic mass
4. Volvulus

Intramural causes
5. Stricture (e.g., as a result of Crohn's disease or radiation therapy)
6. Intramural mass (e.g., metastasis, primary carcinoid)
7. Intussusception (caused by a mass or polyp)

Intraluminal causes
8. Gallstone ileus
9. Foreign body
10. Meconium ileus

What is gallstone ileus?

A gallstone erodes through the wall of the gallbladder, passes into the small bowel (often the duodenum), and then travels to the terminal ileum, where it obstructs the lumen and results in mechanical small bowel obstruction.

Name 10 causes of adynamic ileus.

1. Any surgical procedure
2. Peritonitis
3. Vagotomy
4. Drugs (narcotics, anticholinergics)
5. Trauma
6. Ischemia
7. Radiation therapy
8. Connective tissue diseases
9. Malabsorption syndromes
10. Metabolic disorders (e.g., diabetes, hypothyroidism, hyperkalemia)

List 6 common causes of malabsorption.

1. Celiac disease, such as nontropical sprue (i.e., insensitivity to gluten leading to bowel dilatation and intussusceptions)
2. Scleroderma
3. Whipple's disease
4. Parasitic infestation (e.g., giardiasis, schistosomiasis)
5. Endocrine causes (e.g., VIPoma, Zollinger-Ellison syndrome)
6. Infiltration (e.g., lymphoma, Waldenström's macroglobulinemia)

How does sprue lead to ileus and bowel dilatation?	The malabsorption syndrome causes increased fluid in the bowel.
What are the characteristic findings of sprue on SBFT studies?	Segmentation of the small bowel (i.e., clumps of barium separated by strings of barium) and dilution of barium
What is the appearance of peptic ulcer disease in the duodenum?	Ulcer craters and mounded tissue are usually seen in the duodenal bulb. The mucosal folds may be thickened.
Are duodenal ulcers usually malignant?	No, virtually all are benign.
What is the most common cause of a cloverleaf deformity of the duodenal bulb?	Scarring from peptic ulcer disease
What is Zollinger-Ellison syndrome?	An unregulated gastrin-secreting islet cell tumor of the pancreas leads to hyperacidity, which in turn results in thickening of the duodenal folds and ulceration in the duodenum and proximal jejunum.
What is the main distinctive radiographic feature of Zollinger-Ellison syndrome?	Multiple, post-bulbar ulcers
What entity may result in a barium collection outside of the lumen, mimicking an ulcer?	Duodenal diverticulum
What is a duodenal diverticulum?	A herniation of the mucosa and serosa through the muscular portion of the duodenal wall; usually of no clinical significance
What is the most common site of a duodenal diverticulum?	The medial wall of the second part of the duodenum
What are 6 causes of thickened duodenal folds?	1. Duodenitis (e.g., as a result of peptic ulcer disease or Zollinger-Ellison syndrome) 2. Infection (*Giardia lamblia*, *Strongyloides stercoralis*, *Mycobacterium tuberculosis*)

3. Paraduodenal inflammation (e.g., pancreatitis, cholecystitis)
4. Infiltration (e.g., Whipple's disease)
5. Vascular disorders (e.g., varices, hemorrhage)
6. Neoplasia (e.g., lymphoma)

Name 8 causes of regular thickened small bowel folds.

When the folds are **regular,** perpendicular to the lumen, and parallel to each other, **think fluid** as the cause of the thickening:
Hemorrhage into the bowel wall
1. Coagulation defects (e.g., anticoagulant therapy, liver disease, hemophilia)
2. Trauma
3. Ischemia or infarction
Intestinal edema
4. Hypoproteinemia (seen in cirrhosis, Ménétrier's disease)
5. Ascites
6. Mesenteric lymphatic or venous obstruction
7. Zollinger-Ellison syndrome
8. Giardiasis

What are 4 causes of bowel ischemia?

Atherosclerosis, emboli, hypotension (nonocclusive mesenteric ischemia), venous occlusion

Name 9 causes of irregular thickened small bowel folds.

Think cellular infiltration with **irregular** folds:
1. Lymphoma
2. Metastases
3. Crohn's disease
4. Whipple's disease
5. Cystic fibrosis
6. Mastocytosis
7. Amyloidosis
8. Giardiasis
9. Typhoid

What is Peutz-Jeghers syndrome?

Hamartomas of the small bowel (may also be seen in the stomach or colon)

What are the clinical features of Cronkhite-Canada syndrome?

Skin changes, alopecia, and adenomatous polyps

What is seen in Gardner's syndrome?

Gardner's syndrome is usually characterized by adenomas in the colon, but the small bowel can also be affected.

Name 7 causes of thickened small bowel folds with stomach involvement.

1. Lymphoma
2. Ménétrier's disease
3. Crohn's disease
4. Whipple's disease
5. Zollinger-Ellison syndrome
6. Amyloidosis
7. Eosinophilic gastroenteritis

What is eosinophilic gastro-enteritis?

Eosinophilic gastroenteritis is an uncommon disorder characterized by eosinophilic infiltration of the bowel folds, especially in the duodenum and gastric antrum. Patients usually have peripheral eosinophilia. The clinical course is characterized by remissions and exacerbations.

Name 5 causes of a duo-denal filling defect.

1. Duplication cyst
2. Choledochocele
3. Ectopic pancreas
4. Neoplasm
5. Peptic ulcer disease

What is Crohn's disease?

An idiopathic relapsing enteritis affecting the small bowel and colon

What are 6 radiographic signs of Crohn's disease?

1. Fold thickening or nodules (as a result of bowel wall edema)
2. Aphthous ulcers (can progress to deep ulcers)
3. Fistulas (may lead to abscess formation)
4. "Skip" lesions
5. Stranding (inflammation) in mesenteric fat and fatty proliferation
6. Filiform polyps as the mucosa heals

In what part of the gastro-intestinal tract is Crohn's disease most likely to be seen?

Terminal ileum

What is a fistula called between the small bowel and the:

   Bowel?

Enteroenteric

   Skin?

Enterocutaneous

   Bladder?

Enterovesicular

   Vagina?

Enterovaginal

How is a fistula treated?

Bowel rest (i.e., parenteral nutrition), relief of any downstream obstruction, treatment of any adjacent abscesses (i.e., percutaneous drainage)

List 12 causes of solitary small bowel filling defects.

1. Adenocarcinoma
2. Leiomyoma
3. Leiomyosarcoma
4. Lymphoma (but usually multiple)
5. Metastasis (but usually multiple)
6. Neurofibroma (but usually multiple)
7. Carcinoid tumor
8. Adenoma
9. Kaposi's sarcoma
10. Endometrioma
11. Foreign body
12. Gallstone

What is a carcinoid tumor?

Carcinoid tumors, the most common primary tumors of the small bowel and mesentery, are tumors of neuroendocrine origin.

What is the carcinoid syndrome?

A syndrome characterized by diarrhea, flushing, and bronchospasm that is caused by excess serotonin metabolite

Are carcinoid tumors of the bowel usually associated with carcinoid syndrome?

No. Most carcinoid tumors in the bowel do not produce vasoactive peptides, which are responsible for the carcinoid syndrome.

Where do carcinoid tumors occur most often?

The appendix (40% of cases) and the ileum (30% of cases)

What are the most common sites of metastasis for carcinoid tumors?

The liver (typically a hypervascular metastasis) and the lymph nodes

What is the appearance of a carcinoid tumor on CT or SBFT testing?

A mural mass, often with tethering of the bowel folds and mesentery owing to a desmoplastic reaction.

What is the rule of thirds for carcinoid?

One third multiple, one third carcinoid syndrome, one third metastatic, one third associated with another malignancy

What are the imaging features of small bowel lymphoma?

Masses (may be large, ulcerated, and thick-walled) or nodules, fold thickening, mesenteric or periaortic lymphadenopathy

List 8 causes of multiple small bowel filling defects.

1. Lymphoid hyperplasia
2. Metastases (e.g., melanoma, breast cancer, bronchial tumors, gastrointestinal tumors larger than 4 mm)
3. Lymphoma
4. Leiomyomas (but usually solitary)
5. Neurofibromas
6. Polyposis syndromes (e.g., Peutz-Jegher's syndrome, Cronkhite-Canada syndrome, Gardener's syndrome)
7. Foreign bodies
8. Carcinoid tumor (but usually solitary)

Are most symptomatic small bowel tumors benign or malignant?

75% are malignant.

What are 4 causes of small nodules found in the mucosa of the small bowel?

1. Lymphoma
2. Lymphoid hyperplasia (nodules are 2–4 mm in size)
3. Polyps
4. Metastases

List 4 causes of small bowel nodules in a patient with AIDS.

1. CMV infection
2. *Mycobacterium avium-intracellulare* infection
3. *Cryptosporidium* infection
4. Lymphoma

List 6 causes of multiple small bowel "bull's-eye" lesions.

Metastatic neoplasia (60% of cases)
1. Melanoma
2. Breast, renal, or pulmonary carcinoma

3. Kaposi's sarcoma
Primary neoplasia
4. Carcinoid tumors
5. Lymphoma
6. Neurofibromatosis

What 6 entities cause a solitary small bowel "bull's-eye" lesion?

1. Peptic ulcer (most often in the duodenum)
2. Leiomyoma
3. Leiomyosarcoma
4. Adenocarcinoma
5. Ectopic pancreas
6. Metastasis (melanoma, breast tumor)

Name 6 causes of a wide or distorted duodenal C-loop.

1. Pancreatic disorders (e.g., pancreatitis, pancreatic cancer)
2. Abscess (pancreatic or lesser sac)
3. Enteric duplication cyst
4. Lymphadenopathy
5. Spread of neoplasia from an adjacent structure (e.g., the stomach, colon, or kidney)
6. Lymphoma

List 11 causes of real or apparent separation of bowel loops.

Intrinsic causes
1. Thickened bowel wall
2. Hemorrhage
3. Ischemia
4. Neoplasm (e.g., lymphoma)
5. Inflammation (e.g., Crohn's disease, Whipple's disease, tuberculosis)
Extrinsic causes
6. Ascites (e.g., as a result of liver disease, peritonitis, peritoneal carcinomatosis)
7. Extrinsic neoplasia (e.g., lymphoma, metastatic lesions)
8. Endometriosis
9. Abscess
10. Desmoplastic processes (especially carcinoid)
11. Mesenteric lipomatosis

LARGE BOWEL

List 12 causes of a polypoid colonic filling defect.

1. Hyperplastic polyp (most often multiple and less than 5 mm in diameter)

2. Adenomatous polyp
3. Hamartomatous (inflammatory) polyp
4. Filiform polyp
5. Lipoma (usually solitary)
6. Villous adenoma
7. Metastatic lesion (usually multiple)
8. Carcinoid tumor
9. Lymphoma (usually multiple)
10. Feces
11. Gallstone
12. Foreign body

Which polyps have malignant potential?

Adenomatous polyps

What are 3 types of adenomatous polyps?

1. Tubular (polypoid)
2. Villous (sessile, flat, frond-like)
3. Tubulovillous

Of these 3 types of adenomatous polyps, which has the highest potential for malignancy?

Villous adenomatous polyps

Where in the colon is cancer most likely to develop?

Rectosigmoid colon (60% of cases), left colon to the mid-transverse colon (25% of cases), right colon (15% of cases)

How does the size of an adenomatous polyp correlate with the likelihood of developing cancer?

Polyps with a diameter of less than 1 cm are associated with a 1% risk of cancer; those with a diameter of 1–2 cm are associated with a 10% risk of cancer; and those with a diameter of more than 2 cm are associated with a 25%–50% risk of cancer.

What are the radiographic characteristics of:

Benign colonic polyps? (List 6)

1. Smooth surface
2. Long stalk
3. Normal mucosa
4. Small diameter
5. Stable in growth
6. Spherical shape

Malignant colonic polyps? (List 6)

1. Irregular shape
2. Sessile

3. Puckered mucosa
4. Large diameter
5. May exhibit sudden growth
6. Base broader than height

What 3 factors increase the risk for colon carcinoma?

Polyp size, polyposis syndromes, family history

What is familial polyposis?

Familial polyposis, the most common polyposis syndrome, is an inherited disease characterized by the development of numerous adenomatous polyps throughout the colon and rectum. These polyps usually occur in childhood and undergo malignant degeneration as the patient matures.

What is the treatment for familial polyposis?

Colectomy is curative.

What are the clinical features of Gardner's syndrome?

Gardner's syndrome must be **STOPPED**

Soft tissue tumors
Teeth abnormalities
Osteomas
Polyps (adenomatous)
Pigmentation of the skin
Epidermoid or sebaceous cysts
Desmoid tumors

m

What percentage of colon carcinomas are:

Synchronous (i.e., two separate cancers occurring simultaneously)?

5%

Metachronous (i.e., two separate cancers occurring at different times)?

5%

List 9 causes of multiple colonic filling defects.

1. Hyperplastic polyps (90% of cases)
2. Adenomatous polyps
3. Hamartomatous polyps
4. Multiple adenocarcinomas
5. Lymphoma
6. Metastases (usually from the breast, lung, or ovary)

7. Lymphoid hyperplasia > 4 mm (e.g., as a result of lymphoma, Crohn's disease, or AIDS prodrome)
8. Endometriosis
9. Foreign bodies (e.g., food, tablets, stool)

List 12 causes of a cecal filling defect.

1. Carcinoma
2. Lipoma
3. Metastases (usually from the ovary, stomach, or colon)
4. Carcinoid tumor
5. Appendicitis
6. Appendiceal stump
7. Lipomatous ileocecal valve
8. Mucocele of appendix
9. Periappendiceal abscess
10. Diverticulitis
11. Intussusception
12. Fecal matter

What are 6 causes of colonic narrowing?

1. Carcinoma
2. Diverticulitis
3. Colitis (idiopathic, infectious, ischemic, or as a result of radiation therapy)
4. Endometriosis
5. Pelvic lipomatosis
6. Metastasis

What is the typical route of spread of metastatic tumor through the mesentery to the colon?

Gastric cancer typically spreads to the superior surface of the transverse colon through the gastrocolic ligament. Pancreatic cancer typically spreads to the inferior surface of the transverse colon through the transverse mesocolon.

What are 3 radiographic signs of severe colitis?

1. Loss of haustrations
2. Thickening and irregularity of the colonic mucosa
3. Toxic megacolon

What is ulcerative colitis?

A chronic idiopathic colitis characterized by superficial ulceration in a continuous pattern beginning in the rectum

Compare ulcerative colitis and Crohn's disease:

	Ulcerative Colitis	*Crohn's Disease*
Continuous?	Yes	No
Symmetric?	Yes	No
Portion of gastrointestinal tract most often affected?	Colon only	Ileum, colon
Mucosal, transmural, or submucosal?	Mucosal	Transmural or submucosal
Type of ulceration?	Superficial	Deep and linear
Pathologic finding?	Thumbprinting	Cobblestoning
Risk of colon cancer?	High	Much lower
Bloody stool?	Common	Rare
Complications?	Toxic megacolon, backwash ileitis	Fistulae, fissures, strictures
Prognosis?	Colectomy curative	Risk of recurrence after resection

What causes pseudomembranous colitis?

Overgrowth of *Clostridium difficile* (as a result of antibiotic administration)

What is the pseudomembrane formed of?

Sloughed mucosa and white blood cells (WBCs)

How can a diagnosis of pseudomembranous colitis be confirmed?

Detection of *C. difficile* toxin in a stool sample

How is pseudomembranous colitis treated?

With metronidazole or oral vancomycin

What is typhlitis (neutropenic colitis)?

An inflammatory colitis occurring in neutropenic patients (especially patients with leukemia who are undergoing chemotherapy) that is characterized by thickening of the cecum, ascending colon, or both and carries the risk of perforation and peritonitis.

What are the clinical signs of typhlitis?

Abdominal pain and diarrhea

How may appendicitis be assessed radiographically?

Plain film, ultrasound, CT, or barium enema

What is the CT appearance of appendicitis?

1. Diameter of appendix > 6 mm
2. Stranding in periappendiceal fat
3. Thickened, enhancing walls
4. Periappendiceal abscess may be seen (if appendix has perforated)

What percentage of patients with acute appendicitis have a calcified appendicolith?

10%–15% on plain films; 25% on CT

Are patients with an appendicolith and RLQ pain likely to have a perforated appendix?

Yes.

What is a mucocoele of the appendix?

A distended, obstructed appendix filled with mucus

Name 2 causes of a mucocoele of the appendix.

1. Chronic obstruction from an appendicolith
2. Mucus-secreting tumors of the appendix (e.g., cystadenoma or cystadenocarcinoma)

What dangers are associated with a mucocoele of the appendix?

Rupture can lead to pseudomyxoma peritonei.

Where do most diverticula occur?

The sigmoid colon (65%–70% of cases) and the ascending colon (25%–30% of cases)

On what side of the colon do diverticuli occur?

The antimesenteric side, between the taenia

What modality is best for evaluating diverticular disease?

Barium enema is best for evaluating diverticula; CT is best for evaluating diverticulitis.

What are the CT findings of diverticulitis?

Focal bowel wall thickening, stranding in the pericolonic fat, possibly gas collection adjacent to the wall

List 7 causes of a cone-shaped cecum.

1. Crohn's disease with involvement of the terminal ileum
2. Ulcerative colitis
3. Tuberculosis
4. Amebiasis (cecum involved in 90% of cases)
5. Carcinoma
6. Blastomycosis or actinomycosis
7. Typhlitis (neutropenic colitis)

What is toxic megacolon?

Toxic megacolon is a syndrome of colonic dilatation and abdominal pain, fever, and leukocytosis. Because spontaneous perforation occurs in 50% of cases, toxic megacolon is associated with a high mortality rate.

What are the plain film findings of toxic megacolon?

Distention of the colon, often with an edematous wall

Which portion of the colon is typically affected in toxic megacolon?

The transverse colon

How can obstruction be ruled out as a cause of the distention?

With decubitus films

What are 7 causes of toxic megacolon?

Ulcerative **C**olitis **IS A P**ain, **C**harlie
Ulcerative colitis (75% of cases)
Crohn's disease
Ischemic colitis
Shigellosis
Amebic colitis
Pseudomembranous colitis
Chagas' disease

m

List 9 causes of colonic obstruction.

1. Carcinoma
2. Diverticulitis
3. Volvulus (sigmoid more than cecal)
4. Hernias (internal, external, or diaphragmatic)
5. Invasive pelvic malignancy
6. Intussusception
7. Postinflammatory stricture
8. Endometriosis
9. Fecal impaction

What is Ogilvie's syndrome?

Large bowel pseudo-obstruction (i.e., idiopathic dilatation of the large bowel, especially the cecum, that is often seen in critically ill or bedridden patients)

How is Ogilvie's syndrome treated?

If it doesn't resolve, surgical or endoscopic decompression may be necessary.

List 5 causes of colonic thumbprinting.

Smooth folds (as a result of fluid accumulation)

1. Hemorrhage
2. Ischemic edema
3. Inflammatory edema (e.g., as a result of pseudomembranous colitis, idiopathic colitis, diverticulitis, pancreatitis, typhlitis)

Irregular folds (as a result of cell infiltration)

4. Lymphoma
5. Metastatic lesions

What are 3 components of the AIDS complex that can be seen on CT?

1. Rectal stranding (i.e., edema around the rectum)
2. Adenopathy
3. Splenomegaly

In patients with AIDS, what disorders are most common in the:

Esophagus?

Candidiasis and HSV infection

Stomach and small bowel?

Lymphoma and Kaposi's sarcoma

Small bowel?

Mycobacterium avium-intracellulare and *Cryptosporidium* infection

Large bowel?

CMV infection

Rectum?

Lymphogranuloma venereum

LIVER

List 6 causes of homogeneous increased liver echoes on ultrasound.

1. Fatty infiltration (e.g., as a result of Cushing's disease, steroid therapy, obesity, diabetes, alcoholism, or hyperalimentation)
2. Cirrhosis
3. Hepatitis (although most patients have normal echogenicity)
4. Amyloidosis
5. Leukemic infiltration (often normal to low echogenicity)
6. Hemochromatosis

What is the normal CT density of the liver, as compared with the spleen?

Normally, the CT density of the liver is greater than that of the spleen. If the density of the liver on CT is less than that of the spleen, fatty change is likely.

Name 2 ways fatty infiltration can simulate a lesion in the liver on CT.

Focal fatty infiltration: The low-density region emulates a low-attenuation metastasis. Fat often occurs adjacent to the falciform ligament; don't be fooled.

Fatty sparing: In a fatty infiltrated liver, if part is spared, the normal liver may have the appearance of a hyperdense mass when compared with the fatty infiltrated liver.

What are 6 signs of cirrhosis at imaging?

1. Nodularity of the liver surface
2. Small, shrunken liver
3. Ascites
4. Large caudate lobe
5. Recanalized umbilical vein
6. Irregular enhancement

Is there an increased risk of hepatocellular carcinoma with cirrhosis?

Yes. The risk of malignancy is also increased with several other causes of liver failure, including hemochromatosis, Wilson's disease, aflatoxin, chronic active hepatitis, and thorotrast.

In a cirrhotic liver, what lesion may mimic hepatocellular carcinoma?

A regenerating nodule

What is hemochromatosis?

Iron overload leading to deposition in the liver and spleen

What are the 2 types of hemochromatosis?

Primary: Caused by abnormal absorption in the intestine
Secondary: Caused by multiple transfusions

How can primary hemochromatosis be differentiated from secondary hemochromatosis?

If the pancreas is involved, the hemochromatosis is usually of the primary type.

What are the characteristics of hemochromatosis on:

Ultrasound?

Hyperechoic liver

CT?

Dense liver (> 75 HU)

Magnetic resonance imaging (MRI)?	Liver and spleen are very hypointense owing to paramagnetic effect
What are 2 other causes of increased liver attenuation as seen on CT?	Wilson's disease and amiodarone toxicity
What is most common mass seen in the liver?	Simple hepatic cyst
What is the most common cause of a hyperechoic liver mass on ultrasound?	Hemangioma (i.e., a benign proliferation of vascular tissue)
What is meant by the phrase, "lesion too small to characterize"?	Some lesions less than 1 cm in diameter do not reveal enough of their nature because of their small size, and therefore, cannot be characterized by imaging.
How are these lesions managed?	In patients without a known malignancy, they may be assumed to be benign. In cancer patients, they are problematic; close follow-up or laparoscopy are two options.

List 7 entities in the differential diagnosis of a solitary hepatic mass.

1. Cyst
2. Metastasis
3. Focal nodular hyperplasia (FNH)
4. Adenoma
5. Hepatoma
6. Fatty infiltration
7. Hemangioma

What are the characteristics of a simple hepatic cyst on:

Ultrasound?	Anechoic, sharp rear wall, increased transmitted sound
CT?	Density of less than 20 HU, well-defined margins, no enhancement after contrast administration

What is the appearance of a hemangioma on:

Ultrasound?	Hyperechoic and well-defined
Noncontrast CT?	Low attenuation

Contrast CT?	Focal nodular enhancement (usually peripheral), may appear as bright as the aorta initially, centripetal enhancement from the periphery may be noted if followed to the late phase
Nuclear medicine?	Lesion fills in on red blood cell (RBC) scan
T$_1$-weighted MRI?	Hypointense to liver; with gadolinium-diethylenetriamine penta-acetic acid (Gd-DTPA), peripheral enhancement is seen initially and most lesions "fill in" within 15–30 minutes; enhancement is persistent
T$_2$-weighted MRI?	Hyperintense to liver—as bright as a light bulb, with an intensity as high as that of pure fluid [e.g., cerebrospinal fluid (CSF), bile]
Gradient echo MRI?	Low signal intensity
Do large hemangiomas behave differently from smaller ones?	Yes; if large, they may appear hetero-geneous. There may be thrombosis, or a central stellate scar with a giant hemangioma.
Which study is particularly useful for diagnosing hemangiomas greater than 2 cm in diameter?	Nuclear medicine (tagged RBCs)
In which group of patients is FNH most likely to be seen?	Young women
What is the appearance of FNH on:	
Ultrasound?	Appearance is variable, but low echoes in the center may be seen.
Noncontrast CT?	Lesion has low attenuation compared with the normal liver; a central stellate scar may also show low attenuation
Contrast CT?	Homogenous enhancement, but may enhance early

Nuclear medicine?	Takes up sulfur colloid
T_1-weighted MRI?	Hyperintense to liver; central scar enhances with Gd-DTPA
T_2-weighted MRI?	Isointense to slightly hyperintense to liver; central scar is hyperintense
With which class of prescription drugs is adenoma associated?	Oral contraceptives
What are the clinical features of an adenoma?	Benign, may be seen with pregnancy, may enlarge, has a tendency to bleed

What is the appearance of an adenoma on:

Noncontrast CT?	Low attenuation
Contrast CT?	No marked enhancement, may see hemorrhage
Nuclear medicine?	Does not take up sulfur colloid
T_1-weighted MRI?	Heterogeneous, with areas of increased signal from both fat and hemorrhage
T_2-weighted MRI?	Heterogeneous, with areas of increased signal; on in- and out-of-phase imaging, a decrease in signal on the out-of-phase sequence is seen if the lesion contains fat

A cystic liver mass with internal echoes is noted on ultrasound examination. Name 6 potential diagnoses.

1. Hemorrhagic cyst
2. Abscess
3. Echinococcal cyst
4. Biliary cystadenoma
5. Metastasis
6. Hepatocellular carcinoma with necrosis

What is the most common malignant mass in the liver?

Metastasis

What are the 3 most common sources of metastasis to the liver?

1. Primary tumors of the gastrointestinal tract (e.g., tumors of the colon, pancreas, or stomach)
2. Breast tumors
3. Lung tumors

What is the blood supply to most metastases?

Hepatic artery

What are the hypervascular liver tumors?

2 primary tumors + 5 metastases
   (**MRI CT**)
Hepatocellular carcinoma
FNH
Melanoma
Renal cell carcinoma
Islet cell tumor of the pancreas
Carcinoid tumor
Thyroid cancer

When are hypervascular masses best seen on CT?

During the arterial phase (however, many are also seen well during the portal venous phase)

What is the appearance of most metastases in the portal venous phase?

Most metastatic tumors are hypodense during the portal venous phase of bolus or ynamic CT. Some may have rim enhancement.

Can metastases calcify?

Yes.

What are 5 risk factors for hepatocellular carcinoma?

Hepatocellular carcinoma typically occurs in an abnormal liver. Risk factors include:
1. Cirrhosis of any cause (especially alcoholic cirrhosis)
2. Hemochromatosis
3. Steroid use
4. Hepatitis B or C infection
5. Liver fluke infestation (especially in Southeast Asia)

What are the characteristics of hepatocellular carcinoma?

Single, multiple, or diffuse lesions may be seen. Lesions are often accompanied by hemorrhage and necrosis.

Does hepatocellular carcinoma invade vascular structures?

Yes. It tends to invade the portal and hepatic veins and may cause thrombosis.

What is the appearance of hepatocellular carcinoma on:

   Noncontrast CT?

Hypodense; calcification may be seen

   Contrast CT?

Dense, diffuse nonuniform enhancement; some lesions are hypervascular

T₁-weighted MRI?	Variable signal, reflecting fatty change and fibrosis Hypointense to liver with contrast enhancement (will enhance with Gd-DTPA) Hypervascular lesions enhance early with Gd-DTPA
T₂-weighted MRI?	Typically hyperintense to liver (although the lesion may appear hypointense if hemochromatosis is present) A "capsule" may be seen
What are 4 causes of a calcified liver mass?	1. Granulomatous disease 2. Metastasis from the colon or stomach 3. Hepatocellular carcinoma 4. Hematoma
List 5 causes of portal vein thrombosis.	1. Pancreatitis 2. Cirrhosis 3. Hepatic or biliary surgery 4. Hepatoma with tumor thrombus 5. Hypercoagulable states
What is cavernous transformation of the portal vein?	Recanalization of the periportal collateral vessels following thrombosis of the portal vein
What is Budd-Chiari syndrome?	Hepatic vein obstruction, usually thrombosis, leading to portal hypertension and ascites
What causes Budd-Chiari syndrome?	Most cases are idiopathic, although the syndrome has been associated with hypercoagulable states (e.g., polycythemia vera, malignancy, oral contraceptive use).
How does Budd-Chiari syndrome appear on:	
Ultrasound?	Absent flow in the hepatic veins or IVC; inhomogeneous echoes
CT?	Hepatosplenomegaly and ascites, patchy enhancement
Why is the caudate lobe spared?	Venous drainage from the caudate lobe is directly to the IVC.

BILIARY SYSTEM, PANCREAS, AND SPLEEN

BILIARY SYSTEM

List 9 causes of a nonvisualized gallbladder with shadowing in the gallbladder fossa on ultrasound.

1. Chronic cholecystitis (gallbladder contracted around stones)
2. Emphysematous cholecystitis
3. Porcelain gallbladder
4. Nonfasting patient (normally contracted gallbladder and air in the bowel)
5. Post-cholecystectomy (imaging the duodenum instead)
6. Gallbladder obscured by gas
7. Ectopic gallbladder
8. Carcinoma of the gallbladder
9. Metastases to the gallbladder bed

What is the thickness of the normal gallbladder wall?

≤ 3 mm

Using ultrasound, where should the gallbladder wall be measured?

At the wall adjacent to the liver

What are 6 causes of gallbladder wall thickening?

Gallbladder wall thickening is a non-specific finding; therefore, the clinical setting is critical to making the diagnosis. Potential diagnoses include:
1. Acute cholecystitis
2. Pancreatitis
3. Ascites
4. Liver disease (e.g., hepatitis) or hypoproteinemia
5. Fluid overload [e.g., as a result of congestive heart failure (CHF)]
6. Cancer of the gallbladder

What is the initial study that should be used to evaluate RUQ pain?

Ultrasound

Why?

Ultrasound can easily diagnose acute cholecystitis, gallstones, and other causes of RUQ pain unrelated to the gallbladder.

When is a hepatobiliary scan most helpful?

Nuclear medicine may be very useful if the clinical suspicion is high for gallbladder pathology and ultrasound results are negative.

What are 6 ultrasound findings in acute cholecystitis?

1. Focal gallbladder tenderness
2. Increased gallbladder size [i.e., anterior-posterior (AP) diameter of more than 4 cm]
3. Wall thickening (greater than 3 mm)
4. Impacted stone in gallbladder neck
5. Pericholecystic fluid collection
6. Intraluminal complex echoes

How do gallstones appear on ultrasound?

Echogenic focus, acoustic shadowing (i.e., dark behind stone), mobile (i.e., they move when the patient changes position)

Name 6 causes of non-shadowing intraluminal gallbladder echoes on ultrasound.

1. Small calculi
2. Tumefactive sludge (i.e., calcium bilirubinate and cholesterol crystals)
3. Post-lithotripsy (therapy for gall-stones)
4. Blood clots
5. Inflammatory mass of debris (e.g., fungus balls)
6. Cholesterol crystals

What is the sonographic Murphy's sign?

The patient reports pain as the operator presses on the gallbladder as guided by ultrasound.

What finding is most accurate in excluding acute cholecystitis?

Lack of focal gallbladder tenderness is the most accurate finding for excluding acute cholecystitis—the predictive value of a negative finding is 90%. (In other words, if focal gallbladder tenderness is **not** found, then the chance of a patient having acute cholecystitis is 10%.)

What percentage of patients with cholecystitis have acalculous cholecystitis?

10%

What 3 groups of patients tend to develop acalculous cholecystitis?

1. Patients who are fasting or receiving hyperalimentation [e.g., those in the intensive care unit (ICU)]
2. Patients with AIDS
3. Patients with diabetes

What imaging modality is most useful for diagnosing acalculous cholecystitis?

A nuclear medicine DISIDA or HIDA scan demonstrates nonvisualization of the gallbladder.

What is a porcelain gall-bladder?

Calcification of the gallbladder wall owing to inflammation

What is the concern in these patients?

Gallbladder cancer develops in 25% of patients with porcelain gallbladder.

What is emphysematous cholecystitis?

Gas in the gallbladder wall as a result of infection; usually seen in patients with diabetes

What is adenomyomatosis?

Hyperplasia of the gallbladder wall that leads to outpouching of the wall over the Rokitansky-Aschoff sinuses

How may adenomyomatosis appear on ultrasound?

Multiple intraluminal triangular echoes (comet tail artifact)

What is "milk of calcium" bile?

Bile becomes very concentrated in an obstructed gallbladder and precipitates, forming a layer of high-density material called "milk of calcium" bile.

List the 5 causes of a fixed intraluminal gallbladder mass.

1. Primary carcinoma of the gallbladder
2. Metastatic lesion
3. Polypoid cholesterolosis
4. Adenomyomatosis
5. Papillary adenoma

Is gallbladder cancer common?

It is uncommon, but more common than other types of biliary tract cancer.

Describe 2 mechanisms that can lead to dilatation of the common bile duct.

1. Common bile duct obstruction (e.g., as a result of calculi; tumors of the bile duct, pancreas, or duodenum; post-inflammatory strictures; or inflammatory change in the pancreas, such as a pancreatic pseudocyst)
2. Cholecystectomy (following cholecystectomy, the duct may be as wide as 10 mm)

How can you determine if the duct is truly obstructed (as opposed to atonic)?

Administer cholecystokinin (CCK) or have the patient eat a fatty meal—if the duct is truly obstructed, it will dilate in response to these measures.

Where is intrahepatic biliary duct dilatation best seen in the liver?

Intrahepatic biliary duct dilatation is usually seen easily in the left lobe, and these ducts may dilate earlier if the whole system is obstructed.

What is Mirizzi syndrome?

Extrinsic compression of the common hepatic duct caused by a stone impacted in the gallbladder neck.

What is primary sclerosing cholangitis (PSC)?

An inflammatory process of unknown cause that involves the biliary ducts

What are the risk factors?

Family history, ulcerative colitis

What is the frequency of association with ulcerative colitis?

25%–75% of patients with PSC have ulcerative colitis, but fewer than 5% of patients with ulcerative colitis have PSC.

How does PSC appear on imaging studies?

Multiple irregular dilatations and strictures of the ducts

What is ascending cholangitis?

Bacterial infection (usually by Gram-negative rods) of the biliary tract; often seen in patients with biliary obstruction

What organisms cause cholangitis in patients with AIDS?

CMV, *Cryptosporidium*

What is the most common primary malignancy of the biliary system?

Cholangiocarcinoma

Is cholangiocarcinoma usually intra- or extra-hepatic?

The extrahepatic distal common bile duct is affected in 50%–70% of cases.

What is a Klatskin's tumor?

Cholangiocarcinoma that arises at the bifurcation of the left and right hepatic ducts

What is Caroli's disease?

A congenital disorder characterized by multiple saccular dilatations of the biliary system without obstruction

What are the clinical features of Caroli's disease?

Cholecystitis (may develop as a result of stasis), renal abnormalities (i.e., medullary sponge kidney), and cholangitis

Identify the following appearances on ERCP:

A = Gallstones
B = Obstructing gallstone
C = Cholangiocarcinoma
D = PSC
E = Bacterial cholangitis
F = Pancreatic carcinoma
G = Mirizzi syndrome
H = Postsurgical stenosis

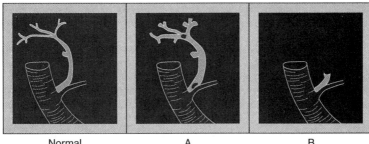

Normal   A   B

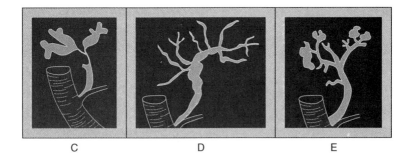

C   D   E

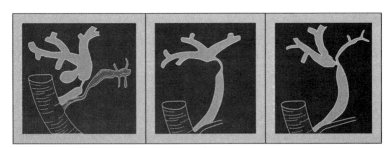

F   G   H

PANCREAS

List 7 causes of a focal pancreatic enlargement.	1. Primary adenocarcinoma 2. Focal pancreatitis 3. Islet cell tumor 4. Metastasis 5. Lymphoma 6. Cystadenoma 7. Cystadenocarcinoma
What are the plain radiographic signs of acute pancreatitis?	Duodenal ileus with gas filling the duodenal C-loop Jejunal ileus (not as specific as duodenal ileus) Colon cut-off sign (not specific for pancreatitis) Thickening of the wall of the transverse colon with loss of haustra Soft tissue mass between the stomach and transverse colon Left pleural effusion, left basilar atelectasis, elevated left diaphragm
What imaging modalities are best for evaluating pancreatitis?	CT and ultrasound, although the latter may have blind spots owing to overlying bowel gas
When should a CT scan be ordered for a patient with suspected pancreatitis?	When complications of pancreatitis (e.g., pancreatic pseudocyst, abscess, or fluid collections) are suspected
Name 2 applications of ultrasound evaluation in a patient with suspected pancreatitis.	1. To look for complications 2. To evaluate for gallstones as the cause of the pancreatitis
What are 4 CT signs of pancreatitis?	1. Enlarged pancreas with loss of normal internal structure 2. Fluid collections 3. Pancreatic duct dilatation and stricture 4. Stranding in peripancreatic fat
Can pancreatitis always be diagnosed on the basis of CT findings?	No. The pancreas may appear normal in mild pancreatitis.
How are fluid collections classified in pancreatitis?	**Acute fluid collections** include peripancreatic fluid collections (infected or

sterile) and pancreatic necrosis. **Chronic fluid collections** (those developing over 4–6 weeks) include abscesses and pseudocysts.

What percentage of fluid collections in pancreatitis resolve spontaneously?

50%

When and how should a fluid collection be drained?

Fluid collections should be drained when they are large, infected, or symptomatic. They may be drained percutaneously or surgically. Percutaneous drainage is associated with a lower morbidity rate and a shorter hospital stay post-procedure.

What percentage of patients with acute pancreatitis develop a pancreatic abscess?

2%–6%

Compare an endoscopic retrograde cholangiogram in a patient with chronic pancreatitis to one taken in a patient with pancreatic cancer.

In a patient with chronic pancreatitis, a beaded, dilated duct with sacculations is seen, whereas in a patient with pancreatic cancer, stenosis with distal dilatations or an abrupt cut-off (*arrow*) is seen.

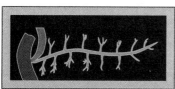

Normal

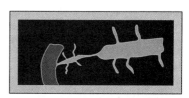

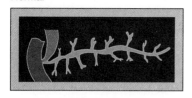

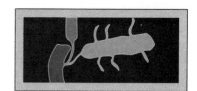

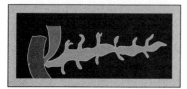

Chronic pancreatitis

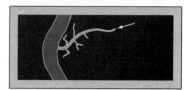

Pancreatic cancer

What is the plain radio graphic sign of chronic pancreatitis?

Pancreatic calcification (multifocal or chunky)

What characteristics help to distinguish pancreatic cancer from focal pancreatitis?

Pancreatic cancer is indicated by metastatic disease, invasion of the fat surrounding the SMA, and adenopathy.

What is the best way of distinguishing pancreatic cancer from focal pancreatitis?

Needle biopsy

Where do most pancreatic cancers arise?

In the pancreatic head, causing atrophy of the tail

What features render a pancreatic tumor unresectable?

Vascular encasement (i.e., of the SMA, celiac artery, SMV, or portal vein), distant metastases, or involvement of the regional lymph nodes

What is the best way of assessing the resectability of a pancreatic cancer?

CT

What is the typical appearance of pancreatic cancer on ultrasound?

A low echogenicity mass (95% of cases) causing bile duct obstruction

What other findings help to make the diagnosis?

Pancreatic duct dilatation (more than 2 mm), metastatic lesions, and adenopathy

What is the most common histologic type of pancreatic neoplasia?

Adenocarcinoma

What are the other subtypes of pancreatic neoplasia?

Serous cystadenoma or mucinous cystadenoma/cystadenocarcinoma
Islet cell tumor
Solid and papillary epithelial neoplasm

What 7 signs of pancreatic adenocarcinoma are seen on CT?

1. Focal mass
2. Atrophy of the gland distal to the mass
3. Bile duct dilatation
4. Pancreatic duct dilatation
5. Metastatic lesions (usually in the nodes, liver, or lung)
6. Fat plane invasion
7. Splenic vein obstruction

Is calcification a common feature of pancreatic adenocarcinoma?

No, unless the tumor arises in a focus of chronic pancreatitis

Is the double duct sign specific for pancreatic cancer?

No, it may also be seen in focal pancreatitis.

What are 3 causes of a cystic pancreatic mass?

1. Complicated pseudocyst
2. Abscess
3. Cystic or necrotic neoplasm

What are the 2 cystic pancreatic neoplasms?

Serous cystadenoma and mucinous cystadenoma/cystadenocarcinoma

Compare microcystic pancreatic neoplasms (i.e., serous cystadenoma) and macrocystic pancreatic neoplasms (i.e., mucinous cystadenoma/adenocarcinoma).

	Microcystic	*Macrocystic*
Gender of patient?	Female > male 3:2	Female > male 6:1
Age of patient?	> 60 years	40–60 years
Benign or malignant?	Benign	Many malignant (10%–20% metastasize)
Number of cysts?	> 6	< 6
Size of cysts?	< 2 cm	> 2 cm
Area of pancreas?	Head	Body and tail
Appearance?	Can appear solid, stellate scar formed of calcium	Always appear cystic

What is a solid and papillary epithelial neoplasm?

An uncommon low-grade malignancy with both solid and cystic components most often found in young women

What are islet cell tumors?

Tumors arising from endocrine pancreatic tissue

List 3 islet cell tumors.

Insulinoma, gastrinoma, glucagonoma

What is the most common secreting islet cell tumor?

Insulinoma

How are insulinomas best imaged?

Insulinomas are small; therefore, they are best seen on intraoperative ultrasound.

They may also be detectable on CT or MRI if dedicated protocols used.

What syndrome does a gastrinoma cause?

Zollinger-Ellison syndrome

What nuclear medicine test can be used for the diagnosis of gastrinoma?

Octreotide scan (octreotide is a somatostatin analog)

What clinical syndromes are associated with pancreatic neoplasms?

von Hippel-Lindau disease may be associated with pancreatic cysts, adenomas, and islet cell tumors. Multiple endocrine neoplasia, type I (MEN-I) may have pituitary, parathyroid, and pancreatic involvement.

In what other condition are pancreatic cysts seen?

Autosomal dominant polycystic kidney disease

SPLEEN

What are the acceptable limits for normal splenic size (long axis):

    On radiographs?

15 cm (owing to magnification)

    On CT or ultrasound?

13–14 cm

What are 8 causes of splenomegaly?

1. Cirrhosis with portal hypertension
2. Right-sided heart failure
3. Lymphoma
4. Leukemia
5. Myeloproliferative disease
6. Infection (including protozoal infection)
7. Erythropoietic diseases (e.g., spherocytosis, thalassemia)
8. Infiltrative and storage disorders (e.g., Gaucher's disease, mucopolysaccharidoses)

List 8 causes of a small spleen.

1. Any autoimmune process
2. Sickle cell disease
3. Essential thrombocythemia
4. Congenital abnormality
5. Irradiation

6. Malabsorption
7. Inflammatory bowel disease
8. Collagen vascular disease

**What is the CT appearance
of splenic infarction:**

   On contrast CT?

A wedge-shaped area of absent
enhancement. The base of the wedge is at
the periphery of the spleen

   On noncontrast CT?

Low attenuation wedge shaped area

**List 4 causes of splenic
infarction.**

1. Septic emboli (bacterial endocarditis)
2. Pancreatitis
3. Sickle cell disease
4. Polycythemia vera

**Which neoplasms may
occur in the spleen?**

Hodgkin's lymphoma
Non-Hodgkin's lymphoma
Metastatic lesions
Primary malignancy (spindle cell or
   vascular sarcomas)
Benign tumors (hamartoma or
   hemangioma)

**What are the typical
appearances of lymphoma?**

Splenomegaly
Often no definable mass
Occasionally hypovascular mass or masses

**List 5 non-neoplastic causes
of a splenic mass.**

1. Cyst (epithelial or epidermoid)
2. Hematoma
3. Infarction
4. Abscess
5. Sarcoidosis

**List 5 differential diagnoses
for a cystic splenic lesion.**

1. Parasitic cyst (most common
   worldwide)
2. Epidermoid cyst
3. Post-traumatic lesion (most common
   in the United States)
4. Abscess
5. Infarct

**What is polysplenia
(bilateral left-sidedness)?**

Multiple spleens

**What is asplenia (bilateral
right-sidedness)?**

No spleen

What are 5 anomalies associated with:

Polysplenia (bilateral left-sidedness)?

1. Cardiac septal defects (acyanotic)
2. Incomplete IVC with azygos continuation
3. Trilobed lungs
4. Abdominal situs inversus
5. Gallbladder absence

Asplenia (bilateral right-sidedness)?

1. Congenital cardiac anomalies (severe)
2. Left-sided IVC
3. Bowel malrotation
4. Situs ambiguous
5. Large transverse liver

What are 7 causes of splenic calcifications?

1. Histoplasmosis
2. Tuberculosis
3. Brucellosis
4. Old infarct
5. Healed abscess
6. Cyst wall calcification
7. *Pneumocystis carinii* pneumonia (PCP)

List the 4 most commonly injured abdominal organs following a motor vehicle crash (MVC).

From most to least, the most commonly injured abdominal organs as a result of an MVC are the spleen, the liver, the pancreas, and the kidney.

What is the test of choice to assess splenic trauma?

CT with rapid infusion of contrast and fast scanning

What is the appearance of a subcapsular hematoma?

A low-attenuation crescentic mass conforming to the shape of the spleen

What is the appearance of splenic laceration?

A nonenhancing linear region with low attenuation

What entities may mimic a splenic laceration?

Accessory spleen, splenic clefts, large left hepatic lobe, splenic infarction

What are the risk factors for poor outcome in patients with splenic injury?

Shattered spleen, active bleeding, extension into the hilum

Are all splenic injuries treated surgically?

No. Splenic lesions may be treated conservatively if the patient is stable.

Salvage of the spleen is often possible and preferable.

Does a normal dynamic CT scan rule out a splenic injury?

No. Some hematomas may be isodense to the surrounding spleen on CT, but this is very rare.

What are 3 nontraumatic causes of splenic rupture?

Infectious mononucleosis, viral hepatitis, and coagulopathies

PERITONEUM

What are 6 causes of ascites?

1. Liver disease (e.g., cirrhosis)
2. Fluid overload (e.g., CHF, renal failure)
3. Massive metastatic disease
4. Peritonitis (malignant or infective)
5. Ovarian neoplasm
6. Trauma leading to intraperitoneal hemorrhage

How do you differentiate loculated fluid from free peritoneal fluid on a CT scan?

Decubitus positioning causes nonloculated fluid to flow to a dependent portion.

What is the appearance of an abscess on CT?

Low density center (may be higher if an infected hematoma)
Rim of enhancement
Gas bubbles may or may not be present, but usually indicate an infected fluid collection

In the diagnosis of an abscess, what are the:

Advantages of CT?

CT can be thought of as a "radiologic exploratory laparotomy"—this modality gives an all-encompassing image, is not affected by bowel gas, can be used to assess a route for drainage, and may locate other abnormalities.

Advantages of ultrasound?

Ultrasound, which is most effective in the right upper quadrant (RUQ), can be performed at the bedside and does not expose the patient to ionizing radiation.

Limitations of ultrasound?	Gas may limit examination of the mid-abdomen, and ultrasound cannot be used to definitively rule out abscess.
What is pseudomyxoma peritonei?	Pseudomyxoma peritonei is filling of the peritoneal space with mucinous material, usually as a result of metastasis from a cystadenocarcinoma of the appendix or ovary. The mucinous material forms gelatinous masses that appear cystic on CT but may calcify.
What is the appearance of pseudomyxoma peritonei on CT?	High attenuation ascites and thickening of the peritoneum Scalloping of the liver surface

ACUTE ABDOMEN

What radiographic views are needed to assess an acute abdomen?	Supine and upright views of the abdomen and an upright posterior-anterior (PA) chest film.
Which view is most sensitive for pneumoperitoneum?	The upright chest film
If the patient is too ill to stand or sit upright, what other view may be used?	A left lateral decubitus view (i.e., taken with the left side down) can be used to look for free air over the liver.
List 4 radiographic signs of pneumoperitoneum.	1. Free air under the diaphragm on an upright film 2. Gas outlining the falciform ligament 3. Gas on both sides of the bowel wall (the double wall sign) 4. Air between the liver and the abdominal wall laterally on a left lateral decubitus film
Name 5 causes of pneumo-peritoneum.	1. Ruptured hollow viscus (duodenal ulcer is the most common cause of ruptured hollow viscus) 2. Surgery 3. Pneumatosis cystoides intestinalis 4. Steroid therapy 5. Air forced through fallopian tubes
Following surgery, how quickly should pneumo-peritoneum resorb?	Within 4–5 days (longer with a large volume of air or in an obese patient)

List 6 causes of pneuma-tosis intestinalis.

1. Bowel necrosis
2. Emphysematous gastritis
3. Mucosal disruption (e.g., as a result of peptic ulcer disease)
4. Immunocompromise (e.g., as a result of AIDS, steroid therapy, or lymphoma)
5. Pulmonary disease [e.g., chronic obstructive pulmonary disease (COPD), asthma, cystic fibrosis]
6. Overdistention as a result of obstruction or endoscopy

Are patients with pneuma-tosis intestinalis typically very ill?

Usually, but not necessarily. The patient with pneumatosis caused by bowel necrosis may be septic and morbidly ill, but if the cause is COPD or immuno-deficiency, the patient may be entirely asymptomatic.

How may gas in the portal veins be distinguished from gas in the bile ducts on:

Plain film radiography?

On plain films, portal venous gas extends to the periphery of the liver and biliary ductal gas is central in the bile ducts. The gas travels in the normal direction of flow in the structure (i.e., portal gas flows to the periphery like portal blood, and biliary gas stays central, where bile flows).

On CT?

On CT, anatomic placement usually makes it apparent whether the portal veins or the biliary ducts are gas-filled. The portal veins are larger and located posterior to the ducts.

What are the causes of portal venous gas?

Portal venous gas is an ominous sign because it usually signals bowel necrosis associated with ischemia. Rarely, portal venous gas can result from a barium enema, peptic ulcer disease, ulcerative colitis, or adynamic ileus.

What is pneumobilia?

Gas in the bile ducts

List 6 causes of pneumobilia.

1. Iatrogenic pneumobilia, as a result of ERCP or sphincterotomy

2. Surgery (e.g., biliary enteric anastomosis)
3. Fistulization between the biliary tract and the bowel, such as occurs with peptic ulcer erosion
4. Malignancy with erosion
5. Gallstone ileus (i.e., erosion of a gallstone into the bowel)
6. Infection by a gas-forming organism (e.g., *Clostridia, Bacteroides fragilis*)

List 5 radiographic signs of ascites.

1. "Floating" of bowel loops to the mid-abdomen on the supine view
2. Displacement of bowel loops (more than 6 mm apart from each other)
3. Generalized abdominal haziness ("ground glass")
4. Displacement of the large bowel from the flank stripe
5. "Dog ears" sign (not usually useful)

Name 4 radiographic signs of mechanical bowel obstruction.

1. The transition point [i.e., large-caliber bowel loops proximal to the site of obstruction (as a result of distention) and small-caliber bowel loops distal to the site of obstruction]
2. A large quantity of fluid in the bowel loops proximal to the obstruction
3. The stairstep sign (i.e., air-fluid levels on an upright film)
4. The "string of pearls" sign

How can bowel obstruction be assessed radiographically?

Plain radiography is the least expensive and least sensitive method, because fluid-filled loops may not be seen. CT is 90% sensitive and shows the transition point in 50%–75% of patients (i.e., dilated bowel turns to collapsed bowel). A barium enema, SBFT study, or enteroclysis may also be used. Enteroclysis is the most sensitive method, but is difficult for patients.

What would be the best approach to take with a patient with suspected bowel obstruction?

1. Obtain plain films first. The "obstruction" might be constipation. Furthermore, barium studies might compromise the quality of a CT scan.
2. If large bowel obstruction is

suspected, a barium enema should be performed. This study will be cleared in 1 day, permitting another study of the small intestine (i.e., enteroclysis) to be performed if necessary. If the small bowel study is done first, the barium may not be readily cleared.

3. If small bowel obstruction is suspected and there is no known cause, a CT scan can be very helpful.

What are the radiographic signs of adynamic (paralytic) ileus?

Paralytic ileus is characterized by multiple distended loops of bowel and usually involves the small intestine and colon.

It may be difficult to differentiate an ileus from an early or partial small bowel obstruction. Name one way of differentiating the two.

Dynamic air-fluid levels suggest obstruction.

Name 4 ways that ileus can be distinguished from low colonic obstruction.

1. Perform a digital rectal examination.
2. Insert a rectal tube or sigmoidoscope.
3. Demonstrate gas in the rectum on prone, lateral, or decubitus radiographs (taken with the right side down).
4. Perform a single-contrast barium enema evaluating just the distal colon.

In a patient with ileus, which segments of the bowel are most typically distended with gas on a supine abdominal radiograph?

The most anterior portions of the bowel (i.e., the transverse colon and small bowel)

Gross distention of which portion of the bowel is the greatest threat to perforate?

The cecum—patients may require endoscopic or surgical decompression, even if the distention is caused by ileus rather than mechanical obstruction.

Why is the cecum most prone to perforation?

The cecum has the largest diameter of the intestinal segments. According to Laplace's law, the surface tension is proportional to the radius of the lumen and the pressure [i.e., the tension (T) equals the pressure (P) multiplied by the radius (R).]

What is the ideal position of a Dobhoff feeding tube if the patient is at risk for aspiration?

The tip of the feeding tube should be located in the distal duodenum or proximal jejunum.

8 Genitourinary Imaging

John P. Schreiber

ANATOMY

KIDNEY AND RENAL COLLECTING SYSTEM

Identify the parts of the kidney and renal collecting system

A = Pelvis
B = Calyx
C = Fornix
D = Cortex
E = Capsule
F = Infundibulum
G = Renal sinus fat
H = Medulla
I = Papilla

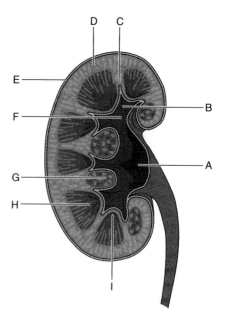

What are the contents of the renal pedicle?

Renal artery
Renal vein

Collecting system and ureter
Lymphatics

What are the contents of the retroperitoneal spaces?

Anterior pararenal space: Duodenum, pancreas, colon (Note that fluid from pancreatitis or ruptured duodenum may accumulate here.)

Perirenal space (Gerota's fascia marks the boundaries): Kidneys, adrenal glands, renal pelvis, ureter, fat (important for staging renal cell cancer)

Posterior pararenal space: Flank stripe (extraperitoneal fat), no organs

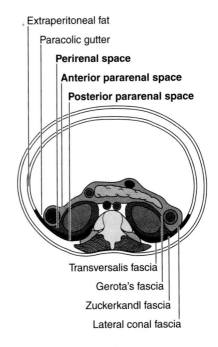

Extraperitoneal fat
Paracolic gutter
Perirenal space
Anterior pararenal space
Posterior pararenal space

Transversalis fascia
Gerota's fascia
Zuckerkandl fascia
Lateral conal fascia

What is the ureteropelvic junction (UPJ)?

The UPJ is where the renal pelvis becomes the ureter.

What is the ureterovesical junction (UVJ)?

The UVJ is the junction of the ureter and bladder.

Why is the UVJ notable?

It is the most common location of impacted kidney stones.

PROSTATE GLAND

What is the zonal anatomy of the prostate gland, and which disease processes typically arise in each zone?

Peripheral zone: Most cancers
Transitional zone: Benign prostatic hypertrophy (BPH)
Central zone: Few cancers

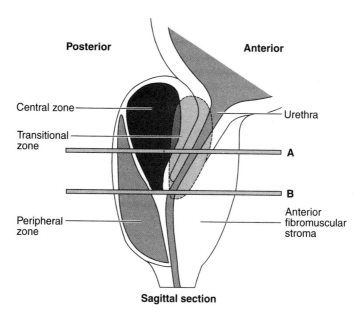

Sagittal section

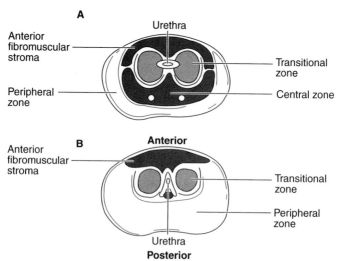

Transverse sections

URETHRA

Describe the anatomy of the urethra.

Posterior urethra = prostatic + membranous portions
Membranous urethra demarcates the urogenital diaphragm
Anterior urethra = bulbous + penile portions

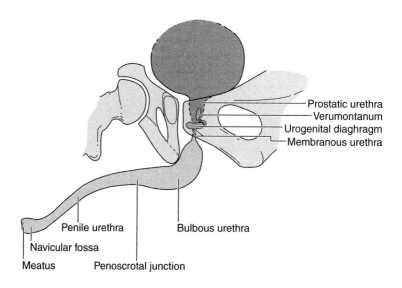

Prostatic urethra
Verumontanum
Urogenital diaghragm
Membranous urethra

Penile urethra   Bulbous urethra
Navicular fossa
Meatus   Penoscrotal junction

What structures enter the urethra at the verumontanum?

The ejaculatory ducts

SCROTUM AND TESTIS

Identify the labeled parts of the scrotal contents:	A = Vas deferens B = Head of epididymis C = Testicle D = Septa E = Tunica albuginea F = Tail of epididymis G = Tunica vaginalis

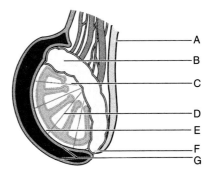

Describe the anatomy of the epididymis.	The epididymis lies **posterolateral** to the testis. It has an expanded head that lies at the upper pole of the testis, a body, and a tail that is directed downward and continues as the vas deferens.
What is the tunica vaginalis?	A serous cavity that surrounds the anterior, medial, and lateral surfaces of the testes
Identify these portions of scrotal anatomy:	A = External oblique muscle B = Peritoneum C = Superior pubic ramus D = Vas deferens E = Pampiniform plexus F = Tunica vaginalis

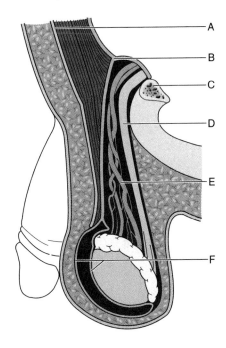

ADRENAL GLANDS

What is the size of the normal adrenal gland?

The limbs are 3–6 mm thick. The length of the entire adrenal gland is 4–6 cm.

How do you find the adrenals on a computed tomography (CT) scan?

Look just superior to the kidneys. The right adrenal is posteromedial to the right lobe of the liver, posterior to the inferior vena cava (IVC), and lateral to the right crus of the diaphragm. The left adrenal is lateral to the aorta and left crus of the diaphragm and posterior to the splenic vessels at the cephalad aspect.

IMAGING TECHNIQUES

USE OF INTRAVENOUS (IV) CONTRAST

What is the risk of contrast-induced nephrotoxicity?

3%–7%

What are the risk factors?

Pre-existing renal insufficiency (serum creatinine ≥ 1.4 mg/dl), diabetes mellitus, dehydration

What factors increase the relative risk of allergic reaction in a patient?

Prior reaction to IV contrast (best predictor), asthma, allergies

What are the incidences of mild, moderate, and severe reactions to ionic IV contrast?

Mild = 5%
Moderate = 1%–2%
Severe (life-threatening) = 0.09%–0.4%

What is the incidence of death due to IV contrast?

~1 in 75,000

How should you evaluate a patient who is having a reaction to IV contrast?

Take the patient's blood pressure and pulse; ask about the patient's symptoms; observe skin for hives

Consider oxygen and IV fluids if the patient has breathing problems or is hypotensive

Most reactions occur within 30 minutes of injection—observe until all symptoms abate

What is the treatment for contrast reactions?

It depends on the severity and type of reaction.

What is the treatment for:

Urticaria?

Treatment is not needed in most cases. If symptoms do not resolve spontaneously, then diphenhydramine (50 mg IV) is given.

Hypotension?

Place the patient in the Trendelenburg position and administer 500 ml of isotonic fluid [normal saline (0.9%) or lactated Ringer's solution].

Hypotension with brady-cardia?

Place the patient in the Trendelenburg position and administer fluids and atropine (0.6–1.0 mg IV). (Vasovagal)

Hypotension with tachy-cardia?

Place the patient in the Trendelenburg position and administer fluids and epinephrine (1–3 ml 1/10,000 IV every 5–10 minutes as needed, up to three times). An electrocardiographic monitor should be used when administering IV epinephrine. Administer oxygen by nasal cannula or mask.

Facial or laryngeal edema?

Call a code. Evaluate the patient's airway and intubate or perform cricothyrotomy, if necessary. Administer oxygen via a nasal cannula or mask. Give epinephrine (1 ml 1/10,000 IV slow push over 3–4 minutes).

Bronchospasm?

Administer oxygen via a nasal cannula or mask. If the patient does not respond, use a β-agonist inhaler (metaproterenol or albuterol). Give epinephrine (0.1–1.0 ml 1/1000 subcutaneously every 15 minutes as needed, up to three times or a total dose of 1 mg).

What is nonionic contrast?

Ionic contrast has sodium or meglumine associated with a carboxyl group off the iodine containing the benzene ring. Nonionic contrast has hydroxyl groups that do not dissociate in solution. The main difference clinically is that the osmolality is much lower, making it similar to blood.

What are the benefits of nonionic compared with ionic contrast?

Nonionic contrast is associated with one-fifth as many mild, moderate, and severe reactions and causes much less patient discomfort.

What are the limitations?

Cost—nonionic contrast is 5–10 times more expensive than ionic contrast.

What medication should be given prophylactically to patients with a true history of contrast allergy?

Methylprednisolone (32 mg orally, 12 hours and 2 hours prior to injection) or dexamethasone (4 mg orally every 6 hours for 24 hours prior to injection). The patient should get *nonionic* contrast. Ask yourself:

- Does the patient **really** need this study?
- Are other modalities available [e.g., ultrasound, magnetic resonance imaging (MRI)]?

Why does metformin, an oral hypoglycemic agent, affect the decision to give IV contrast?

IV contrast could cause renal failure, compromising the patient's ability to excrete metformin, so the patient could become profoundly hypoglycemic.

What is the recommendation?	Discontinue metformin at the time of the study and for 48 hours after IV contrast. Check renal function prior to reinstating metformin.
What is extravasation?	Injection of contrast into the tissues around the vein
What is the concern if this happens to a patient?	The skin may develop blisters and could potentially slough.
How much extravasated contrast should cause concern?	Be concerned if more than 30 ml of ionic contrast or more than 100 ml of nonionic contrast are extravasated.
What is the recommended treatment?	**Elevate** the extremity above the level of the heart; maintain this position, if possible, for approximately 24 hours. The patient should apply **ice packs** or **cold compresses** 3 times daily until the area is normal. Maintain contact with the patient by phone until the problem is resolved.
What is vicarious excretion?	Normally, only 1% of IV contrast is excreted by the liver and gastrointestinal tract. In patients with compromised renal function or large contrast loads, more contrast must be excreted by extrarenal means. Vicarious excretion is usually seen as a fluid-contrast level in the gallbladder 1–2 days after the contrast load.
How is the concentration of IV contrast measured?	In milligrams of iodine per milliliter of contrast. This makes the total dose to the patient calculable: 100 ml of 300 mg I/ml = 30 g I, and 100 ml of 350 mg I/ml = 35 g I. Usually, the dose in any 24-hour period is limited to 60 g I, if possible.

RADIOLOGY AND INTRAVENOUS PYELOGRAPHY (IVP)

What can IVP evaluate in the genitourinary system?	IVP provides both functional and anatomical information and is relatively inexpensive. The whole urinary tract can be seen on just a few films.
How much contrast is administered for an IVP?	20–30 g of iodine for the average adult patient (100 ml of 300 mgI/ml = 30 g)

What is a KUB?

A coned plain radiograph of the abdomen centered lower to include the kidneys, ureters, and bladder (KUB). A KUB is the first film taken in IVP.

In IVP, describe the path of contrast medium to the collecting system.

The contrast medium is injected intravenously and is carried in the blood to the kidneys, where it passes into the glomerular filtrate. Contrast is not absorbed by the tubules, so substantial concentration is achieved in the urine.

On what factors are the density of the nephrogram and the density of the pyelogram dependent?

Visualization of the renal substance (the nephrogram) depends on the amount of contrast reaching the kidneys.
Visualization of the collecting systems (the pyelogram) depends mainly on the ability of the kidneys to concentrate the urine.

What films are routinely obtained during IVP?

Preliminary film
1-minute nephrogram film (possible tomograms if question of hematuria or mass)
5-minute film in Trendelenburg position (a compression band is used after the 5-minute film to compress the ureters and distend the collecting system if there is a question of a calyceal or ureteral lesion)
10-minute film of the collecting system
Delayed film of the bladder
Post-void film of the bladder

How does one evaluate IVP films?

Preliminary film. The scout film is in essence a plain film of the abdomen centered lower (i.e., a KUB). Think, **"gas, mass, stones, bones."**

- Find renal shadows and evaluate the size and axis (should parallel the axis of the psoas muscles).
- Evaluate renal shadows and the course of the ureters and bladder for calcifications, which can be obscured by contrast medium.
- Look for bowel pathology (evaluate the caliber and wall thickness).

- Examine the bony structures.
- Check the corners of the film (lung bases).

Nephrogram. Evaluate the following:

- **Size:** Normal adult kidney = 10–16 cm
- **Shape:** Reniform?
- **Symmetry:** Prompt, bilateral, symmetrical nephrograms?
- **Contour:** Any local indentations or bulges?
- **Orientation:** Axes parallel to the outer margins of the psoas muscles?

Pyelogram. Evaluate the following:

- **Calices** should be evenly distributed and reasonably symmetrical. The normal calyx is "cupped," and the dilated calyx is "clubbed." The renal pelvis is extremely variable in location, size, and shape (look for filling defects within the renal pelvis).
- **Ureters** usually are seen in only part of their length on any one plain film because of obliteration of the lumen by peristalsis. No portion of either ureter should be more than 7 mm in diameter. Note any displacement of these structures.
- **Bladder** should have a smooth outline. After micturition, the bladder should be empty; otherwise, there is a post-void residual.

List 9 causes of unilateral nonvisualization (i.e., no contrast in or out; no urine out) on IVP.

1. Ureteral obstruction
2. Renal artery obstruction
3. Renal vein thrombosis
4. Fractured kidney
5. Neoplasm
6. Ectopic kidney
7. Absent kidney (agenesis associated with duplication of uterus or vagina)
8. Severe infection (tuberculosis or xanthogranulomatous pyelonephritis)
9. Multicystic kidney

What is a persistent nephrogram?

The nephrogram should fade as the contrast is excreted into the calices. If this doesn't happen, and the nephrogram is seen past 10 minutes, it is persistent.

What is the hypotensive nephrogram sign?

The appearance of **bilateral persistent nephrograms** during an excretory urogram suggests arterial hypotension and indicates the need for an immediate blood pressure determination.

List 7 causes of a persistent nephrogram on IVP.

1. Ureteral obstruction
2. Hypotension
3. Ischemia
4. Acute renal failure
5. Glomerulonephritis
6. Acute tubular necrosis
7. Renal vein thrombosis

What is a striated nephrogram?

A striated nephrogram has striations or stripes through the renal cortex instead of a homogeneous enhancement:

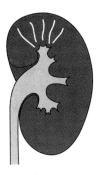

List 5 causes of a striated nephrogram.

1. Acute obstruction
2. Renal vein thrombosis
3. Acute pyelonephritis
4. Infantile polycystic kidney disease
5. Medullary sponge kidney (contrast in dilated tubules)

ULTRASOUND

Describe typical findings on an ultrasound of the urinary tract.

Kidneys: Smooth in outline; 9–12 cm long in adults

Renal cortex: Homogenous echoes that are less echoic than the adjacent liver or spleen

Renal pyramids: Triangular sonolucent areas adjacent to the renal sinus

Ureters: Not usually visualized (a calculus may be visualized in the UVJ)

Urinary bladder: Examine while distended; the walls should be sharply defined and barely perceptible

D = diaphragm; L = liver; U = upper pole of the kidney; C = renal cortex; E = central echo complex (surrounded by parenchyma; contains fat, vessels, and the collecting system); P = renal pyramid

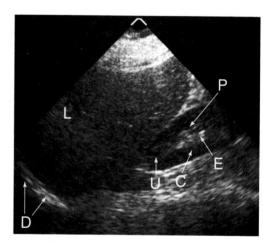

COMPUTED TOMOGRAPHY (CT)

How is CT used to evaluate the genitourinary system?

CT is great for focal parenchymal problems such as **renal masses.** Another major advantage is the delineation of the adjacent **retroperitoneum,** which can be useful for evaluating tumors, abscesses, and lymphadenopathy. Spiral CT also is excellent for diagnosing **calculi without IV contrast.**

What should you look for in a CT of the urinary tract?

Kidneys: Smooth outline; uniform and symmetrical opacity after administration of IV contrast

Pelvicaliceal system: Cupped calices with uniform width of renal parenchyma from calix to renal edge

Ureters: Seen in cross-section as dots lying on the psoas muscles and not necessarily visible at all levels; may not be opacified if scanned early (i.e., within 2 minutes)

Bladder: Smooth outline; wall is thin and of reasonably uniform diameter; the dependent portion is usually more opacified because contrast medium is heavier than urine

How is CT performed for evaluation of possible renal mass?	Noncontrast images are obtained. Routine abdominal CT scans are optimized for the liver at 70-second delay in the renal corticomedullary phase. Thin slices (5 mm) are performed during the diffuse nephrogram phase (≥ 100 seconds after injection).
What are the major uses for MRI in the genitourinary tract?	Evaluation of adrenal masses not diagnosed by CT Evaluation of renal masses in patients allergic to iodine or who have diminished renal function Staging of renal cell cancer

RETROGRADE PYELOGRAPHY

What are the indications for retrograde pyelography?	It is used when the information cannot be obtained by less invasive means (e.g., IVP, ultrasound). It also gives excellent resolution of the mucosal surfaces of the urothelium and dynamic information regarding flow and distensibility (e.g., with strictures).
What is the technique for antegrade and retrograde pyelography?	Both are performed by directly injecting contrast material into the pelvicaliceal system and ureters. For retrograde pyelography, a catheter is placed via cystoscopy into the ureter. For antegrade pyelography, the catheter is placed percutaneously into the kidney via the flank.

VOIDING CYSTOURETHROGRAPHY (VCUG)

List 5 applications for VCUG.	1. To identify and quantitate vesicoureteric reflux

2. To investigate the anatomy of the bladder neck and urethra
3. To show obstructions, such as strictures or urethral valves
4. To demonstrate the emptying of the bladder and the control of micturition
5. To evaluate voiding dysfunction and neurogenic bladder

How is VCUG performed?   Contrast medium is instilled into the empty bladder through a catheter. The bladder is filled to capacity, and films are taken during voiding. The process should be observed fluoroscopically so that any vesicoureteric reflux can be observed, and bladder contractility can be assessed.

RETROGRADE URETHROGRAPHY (RUG)

List 3 indications for RUG.
1. To identify urethral strictures
2. To check for extravasation from the urethra or bladder neck following trauma or surgery (prostatectomy)
3. Prior to placement of a Foley catheter in a trauma patient with gross hematuria

How is RUG performed?   RUG can be part of cystography, and it can be performed by a retrograde injection technique (i.e., a retrograde urethrogram).

NUCLEAR MEDICINE

What are the types of renal scanning?   Dynamic (functional) renal imaging and cortical imaging

List 4 indications for dynamic (functional) renal imaging.
1. Suspected renal obstruction (furosemide renogram)
2. Suspected renal artery stenosis with resultant hypertension (captopril renogram)
3. Suspected complications from renal transplantation (e.g., acute tubular necrosis, cyclosporin toxicity, rejection)
4. Suspected urine leak in the setting of renal transplantation

List 3 indications for renal cortical imaging.

1. Suspected pyelonephritis
2. Evaluation of renal scarring
3. Evaluation of suspected column of Bertin versus renal cell cancer

What information is provided by a renogram?

Quantitative assessment with a computer enables a renogram curve to be produced and the relative function of each kidney calculated.

List 3 indications for a furosemide renogram.

1. Suspected renal obstruction, often with hydronephrosis demonstrated on cross-sectional imaging such as ultrasound or CT
2. Quantitation of renal obstruction
3. Follow-up of patients with known obstruction, with or without previous intervention

PATHOLOGY

List 8 conditions leading to bilateral large kidneys.

A PAL OMAR
Acute glomerulonephritis
Polycystic kidney disease
Acute tubular necrosis
Leukemia
Obstruction
Myeloma
Amyloid or **A**cromegaly
Renal vein thrombosis

m

What 10 conditions lead to a unilateral large kidney?

1. Obstructive uropathy
2. Acute pyelonephritis
3. Xanthogranulomatous pyelonephritis (XGPN)
4. Acute arterial infarction
5. Renal vein thrombosis (especially in neonates secondary to dehydration)
6. Compensatory hypertrophy
7. Duplicated collecting system
8. Cyst
9. Tumor (particularly renal cell carcinoma)
10. Multicystic dysplastic kidney

List 6 causes of bilateral smooth small kidneys.

1. Chronic glomerulonephritis (after acute glomerulonephritis)
2. Generalized arteriosclerosis

3. Atheroembolic renal disease
4. Papillary necrosis
5. Hereditary chronic nephritis (Alport's syndrome)
6. Arterial hypotension (prolonged, dense nephrogram that reverts to normal if hypotension is reversed)

List 4 causes of a unilateral smooth small kidney.

1. Renal artery stenosis (atherosclerosis, fibromuscular hyperplasia)
2. Congenital hypoplasia (< 5 calices, contralateral enlargement)
3. Radiation nephritis (latent period of 6–12 months)
4. Postobstructive atrophy (dilated calices, contralateral compensatory hypertrophy)

List 3 causes of a unilateral small scarred kidney.

1. Reflux nephropathy (cortical destruction over retracted papilla with dilated calix; polar initially)
2. Lobar infarction [broad based, over normal papilla; embolic, usually cardiac in origin (e.g., atrial fibrillation, subacute bacterial endocarditis)]
3. Tuberculosis (scarring with retraction of underlying papilla)

DISORDERS OF THE KIDNEYS

RENAL CYSTIC DISEASE

Are renal cysts common?

Yes. Roughly 50% of patients older than 50 years have at least one.

What are risk factors for renal cysts?

Age, dialysis (also increases risk of renal cell cancer), von Hippel-Lindau disease, adult polycystic kidney disease (APKD)

Are most renal cysts a problem for the patient?

No. Most cysts are simple cysts and can be diagnosed as such by imaging. Many are found incidentally.

Why is it important to classify renal cysts?

Because some cystic lesions are renal neoplasms, cysts are classified to determine whether they can be dismissed, followed, or biopsied. The Bosniak classification helps sort this out.

What are the Bosniak cyst categories and their criteria?

Bosniak Cyst Categories and Criteria

Category	*Criteria*
Simple cyst (I)	Thin wall, no septae or calcification—**benign**
Mildly complex cyst (II)	Thin septation or calcium in wall
Indeterminate lesion (III)	Multiple septae, mural nodules, thick septae, or internal echoes
Malignant lesion (IV)	Solid component—**malignant**

What work-up is appropriate for a:

Bosniak category II lesion?	3–6 month CT or ultrasound follow-up (a significant percentage are malignant)
Bosniak category III lesion?	Biopsy or partial nephrectomy; follow-up if high risk

What are the ultrasound criteria for a mass to be considered "cystic"?

Smooth, sharply defined walls (especially the back wall):
C = Anechoic interior
E = Distal acoustical enhancement

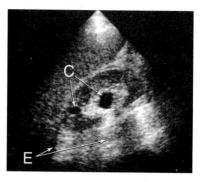

Name 6 lesions that can mimic renal cysts on ultrasound.

Hypoechoic structures—such as renal pyramids, urine collections [e.g., urinoma (localized hydronephrosis)], abscesses, hematomas, intrarenal vascular malformations, and lymphomas—can mimic renal cysts on ultrasound.

List 4 CT findings associated with a simple renal cyst.	1. Smooth margin 2. Paper-thin wall 3. CT Hounsfield units (HU) < 15 4. Little (< 5 HU) or no enhancement after IV contrast administration
What is the definition of a complex cyst?	Does not meet the criteria for simple cysts (Bosniak category II or III): High attenuation material in cyst (> 15 HU) Thick (i.e., not paper thin), irregular wall Thick or multiple septa
What is the beak sign?	As a mass increases in size, it elevates the adjacent edges of the cortex. This cortical margin appears as a very thin, smooth radiopaque rim about the bulging cyst.
Can it be seen in malignant lesions?	Yes, particularly those that are slow growing.

ADULT POLYCYSTIC KIDNEY DISEASE (APKD)

What is the common clinical presentation of patients with APKD?	APKD presents between the ages of 35 and 55 years with features of hypertension, renal failure, hematuria, or bilaterally enlarged kidneys. It is autosomal dominant.
What are the imaging features of APKD?	Large kidneys with multiple cysts that are too numerous to count; the cysts have variable imaging characteristics owing to hemorrhage or proteinaceous fluid, and calcification of the cyst wall is common.
Are there associated findings in other organs?	"Berry" aneurysms of the intracranial arteries Hepatic cysts Pancreatic cysts Splenic cysts

MEDULLARY CYSTIC DISEASE

What are the radiographic features of medullary cystic disease?	Small kidneys Thin cortex; no cortical cysts Multiple small medullary cysts No calcifications

RENAL NEOPLASMS

List 6 causes of a solid renal mass in an adult.	**Renal parenchymal tumors** Renal cell carcinoma (adenocarcinoma), 80% Oncocytoma **Mesenchymal tumors** Angiomyolipoma (fat density) **Renal pelvis tumors** Transitional cell carcinoma, < 10% **Secondary tumors** Metastasis Lymphoma

Renal cell carcinoma (RCC)

What is the classic clinical triad for RCC?	Hematuria, flank pain, palpable mass
What is the most useful imaging study in a patient with suspected RCC?	CT with and without IV contrast can usually diagnose and stage RCC in one setting.
Describe the CT findings of RCC.	Decreased attenuation on noncontrast CT when compared with normal kidney Possible early hypervascularity and enhancement on arterial phase scans Less-than-normal enhancement on nonequilibrium and nephrogram phase scans, usually heterogeneous Thick wall, irregular margin Calcified in 10%–20% of patients (87% nonperipheral calcification) Possible renal vein or IVC thrombus— neoplastic (i.e., tumor) or nonneoplastic (i.e., bland) Possible periaortic adenopathy Liver metastases possibly hypervascular (do biphasic liver CT) Bilateral in a small percentage of patients (incidence increased in patients with von Hippel-Lindau disease)
In what ways is MRI useful for diagnosing RCC?	Good for staging (multiplanar imaging better for evaluation of perirenal extension) Can evaluate venous structures for thrombosis

Gadolinium-enhanced images may be
useful for diagnosis in patients allergic
to iodinated contrast

Describe the angiographic appearance of RCC.

Hypervascular (in most cases)
Arteriovenous shunting, venous lakes
Irregular tumor vessels, neovascularity

How can angiography be useful in the diagnosis and management of RCC?

Angiography may facilitate detection in
complicated and equivocal cases.
Preoperative embolization with alcohol or
polyvinyl alcohol may aid removal of
mass.

What is the traditional system of staging for RCC?

Robson system
I: Confined to renal capsule
II: Perirenal extension within Gerota's
fascia
IIIa: Perirenal extension with renal vein
or IVC invasion
IIIb: Perirenal extension with local nodal
enlargement
IIIc: Perirenal extension with nodal
enlargement and venous invasion
IV: Distant metastases or adjacent spread
beyond Gerota's fascia

What is another system of staging for RCC?

Tumor, node, metastases (TNM) staging
T_1: Small tumor, no enlargement of
kidney
T_2: Large tumor, cortex not broken
T_{3a}: Perinephric or hilar extension
T_{3b}: Renal vein or IVC involvement
T_4: Extension to neighboring organs
N_1: Single homolateral regional node
N_2: Contra- or bilateral/multiple regional
nodes
N_3: Fixed regional nodes
N_4: Juxtaregional nodes
$M+$: Distant metastases

To what sites does RCC tend to metastasize?

Lymph nodes (periaortic, interaortocaval,
and pericaval)
Lung
Liver
Bone
Brain
Contralateral kidney

What is the appearance of renal vein or IVC thrombosis on CT?

Intravascular filling defect
Enlargement of vessel, which helps to
    confirm if uncertain

Is there an imaging characteristic that helps to distinguish bland thrombi from tumor thrombi?

Tumor thrombi tend to enhance on CT
after contrast administration.

What imaging modalities can be used to make the diagnosis of IVC thrombosis?

CT, magnetic resonance venography
(MRV), ultrasonography, venography

Angiomyolipoma

What is an angiomyolipoma?

A renal hamartoma containing blood
vessels (*angio*), smooth muscle (*myo*), and
fat (*lipoma*)

How does the patient usually present?

Patients are most often asymptomatic;
may present with acute retroperitoneal
hemorrhage from tumor requiring
embolization or surgery

What are the radiologic findings in angiomyolipoma?

Identifying fat is key to confirming the
diagnosis. Calcifications are nonexistent.
Ultrasound shows a hyperechoic mass,
    which is nonspecific.
Plain radiography. Lucency may be
    appreciable on a plain radiograph if
    there is a large amount of fat.
CT shows negative HU numbers,
    indicating fat. This finding is specific
    for angiomyolipoma; thin slices may
    be necessary to demonstrate fat.
MRI can confirm fat as well; it appears
    bright on T_1-weighted images.
Angiography features are nonspecific; a
    sunburst pattern is typical.

What are the clinical features of angiomyolipoma seen in patients with and without tuberous sclerosis?

With tuberous sclerosis (incidence 80%):
    50% Bilateral, small, asymptomatic
Without tuberous sclerosis: Single, large,
    4:1 female, symptomatic

Renal lymphoma

Describe the 3 patterns of renal involvement in lymphoma.

1. Multiple lymphomatous masses
2. Diffuse involvement of one or both
   kidneys
3. Adenopathy with contiguous extension

What is the appearance of focal renal involvement on:

    Enhanced CT?   Hypodense-to-normal kidney

    Ultrasound?   Hypoechoic solid masses

Multilocular cystic nephroma (MLCN)

Is MLCN found in adults?   Yes.

What are the radiologic findings?   Cystic septated mass; septations may be calcified

What is the treatment?   Partial or complete nephrectomy; may be difficult to exclude renal cell cancer by imaging

Renal metastasis

What percent of cancer patients have metastases to a kidney on autopsy?   20%

List the 5 most common primary tumors that metastasize to the kidney.   Lung, breast, colon, lymphoma, melanoma

Lesions that simulate renal masses

What is fetal lobulation?   Fetal lobulation is a developmental variation of kidney shape. The surface is lobulated; the indentations generally fall between the calices.

What is a dromedary hump?   This is a hump on the lateral portion of the left kidney sometimes caused by the impression of the normal spleen on the superior pole. The renal tissue is histologically normal.

What is a column of Bertin?   A column of Bertin is a prominent formation of normal renal cortex that may simulate a mass. However, it has normal enhancement on IVP and CT and normal echotexture on ultrasound. Nuclear cortical scanning demonstrates normal renal tissue.

RENAL FAILURE

What are the causes of renal failure, and how are they categorized?	**Prerenal** Hypoperfusion Hypotension Dehydration Congestive heart failure (CHF) **Renal** Nephrotoxicity (e.g., chemotherapeutic agents, antibiotics, iodinated contrast) Infection (e.g., glomerulonephritis) Renal artery occlusion Renal neoplasm or cysts **Postrenal** Obstruction of the ureter or bladder
What is the first step in evaluating a patient with renal failure?	Confirm or exclude urinary tract obstruction, which is often treatable
What diagnostic test is most commonly used to rule out obstruction?	Ultrasound. It is relatively inexpensive, easy for the patient, and quick.
What are the imaging features of acute tubular necrosis?	Smooth, large kidneys Normal renal perfusion Diminished or absent opacification Persistent dense nephrogram Increased cortical and decreased medullary echogenicity
Describe the most common appearance of the end-stage kidney ("medical renal disease") on ultrasound.	Most will be small or normal in size with smooth outlines and normal calices. The kidney is hyperechoic and corticomedullary differentiation is absent.
What is the treatment for renal failure with end-stage kidneys?	Dialysis and transplantation

REFLUX NEPHROPATHY (CHRONIC PYELONEPHRITIS)

What is reflux nephropathy?	A condition caused by reflux of infected urine from the bladder into the kidneys, leading to destruction and scarring of the renal substance.

What is the clinical course of reflux nephropathy?	Most damage occurs in the first year of life, and the severity of the reflux decreases as the child gets older.
What is the most common cause of reflux nephropathy?	A congenital abnormality of the UVJ, with a shorter-than-normal intramural section of ureter leading to vesicoureteral reflux
How is reflux nephropathy most easily demonstrated?	VCUG
List 5 signs of reflux nephropathy.	1. Local reduction in renal parenchymal width 2. Dilation of the calices in the scarred areas 3. Overall reduction in renal size 4. Dilation of the affected collecting system 5. Indentations of the renal contour occur over the calyces, not between them (as in fetal lobulation).

RENAL INFECTION

What are the renal radiologic findings in a patient with acute pyelonephritis on:	
IVP?	Kidney may be enlarged with a striated nephrogram Usually normal even during an acute attack
Ultrasound?	Kidney may appear significantly enlarged and show diminished echoes owing to cortical edema
CT?	Precontrast scans are usually normal but may reveal patchy diminished density. After contrast enhancement, affected portions of the renal cortex show patchy, striated areas of diminished density.
What are the best imaging modalities for diagnosis of renal and perinephric abscesses?	Ultrasound or CT

Describe the typical appearance of a renal abscess.

Most have thick walls and show both cystic and solid components. CT may show enhancement of the wall of the abscess after contrast. The center may not be liquefied sufficiently to drain; it may be aspirated for culture.

Describe the typical appearance of a perinephric abscess.

They frequently conform to the shape of the underlying kidney—subcapsular or perinephric. The CT and ultrasound characteristics are variable, usually showing both cystic and solid elements. The cystic portions frequently contain internal echoes at ultrasound due to debris. An underlying renal abnormality is often demonstrable.

Can simple cysts become secondarily infected?

Yes.

What is the most sensitive imaging modality for pyonephrosis?

Ultrasound. In addition to showing the hydronephrosis, it may demonstrate multiple echoes within the urine due to infected debris.

What are the radiographic findings in XGPN?

Staghorn calculus
Inflammatory mass (may be aggressive and extend into flank and colon)
No or poor function on IVP (may see some function on CT)

Which bacteria commonly cause XGPN?

Proteus species, occasionally *Escherichia coli*

What is emphysematous pyelonephritis?

The presence of gas in the renal parenchyma and collecting system caused by Gram-negative organisms, most often occurring in diabetic patients. Emphysematous pyelonephritis is potentially life threatening and requires percutaneous drainage or nephrectomy.

How does emphysematous pyelitis differ from emphysematous pyelonephritis?

With emphysematous pyelitis, gas is restricted to the lumen of the collecting system, and the patient has a better prognosis.

What is the most common renal fungal infection?	Candidiasis
In what patient population is this infection most common?	Diabetics
What are the radiographic features of renal candidiasis?	Fungal debris in the collecting system, filling defects, papillary necrosis
List 4 renal manifestations of AIDS.	1. AIDS-associated nephropathy 2. Acute tubular necrosis 3. Focal nephrocalcinosis 4. Interstitial nephritis
What radiologic findings are associated with tuberculosis of the urinary system?	**Multifocal** involvement but most often unilateral "Soft" calcification on KUB film (50%) Calyceal erosion or destruction Papillary necrosis (irregular and extensive) Irregular, "beaded," strictured calyceal system and ureters, straightened ureters Wasted parenchyma (autonephrectomy, "putty kidney") Small contracted bladder owing to mural fibrosis Chest radiograph (CXR) abnormal in 50% of patients
Where does tuberculosis initially manifest in the urinary tract?	Tuberculosis generally proceeds from the kidney toward the bladder (as opposed to schistosomiasis, which proceeds from the bladder to the kidney).
What causes symptoms in patients with tuberculosis of the urinary system?	Symptoms are often caused by tuberculosis cystitis.

NEPHROCALCINOSIS

Define nephrocalcinosis.	Nephrocalcinosis is the term used to describe numerous irregular foci of calcium deposited diffusely in the parenchyma of both kidneys.
Where is nephrocalcinosis most commonly found?	95% of calcinosis is **medullary;** 5% is cortical

List 11 causes of medullary nephrocalcinosis.

1. Medullary sponge kidney
2. Renal tubular acidosis (distal type)
3. Hypercalcemia (primary hyperparathyroidism)
4. Lytic bony metastasis
5. Paraneoplastic syndrome (lung, kidney)
6. Milk-alkali syndrome
7. Sarcoidosis
8. Hypervitaminosis D
9. Nephrotoxic acute tubular necrosis
10. Tuberculosis
11. Hyperoxaluria

Name 2 causes of cortical nephrocalcinosis.

Chronic glomerulonephritis and cortical necrosis (dystrophic calcification)

PAPILLARY NECROSIS

What is papillary necrosis?

Part or all of the renal papilla dies, is sloughed, and may fall into the pelvicaliceal system. These necrotic papillae may remain with the pelvicaliceal system, sometimes causing obstruction, or they may be voided.

What does complete papillary necrosis look like on IVP?

"Golf ball on a tee"

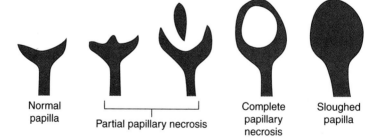

Normal papilla

Partial papillary necrosis

Complete papillary necrosis

Sloughed papilla

List 8 causes of papillary necrosis.

AD SPORT C (The common mnemonic **POSTCARD** does not put the causes in a useful order of incidence.)
Analgesic abuse (e.g., phenacetin)
Diabetes mellitus
Sickle cell disease

Pyelonephritis (especially in children)
Obstruction
Renal vein thrombosis
Tuberculosis (not usually confined to
     papillae)
Cirrhosis

List 5 other conditions that also lead to calyceal clubbing.	1. Hydronephrosis 2. Reflux nephropathy 3. Pyelonephritis 4. Tuberculosis 5. Megacalices

RENAL VASCULAR DISEASE

What 3 conditions may lead to wedge enhancement defects in the kidney on CT?	1. Infarction (cortical rim sign due to perfusion by capsular collaterals) 2. Pyelonephritis 3. Lymphoma
What is the cortical rim sign?	A thin, dense rim surrounding the kidney seen on excretory urography in patients with unilateral renal artery occlusion
What does this sign represent?	It probably represents a nephrogram phase in the preserved outer rim of the viable renal cortex supplied by capsular arterial branches.
In what other conditions can this sign be recognized?	Renal vein thrombosis and acute tubular necrosis
List 5 causes of renal vein thrombosis.	1. RCC with renal vein invasion 2. Hypercoaguable conditions 3. Pancreatic carcinoma with renal vein compression 4. Nephrotic syndrome with membranous glomerulonephritis 5. Amyloidosis
What is the clinical symptom in a patient with a Page kidney?	Hypertension
What is the cause of Page kidney?	Most cases develop following healing of subcapsular or perirenal hematomas. Dense fibrous encasement of the kidney causes compression of the renal paren-

chyma and increased renin production, leading to hypertension.

What is the radiographic appearance of the Page kidney?	Excretory urography demonstrates a functioning, often enlarged kidney with a mass effect and distortion of the collecting system.

RENAL TRAUMA

What are the categories of renal trauma?	**Minor injuries:** 85% (conservative treatment) Hematomas Contusion Small lacerations **Major injuries:** 15% (surgical treatment) Multiple renal lacerations (rupture) Pedicle injury (avulsion, thrombosis)
What nonangiographic studies are commonly employed in patients with renal trauma?	**One-shot IVP:** Allows visualization of both kidneys, excludes pedicle avulsion, performed in the emergency department (ED) **Contrast-enhanced CT:** Study of choice; gives more information
What are the indications for angiography in these patients?	Nonvisualization of kidney on IVP in a patient with abdominal trauma Persistent hematuria in a patient with abdominal trauma Hypo- or hypertension or persistent hematuria following an interventional urologic procedure
What are the potential manifestations of renal trauma?	Renal infarction (segmental branch, vascular pedicle avulsion) Hemorrhage (renal laceration or rupture) Ruptured collecting system, urinoma

RENAL TRANSPLANT

In what percentage of patients with kidney transplant are perirenal fluid collections seen?	40%
In what percentage does this collection persist?	15%

List 4 fluid collections that are associated with decreased transplant function.

HAUL (in order of occurrence after transplant)
Hematoma
Abscess
Urinoma
Lymphocele

m

What are the distinguishing characteristics of the 4 fluid collections?

Hematoma: Commonly seen within 24 hours of surgery, hyperechoic on ultrasound, increased attenuation on CT ($\sim$ 50 HU), pain, hematocrit drop

Abscess: Develops within weeks, complex fluid collection on ultrasound or CT, fever

Urinoma: Develops during the first month, hydronephrosis may or may not be present, "hot" on technetium 99m (Tc-99m) MAG3

Lymphocele: Occurs 5–6 weeks after surgery, low attenuation on CT, linear septations seen on ultrasound in 80% of patients

How is rejection detected by ultrasound?

Enlarged transplant kidney
Increased cortical echogenicity
Poor corticomedullary distinction
Increased resistive index:

$$\frac{\text{Peak systolic velocity} - \text{peak diastolic velocity}}{\text{Peak systolic velocity}}$$

Moderate: > 0.7–0.8
Severe: 0.8–1.0

What are the indications for a nuclear renal scan in the setting of renal transplantation?

Poor function in the immediate postoperative period
Clinically suspected urine leak in the immediate postoperative period

What is the appearance of a normal renal transplant?

Blood flow images should demonstrate activity within the transplant at the same time activity is seen in the iliac arteries. Cortical and clearance phases should be identical to standard dynamic (functional) studies. The cortex should demonstrate uniform uptake during the cortical phase.

List 3 causes of decreased or absent activity in all or part of the transplant.

1. Renal artery occlusion with ischemia (area of absent uptake corresponding to transplant)

2. Occlusion or nonanastomosis of an accessory renal artery (portion of the transplant demonstrates decreased or absent perfusion)
3. Ischemic injury during harvesting, transplantation, or both (may demonstrate improvement on serial scans)

What are the leading causes of a persistent cortical phase with poor clearance, with or without delayed perfusion, in the immediate post-transplant period?

Acute tubular necrosis and cyclosporin toxicity (if immunosuppression was begun pre-transplant)

What is the renal scan appearance of acute tubular necrosis?

There is persistent cortical phase activity with poor clearance (i.e., poor renal function) but relatively preserved renal perfusion. Improvement occurs in days to weeks, depending on severity. Cyclosporin toxicity has a similar appearance in the setting of therapeutic serum levels.

What is the best method of differentiating acute tubular necrosis from cyclosporin toxicity?

Because they appear identical on a single scan, serial scans may be necessary. Acute tubular necrosis improves over days to weeks without intervention and is almost always seen with cadaveric transplantation; it is infrequent and less severe with a living related donor. Cyclosporin toxicity improves with alteration in drug dosage.

What is the renal scan appearance of rejection?

There is decreased renal perfusion and poor renal function.

What is the appearance of a urine leak?

Radioactive urine is detected outside of the collecting system or bladder; an area of decreased activity (e.g., urinoma) fills with activity on delayed images. Ideally, the patient's Foley catheter should be clamped for study. (*Always* consult the transplant surgeon before clamping a patient's catheter in the immediate post-transplant period.) Late images at approximately 2 hours postinjection should always be obtained.

CONGENITAL ANOMALIES

Where is an ectopic kidney usually found?

It is usually in the lower abdomen or pelvis and rotated so that the pelvis of the kidney points forward. The ureter is short and travels directly to the bladder:

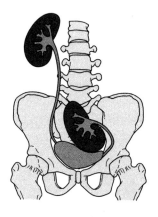

List 3 complications seen in patients with an ectopic kidney.

Chronic pyelonephritis, hydronephrosis, calculi

What is cross-fused renal ectopia?

The renal parenchyma is absent from the renal fossa on one side. It is found fused to the other kidney, usually to the lower pole. Left to right is more common than right to left. Note that the ureter inserts normally in the bladder:

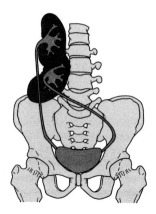

What is a horseshoe kidney?   The kidneys fail to separate at the lower pole, which results in a horseshoe-shaped kidney. The tissue anterior to the aorta may be mostly fibrotic.

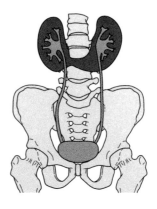

What are some of the problems associated with horseshoe kidney?   Horseshoe kidney can lead to obstruction of the collecting systems and calculus formation, and is more prone to trauma.

What is renal agenesis?   No renal tissue can be identified with ultrasound or CT examination, and the contralateral kidney usually shows compensatory hypertrophy.

HEREDITARY SYNDROMES

Which inherited syndromes are most prominently related to the genitourinary system? Name the associated findings.

1. **von Hippel-Lindau disease (oculocerebellar angiomatosis)**
   Renal cysts or adenomas 10%–35% increase in the incidence of RCC (often multiple tumors)
   Pheochromocytoma (also seen in neurofibromatosis, multiple endocrine neoplasia types II and III)
   Cerebellar hemangioma
   Autosomal dominant
2. **Tuberous sclerosis**
   Multiple bilateral angiomyolipomas in 80% of patients
   Renal cysts
   Central nervous system (CNS) hamartomas or subependymal nodules
   Autosomal dominant with incomplete expression

3. **Turner syndrome**
   Horseshoe kidney
   Coarctation of the aorta
   Webbed neck
   Phenotypic female with XO genotype

DISORDERS OF THE URETERS AND COLLECTING SYSTEM

URINARY OBSTRUCTION

What is the principle feature of urinary obstruction?

Hydronephrosis (i.e., dilatation of the collecting system). The obstructed collecting system is dilated down to the level of the obstructing pathology. Demonstrating this level is a prime diagnostic objective.

How is hydronephrosis graded?

Mild, moderate, or severe, depending on the degree of dilatation of the collecting system:

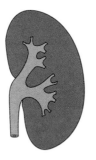 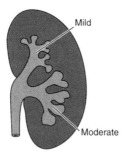 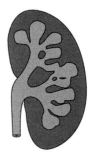

A. Normal   **B.** Mild/Moderate   **C.** Severe

What examinations play the major roles in evaluating urinary obstruction?

IVP and ultrasound; furosemide renogram may be used in patients with acute obstruction and a greatly delayed pyelogram

Describe the findings on IVP in patients with urinary obstruction.

Very dense persistent nephrogram in acute obstruction and a greatly delayed pyelogram

Opacification of urine in an obstructed system usually takes a long time (hours)

Prolonged obstruction causes atrophy of the kidney, which is recognized by observing reduction of the renal parenchymal width

Describe the findings on ultrasound examination in urinary obstruction.

The central echo complex spreads apart. Dilated calices can resemble multiple renal cysts but, unlike cysts, they show continuity with the renal pelvis. Proximal ureteric dilation is often seen, but dilation of the distal ureter is often obscured by overlying bowel. It often is not possible to determine the cause of urinary tract obstruction during ultrasound examination.

List 8 causes of ureteral obstruction.

1. Calculi
2. Clot
3. Cancer
4. Compression (extrinsic owing to tumor, hematoma)
5. Complication of surgery
6. Sloughed papilla
7. Retroperitoneal fibrosis
8. Endometriosis

What treatment is available for ureteral obstruction?

Depending on the cause, the following can be used:
Percutaneous nephrostomy
Ureteral stent
Lithotripsy, if caused by ureteral stone

How does the kidney appear on IVP or ultrasound in a patient with chronic ureteral obstruction?

Thin cortex
Dilated calices and renal pelvis
Poor function

URINARY CALCULI

List 8 causes of pelvic calcifications.

1. Vascular phlebolith (most common entity confused with calculus)
2. Urinary calculus
3. Arterial atherosclerotic calcification
4. Uterine leiomyoma
5. Prostatic calculi
6. Dermoid cyst
7. Fecalith (appendicolith)
8. Foreign material [e.g., barium, bismuth, iophendylate (Pantopaque), pills]

What is a phlebolith?

A calcification in the venous system, usually in the pelvic veins

What is the typical appearance of a phlebolith?

Phleboliths usually appear round with a central lucency. If found caudal to the ischial spine level, confusion with a calculus is less likely because the UVJ is usually above this level.

What is the typical appearance of obstruction by a renal calculus on IVP?

Density (stone) seen on preliminary film, most commonly in the UVJ
Unilateral (ipsilateral) delayed, persistent nephrogram

List the 6 types of renal calculi.

1. Calcium oxalate
2. Calcium phosphate (hydroxyapatite)
3. Struvite
4. Uric acid
5. Cystine
6. Xanthine

What percentage of renal calculi are radiopaque on plain films?

More than 90%

Which of the six types of renal calculi are opaque on plain films?

Calcium oxalate and phosphate calculi
Struvite calculi (staghorn calculi are often struvite)
Cystine calculi (less dense)

Which types of renal calculi are nonopaque on plain films?

Uric acid and xanthine calculi

What percentage of renal calculi are dense on CT?

Essentially **all** are dense on CT.

What are the advantages and limitations of IVP when studying renal calculi?

IVP shows the precise site of obstruction and also can help identify any mechanical obstruction or deranged anatomy that may have predisposed to stone formation. However, it may take a long time for the ureter to opacify if it is completely obstructed.

What size renal calculi can be detected by ultrasound?

Calculi larger than 5 mm are easily detected by ultrasound; smaller calculi may be missed.

Describe the ultrasound characteristics of renal calculi.

Renal calculi produce intense echoes and cast acoustic shadows.

What modality is most sensitive and specific for renal calculi?

Noncontrast CT (97% sensitivity; 96% specificity)

How is CT performed for renal calculi?

Thin slices (~5 mm) are obtained using a spiral CT scanner (pitch 1.25–1.5). These are usually reconstructed at 4-mm intervals (overlapping). No contrast is needed.

What are the CT findings of calculus?

Calcification in the ureter (often in the distal ureter, near the UVJ, a site of narrowing) *must* be demonstrated. Other confirmatory findings include hydroureter and hydronephrosis, stranding in peri-ureteral and perirenal fat, and renal enlargement.

What is the "comet tail" sign?

A curvilinear soft tissue band that extends from the suspected calculus and represents the vein containing the phlebolith

What options are available for treatment of ureteral calculi?

Hydration and expectant management; sometimes a calculus passes spontaneously
Extracorporeal shock wave lithotripsy (ESWL)
Retrograde basket extraction

List 11 causes of a focal calcification over renal shadows other than stones.

1. Renal cell carcinoma (10%–20% calcify)
2. Cyst
3. Infection [e.g., tuberculosis (25% calcify), histoplasmosis, XGPN]
4. Hematoma
5. Metastasis
6. Angiomyolipoma
7. Multicystic dysplastic in adult (curvilinear calcification)
8. Renal artery aneurysm (ring-like)
9. Gallstone
10. Splenic artery calcification
11. Pills in gut

List 4 causes of a filling defect in the renal collecting system.

4 Cs
Calculus
Clot
Carcinoma (transitional cell)
Candida (fungus ball)

List 8 causes of nonobstructive dilation of the renal pelvis.

1. Reflux
2. Infection
3. Diuresis
4. Distended bladder
5. Large extrarenal pelvis
6. Megacalices
7. Papillary necrosis
8. Corrected obstruction

List 6 conditions that can mimic hydronephrosis.

1. Parapelvic cysts
2. Prominent renal pyramids
3. Sinus lipomatosis
4. Central renal cysts
5. Multicystic kidney
6. Lymphoma

List 11 causes of ureteral stricture.

Mucosal
  1. Transitional cell carcinoma
Mural
  2. Endometriosis
  3. Tuberculosis with renal mass
  4. Traumatic or iatrogenic
  5. Amyloid
Extrinsic
  6. Lymphadenopathy
  7. Radiation fibrosis
  8. Retroperitoneal fibrosis
  9. Tubovarian abscess
  10. Gastrointestinal inflammatory disease
  11. Iliac artery aneurysm

URETERAL DISPLACEMENT AND ANOMALIES

List 7 causes of medially displaced ureters.

1. Retroperitoneal fibrosis (acute angle in mid-to-upper ureter)
2. Pelvic lipomatosis
3. Parailiac adenopathy
4. Retrocaval ureter (right side only)
5. Abdominoperineal resection (postoperative "hockey sticking" of lower ureters)
6. Urinoma or lymphocele

7. Horseshoe kidney or cross-fused renal ectopia

Identify each of the following conditions:

Retroperitoneal fibrosis

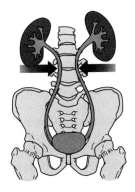

Pelvic tumor

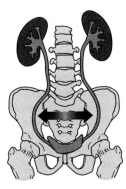

Lymphadenopathy

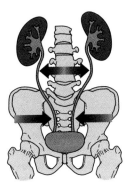

List 4 causes of retroperitoneal fibrosis.	**DIRT** **D**rugs (especially methylsergide) **I**diopathic **R**adiation therapy **T**uberculosis

In retroperitoneal fibrosis, what are the:

CT findings?

Soft tissue mass surrounding the aorta and IVC; eventually causes ureteral obstruction

MRI findings?

Soft tissue mass; dark on T_1- and T_2-weighted images

What is a circumcaval (retrocaval) ureter?

Circumcaval ureter is caused by persistence of the right subcardinal vein. The course of the ureter is "S"-shaped.

What is the most common complication associated with circumcaval ureter?

Obstruction occurs but is not common.

Which ureter is likely to show a vascular impression in the case of a dilated or thrombosed ovarian vein?

The right, because the right ovarian vein crosses the ureter to drain into the IVC.

What are bifid collecting systems?

The most common congenital variations of the ureter, they can be unilateral or bilateral. Two ureters may be separate throughout their length and have separate openings into the bladder. The ureter draining the upper moiety may drain outside the bladder (e.g., into the vagina or urethra). These ectopic ureters are frequently obstructed. The distal end of the dilated ureter may cause a smooth filling defect in the bladder (ureterocele), which can have the appearance of a "cobra head."

What is the Weigert-Meyer rule?

In duplication, the upper moiety obstructs, causing a mass effect on the lower moiety (i.e., the "drooping lily" sign). The lower moiety is prone to reflux. The upper moiety may not be seen on IVP because it is obstructed (*A*). *B* shows the appearance of both right ureters.

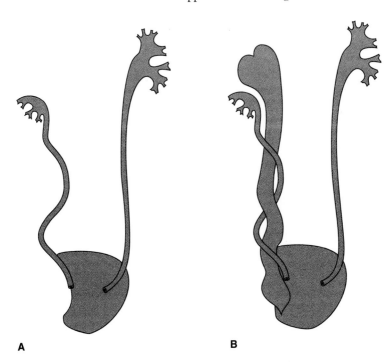

A   **B**

What is the "cobra head" sign, and how is it demonstrated?

Excretory urogram demonstrates an oval density of opacified urine in the dilated distal segment of the ureter. This is surrounded by a thin radiolucent halo (arrows), producing the cobra head sign of a simple ureterocele: (see figure on next page)

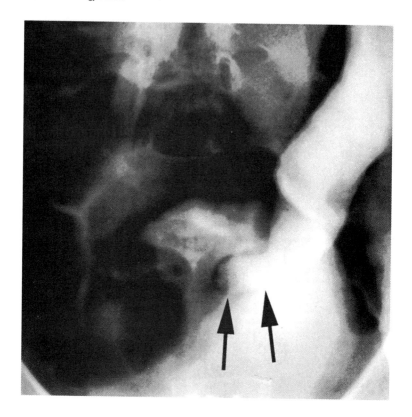

URETERAL TUMORS

What are the most common histologic types of ureteral tumor?	Transitional cell carcinoma > squamous cell carcinoma > metastases
What percentage of ureteral tumors are unilateral?	75%
Is transitional cell cancer usually multifocal?	Yes
What percentage of patients with ureteral tumors develop bladder cancer?	50%
What percentage of patients with bladder cancer develop ureteral cancer?	5%

What is ureteritis (pyelitis, cystitis) cystica?	Asymptomatic cysts ~3 mm in diameter involving the urothelium, usually related to recurrent infection
When is this condition most common?	Most common in sixth decade and usually unilateral but uncommon overall

DISORDERS OF THE BLADDER

INFECTION

What are the imaging findings in acute cystitis?	Mucosal thickening and decreased bladder capacity
List 4 causes of chronic bacterial cystitis.	1. Reflux 2. Bladder calculus 3. Bladder diverticulum 4. Bladder outlet obstruction
List 3 other causes of cystitis.	1. Radiation 2. Cyclophosphamide treatment 3. Eosinophilic cystitis
List 4 conditions that can lead to the finding of gas in the bladder.	1. Emphysematous cystitis—*E. coli* infection (usually in diabetics); gas also in bladder wall 2. Iatrogenic (e.g., catheterization, cystoscopy) 3. Trauma 4. Bladder bowel fistula
Why should emphysematous cystitis be differentiated from emphysematous pyelo-nephritis?	They affect the same group of patients, but emphysematous cystitis is treated with antibiotics, whereas emphysematous pyelonephritis is a surgical emergency requiring percutaneous drainage or nephrectomy.
List 5 causes of a pelvic calcification projected over the bladder.	1. Calculus in bladder 2. Bladder wall calcification 3. Postradiation cystitis 4. *Schistosoma haematobium* infection (Africa) 5. Tuberculosis
List 7 causes of a bladder fistula.	1. Diverticulitis 2. Malignancy of colon, uterus, or bladder

3. Post-op or postpartum
4. Radiation therapy
5. Crohn's disease
6. Trauma
7. Appendicitis

OBSTRUCTION, FILLING DEFECTS, AND DEFORMITY

List 5 causes of bladder obstruction in an adult.

1. BPH
2. Prostate carcinoma
3. Bladder lesions (e.g., tumor, calculus, ureterocele)
4. Urethral stricture
5. Neurogenic bladder

What are the imaging features in bladder outlet obstruction?

Distended bladder with incomplete emptying (postvoid residual)
Upper urinary tract changes may include reflux and dilated ureter
Increased bladder pressure, which causes formation of trabeculae and diverticulae

How can bladder outlet obstruction be diagnosed using ultrasound?

By evaluating the postvoid residual using ultrasound or IVP

What are the 2 basic types of neurogenic bladder?

1. The large **atonic** smooth-walled bladder has poor or absent contractions and a large residual volume.
2. The **hypertrophic** type can be regarded as neurologically induced bladder outflow obstruction. The bladder is of small volume and has a very thick, grossly trabeculated wall.

List 5 causes of bladder wall thickening.

1. Chronic obstruction
2. Neurogenic bladder
3. Infiltrating carcinoma
4. Cystitis
5. Postradiation therapy

List 8 causes of a bladder filling defect.

1. Calculus (think paraplegia or bladder outlet obstruction)
2. Clot
3. Cancer (transitional cell cancer, adjacent spread from tumor of the colon or cervix)

4. Ureterocele (halo sign)
5. Prostatic enlargement
6. Foreign body
7. Fungus ball
8. Cystitis

List 9 causes of an extrinsic bladder deformity.

1. Uterus (normal or tumor)
2. Pregnancy
3. Ovarian tumor
4. Prostatic enlargement
5. Hematoma
6. Colonic distention
7. Lymphadenopathy
8. Pelvic lipomatosis
9. Urachal cyst

What should you do if you are unsure whether the lesion is extrinsic or intrinsic?

Get oblique views or a CT scan.

What is pelvic lipomatosis?

An unusual condition in which fat fills the pelvis, displacing and deforming normal structures such as the bladder and bowel

What is the appearance of a bladder diverticulum?

A smooth-walled diverticulum with a neck that contains all layers of bladder; may permit filling with contrast on CT or IVP

What are the causes and consequences of bladder diverticula?

Bladder diverticula may be congenital in origin, but are usually caused by chronic obstruction of bladder outflow. They predispose to infection and stone formation.

How are diverticula best demonstrated radiographically?

VCUG and post-void views during IVP

BLADDER TUMORS

What cell type are bladder cancers?

Almost all are transitional cell carcinomas (≥90%). Other cell types include squamous cell (6%) and adenocarcinoma (1%).

What are the imaging findings of bladder cancer during IVP?

IVP shows a filling defect in the bladder. The nature and extent of a tumor in the bladder is best observed during cystoscopy. The main value of the IVP is demonstrating ureteric obstruction.

What are the imaging findings of bladder cancer during CT?

A bladder tumor is seen as a soft tissue mass projecting from the wall. The role of CT in this case is to determine the extent of spread of the tumor and lymphadenopathy.

Describe the staging system for malignant bladder neoplasms.

T_{is}: Carcinoma in situ
T_1: Mucosa and submucosa involved
T_2: Superficial muscle layer is involved
T_{3a}: Deep muscular wall is involved
T_{3b}: Perivesicular fat involved
T_4: Other organs invaded

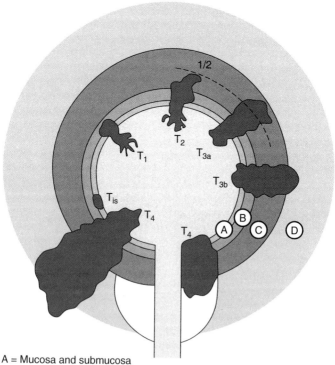

A = Mucosa and submucosa
B = Superficial muscular layer
C = Deep muscular layer
D = Perivesical fat

Describe urachal carcinoma.	Rare tumor Arises from urachal remnant Most often occurs in young patients Adenocarcinoma in almost all—poor prognosis
Where are these tumors located?	Usually anterior and superior to the dome of the bladder
What percentage of these tumors calcify?	70%

TRAUMA

What are the two types of bladder rupture?	Extraperitoneal and intraperitoneal
What are the causes of extraperitoneal rupture?	Pelvic fractures and avulsion (tear)
Where are these injuries located?	Anterior and at the base of the bladder
What are the imaging findings?	Pear-shaped bladder Contrast extravasation (streaky, irregular fluid in the perivesicular fat; fluid may extend into the scrotum) Paralytic ileus
What are the causes of intraperitoneal rupture?	Blunt trauma, iatrogenic (caused by bladder biopsy)
Where are ruptures located?	Dome of the bladder
What are the imaging findings?	Contrast extravasation into the peritoneum (urine ascites). Contrast surrounds bowel loops and is seen in Morrison's pouch and the paracolic gutters.
What is the cause of a pear-shaped or teardrop bladder?	Fluid or blood collecting within the pelvis compresses the bladder bilaterally and symmetrically and lifts it up from the pelvic floor.
In what condition is this finding primarily seen?	In patients with pelvic hematoma due primarily to trauma

List 5 other situations in which pear-shaped or teardrop bladder occurs.

1. Pelvic lipomatosis
2. IVC occlusion
3. Lymphocele
4. Pelvic lymphadenopathy
5. Healthy patient with iliac muscle hypertrophy and a narrow pelvis

DISORDERS OF THE URETHRA

What imaging study is used to image the urethra?

RUG

When is this examination most commonly used?

RUG is used in patients with pelvic trauma, particularly when blood is present at the urethral meatus. It should be performed before the Foley catheter is placed.

What is the most common mechanism of injury to the urethra?

Complex trauma with pelvic fractures

What are the types of urethral injury?

Type I: Urethra intact but narrowed by periurethral hematoma
Type II: Rupture above urogenital diaphragm
Type III: Rupture at the urogenital diaphragm ("pie in the sky")

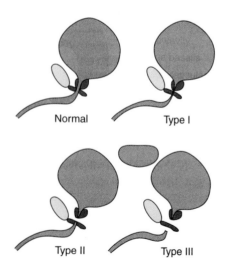

Normal   Type I

Type II   Type III

What is the term for soft tissue injury to the penile or bulbous urethra?	Straddle injury
What is the initial treatment?	Placement of suprapubic catheter
What are the common complications of urethral injury?	Stricture and impotence

List 7 causes of urethral stricture.

Infection
1. *Neisseria gonorrhoeae* infection (most common)
2. Tuberculosis

Trauma
3. Instrumentation [e.g., transurethral prostatectomy (TURP)]
4. Catheter placement

Neoplasia (rare)
5. Polyps (inflammatory, transitional cell papilloma)
6. Malignant primaries [transitional cell cancer (80%), squamous cell cancer (15%)]
7. Prostate cancer

DISORDERS OF THE PROSTATE GLAND

What 2 techniques are primarily used in prostate imaging?	Ultrasound and MRI
For what is ultrasound primarily used?	Guiding prostate biopsy
What are the imaging features associated with an enlarged prostate on CT and ultrasound?	Rounded central filling defect at base of bladder Increased diameter of prostate gland
How may an enlarged prostate gland be detected on intravenous urogram?	Hooking of the ureters may be seen with a massively enlarged prostate. An elevation or indentation of the base of the contrast-filled bladder may be seen.
What are the 2 main causes of prostatic enlargement?	BPH (by far the most common) and prostate cancer

What technique can be used to distinguish these entities?	Transrectal ultrasound with biopsy is usually done if prostate-specific antigen (PSA) is elevated.
What is the appearance of prostate cancer on ultrasound?	Hypoechoic mass in peripheral zone
How is the presence or absence of invasion of other pelvic structures best identified?	MRI
How does metastatic disease from prostate cancer manifest?	Bone metastases—best diagnosed by nuclear bone scans or MRI Lymphadenopathy—obturator nodes; eventually can go to the periaortic nodes Pulmonary metastases—uncommon
How is prostate cancer staged?	**A:** Occult cancer **B:** Cancer confined to the capsule; can do radical prostatectomy **C:** Extracapsular spread **D:** Distant metastases

DISORDERS OF THE SCROTUM AND TESTIS

What is the procedure of choice for scrotal imaging?	Ultrasound
What conditions can scrotal ultrasound identify?	Testicular tumors Testicular torsion Testicular trauma Epididymitis Orchitis Hernias involving the scrotal sac Fluid collections such as hydroceles, hematoceles, and abscesses
List the 4 typical causes of acute scrotal pain.	1. Epididymitis 2. Orchitis 3. Trauma 4. Torsion
What is the appearance of epididymitis on ultrasound?	The epididymis appears enlarged and hypoechoic on ultrasound. Color Doppler ultrasound shows normal-to-increased blood flow to the epididymis.

How is testicular torsion diagnosed:

   On ultrasound?

Early: Absent flow on Doppler ultrasound, no color, normal echotexture

Late: Absent flow, swollen, low echotexture (missed torsion)

   Using nuclear medicine?

Early: No flow

Late: No flow to testis, increased flow to surrounding tissues, doughnut sign

Why is it important to diagnose testicular torsion early?

The salvage rate is 20% at 12 hours, 0% at 24 hours.

What is the result of untreated testicular torsion?

Testicular infarction

How can ultrasound examination be helpful after testicular trauma?

It can differentiate between intra- and extratesticular injuries and promptly identify patients who need surgical management.

What are the types of intratesticular trauma?

Laceration and testicular rupture

List 5 causes of acute scrotal enlargement.

1. Orchitis
2. Testicular torsion
3. Hematocele
4. Pyocele
5. Hernia

How do the ultrasound appearances of hematocele and pyocele differ from that of hydrocele?

Hematocele and pyocele appear as echogenic or complex fluid collections, whereas a hydrocele is anechoic.

List 3 causes of fluid-filled intrascrotal masses.

1. Varicocele [dilated testicular veins of pampiniform plexus ("bag of worms")]
2. Hydrocele (fluid within the tunica vaginalis)
3. Herniation of bowel into the scrotum

What is the clinical problem associated with varicocele?

Infertility (decreased spermatogenesis leads to decreased sperm counts)

Is varicocele more common on one side?

Left > right

TESTICULAR MASSES

How is ultrasound helpful with new scrotal masses?	Ultrasound can differentiate between intratesticular masses, which are generally malignant, and extratesticular masses, which are generally benign.
What other conditions may present as a scrotal mass?	Cyst, abscess, varicocele
Where can intrascrotal cysts be located?	Within the testicle, epididymis, or tunica vaginalis
What is the typical appearance of testicular cancer on ultrasound?	Hypoechoic mass within an otherwise normal testicle
List the 4 cell types that comprise the tumors of the testis.	1. Seminoma (50%) 2. Teratocarcinoma (25%) 3. Embryonal cell carcinoma (20%) 4. Teratoma (5%)
What imaging studies are useful for staging and follow-up of testicular cancer?	CT for periaortic lymphadenopathy CXR for pulmonary metastases
What lymph nodes are affected by testicular cancer?	**Retroperitoneal nodes** at the level of the renal hila **Periaortic, aortocaval,** and **pericaval nodes.** Right testicular tumors may metastasize to the pericaval (*arrow*), aortocaval (*arrow*), and periaortic nodes; left testicular tumors tend to metastasize to the periaortic nodes:

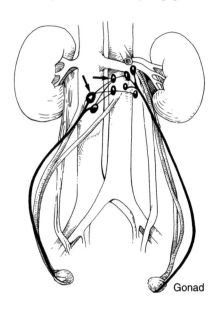

Gonad

What extratesticular tumors may involve the testicle?	Lymphoma or leukemia
How does the testicle appear clinically?	Diffuse enlargement

DISORDERS OF THE ADRENAL GLANDS

List 6 causes of a unilateral adrenal mass in an adult.	1. Adenoma 2. Metastasis 3. Myelolipoma 4. Pheochromocytoma 5. Hemorrhage 6. Adenocarcinoma
List 6 causes of bilateral adrenal masses.	1. Metastasis 2. Pheochromocytoma 3. Hyperplasia (Cushing's disease) 4. Histoplasmosis 5. Lymphoma 6. Hemorrhage (anticoagulant therapy)
Is size helpful in differentiating benign versus malignant tumors?	Yes. Tumors larger than 3 cm are more likely to be malignant.
Is CT attenuation useful?	Yes.

Is calcification useful in differentiating benign versus malignant adrenal tumors?

No. Approximately one-third of adrenal carcinomas are calcified.

ADRENAL ADENOMA

Is an adrenal adenoma a common lesion?

Yes. It is found in 2%–10% of normal people at autopsy.

How can the diagnosis of adrenal adenoma be confirmed on:

    Unenhanced CT?

Less than 10 HU on nonenhanced CT scan (73% sensitive, 96% specific)

    Enhanced CT?

If a lesion is found on bolus spiral scans, a 20-minute delayed scan can confirm that it is a benign lesion if it measures < 30 HU on delayed CT after contrast.

How is MRI used to differentiate adrenal masses?

Adenomas have the same signal intensity as adrenal tissue on T_1- and T_2-weighted images. Metastases have a higher signal intensity than adenomas on T_2-weighted images. Pheochromocytomas have a very high signal intensity on T_2-weighted images.

Are there other sequences to evaluate adenomas?

Yes. A special sequence, called phase-opposed imaging, shows the adenoma to lose signal on the opposed phase image. This is owing to chemical shift artifact, because adenomas contain a small amount of fat (very specific).

Are most adrenal adenomas functioning or nonfunctioning?

Nonfunctioning

ADRENOCORTICAL CARCINOMA

What are the radiographic features of adrenocortical carcinoma?

Large. The mass is often large (> 5 cm) at the time of diagnosis.
CT shows heterogenous enhancement because of areas of necrosis and hemorrhage, and possibly calcification.

With MRI, the tumor appears hyper-intense relative to the liver but is less hyperintense and usually much larger than a pheochromocytoma. Venous extension occurs.

MYELOLIPOMA

What is a myelolipoma of the adrenal gland?	A fatty tumor of the adrenal gland
Is it malignant?	No, it is benign.
What does it contain?	Red blood cell (RBC) precursors and fat
How can the diagnosis of myelolipoma be made?	Negative HUs

PHEOCHROMOCYTOMA

What imaging studies are used to detect a pheochro-mocytoma involving the adrenal glands?	CT or MRI can detect up to 90% of functional tumors. A metaiodobenzyl-guanidine (MIBG) scan can detect approximately 80%.
What is the rule of tens for pheochromocytoma?	10% Bilateral 10% Malignant 10% Extra-adrenal 10% Familial
Where are extra-adrenal pheochromocytomas found?	Organ of Zuckerkandl and the sympathetic chain
What is the role of MIBG nuclear medicine scanning in evaluation of pheochro-mocytomas?	MIBG scans survey the whole body for extra-adrenal pheochromocytoma when the site is not located by cross-sectional imaging. They also confirm small soft-tissue masses seen on CT or MRI as the source of the pheochromocytoma.

ADRENAL METASTASES

What is the most common primary tumor to metasta-size to the adrenal gland?	Lung tumor (seen in 10% of patients at the time of staging)
List the 5 most common primary tumors that metas-tasize to the adrenal glands.	1. Lung 2. Breast 3. Stomach

4. Colon
5. Kidney

What are the CT features of hyperaldosteronism (Conn's disease)?

Small tumors (< 2 cm)

When the clinical indication for an imaging study is adrenal insufficiency, what must the physician look for?

Evidence of bilateral adrenal disease
Metastases
Tuberculosis
Hemorrhage

List 2 causes of adrenal calcification.

1. Granulomatous disease (histoplasmosis, tuberculosis)
2. Hemorrhage

9   Breast Imaging

Katrina T. Vanderveen

ANATOMY

Identify the structures on this cross sectional sketch of a normal breast:

A = Adipose tissue
B = Pectoralis major muscle
C = Cooper's ligaments
D = Subsegmental duct
E = Segmental duct
F = Connective tissue
G = Lactiferous sinus
H = Collecting duct
I = Lobule
J = Superficial fascia

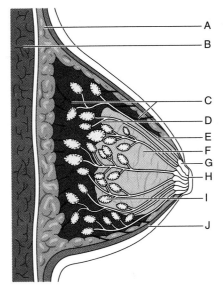

What are Cooper's ligaments?

Suspensory ligaments of the breast (colloquially referred to as "Cooper's droopers" when they fail to support the breast)

What structures comprise the terminal duct lobular unit (TDLU)?

The ductule, the intralobular terminal duct, and the extralobular terminal duct

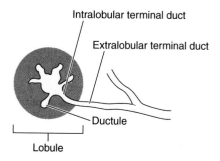

Why is the TDLU important?

Most epithelial tumors originate in the TDLU

IMAGING STUDIES

In addition to mammography, which 4 modalities can be used to evaluate breast tissue?

Magnetic resonance imaging (MRI), ultrasound, nuclear medicine, computed tomography (CT)

MAMMOGRAPHY

What federal law governs mammography standards in the United States?

The Mammography Quality Standards Act (MQSA) of 1993

All mammography facilities must be accredited by which federal agency in order to operate?

The Food and Drug Administration (FDA)

What is the difference between screening and diagnostic mammography?

A screening mammogram is done for a healthy woman with no signs or symptoms of breast cancer. A diagnostic mammogram is obtained under the supervision of a radiologist and is indicated for patients with signs or symptoms related to the breast; enough views are obtained to elucidate the problem.

What percentage of malignancies are not seen on screening mammograms?

10%–20%

What concerns are associated with screening mammograms?

Because screening mammograms are associated with a low yield and involve exposing healthy people to radiation repeatedly, there is the concern that they may cause more malignancies than they detect. Therefore, ensuring that a low dose of radiation is used with each study is extremely important.

What is the radiation dose for mammography?

The average mid-breast dose for 2 views is 0.35 rads.

Why is the breast compressed during mammography? (List 5 reasons)

Compression:
1. Reduces the patient's dose of radiation by decreasing scatter radiation
2. Improves image quality by improving contrast
3. Decreases the occurrence of motion artifacts by immobilizing the breast
4. Reduces geometric blur
5. Reduces change of radiographic density by rendering a more uniform breast thickness

Views

What are the standard views for a screening mammogram?

Mediolateral oblique (MLO) and craniocaudal (CC)

How is the MLO view obtained?

The film cassette is placed in the bucky (film holder), which is positioned obliquely from the axilla to the lower sternum. The breast is compressed with a Lucite plate. The x-ray beam enters the breast from the medial side and exits from the lateral side in an oblique position.

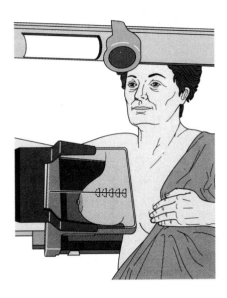

**How is the CC view
obtained?**

The film cassette is placed in the bucky, which is positioned beneath the breast. The breast is compressed from the top with a Lucite plate. The x-ray beam enters from the top of the breast (*cranio*) and exits through the bottom (*caudal*).

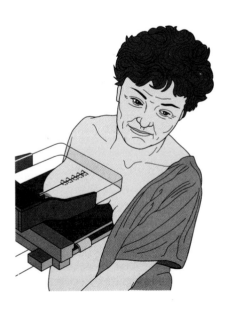

Identify A, B, C, and D (each letter identifies the same structure on both views):

A = Nipple
B = Glandular tissue
C = Fatty tissue
D = Pectoralis muscle margin

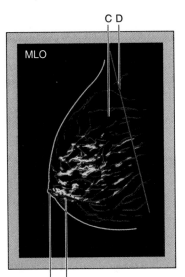

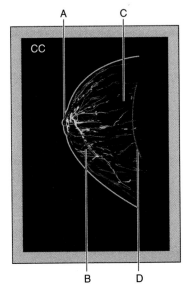

List 7 special views that are sometimes obtained and describe when they are used.

1. Spot compression view (used when the radiologist is uncertain whether a particular area contains a mass)
2. Magnification view (used to evaluate calcifications)
3. True lateral view (used to reveal "milk of calcium" lesions)
4. Axillary tail view (used to examine the breast tissue in the axilla)
5. Cleavage view (used when optimum visualization of the medial breast tissue is required)
6. Rolled (slight oblique) view (used to separate overlapping tissue and may help localize an abnormal finding)
7. Exaggerated CC lateral view (used for visualizing the lateral breast tissue)

What are the advantages of the:

CC view over the MLO view?

The CC view is better than the MLO view for evaluating the medial breast tissue.

MLO view over the CC view and true lateral view?	The MLO view permits visualization of more breast tissue than the CC view and provides better visualization of the axillary tail than the true lateral view.
Why are two views obtained for screening mammograms?	10%–20% of cancers are missed when only single-view mammography is done.
What 4 views are used for screening mammograms in patients with implants?	CC view, MLO view, implant-displaced CC view, and an implant-displaced MLO view
What is the technique of displacing the implant for the purposes of mammography called?	Eklund technique
Why is it important to obtain implant-displaced views when evaluating a patient with implants?	Implant-displaced views allow more complete visualization of the breast tissue.
If the implant cannot be adequately displaced, what view can be useful for screening?	A true lateral view can be added to evaluate the posterior tissue superior and inferior to the implant.

ULTRASOUND

When is ultrasound most useful for evaluation of the breast?	When it is necessary to determine if a mass is **solid** or **cystic**
What type of transducer should be used for breast ultrasound?	A linear, high-frequency transducer (7–10 MHZ)
Why is ultrasound not used as a screening modality?	1. Ultrasound cannot pick up micro-calcifications 2. Occasionally, fairly large masses blend into the background pattern and are not visible as discrete entities on ultrasound.
What are the limitations of breast ultrasound? (List 3)	1. The superficial location of the breast allows the use of a high-frequency transducer, but the ability to penetrate the breast is diminished. Therefore, it

may be necessary to use a lower-frequency transducer (e.g., 5 MHZ) to penetrate large breasts.

2. The appearance of benign and malignant solid tissues can be similar.

3. Breast ultrasound is unable to image microcalcifications.

List 8 ultrasound characteristics of a malignant lesion.

1. Spiculation
2. Angular margins
3. Marked hypoechogenicity
4. Shadowing
5. Calcifications
6. Extension into a duct
7. Branch pattern
8. Microlobulation

List 5 ultrasound characteristics of a benign lesion.

1. Absence of malignant features
2. Hyperechogenicity
3. Ellipsoid shape
4. Gentle bi- or trilobations
5. Thin echogenic pseudocapsule

How often are carcinomas associated with shadowing on ultrasound?

50% of carcinomas demonstrate shadowing. Cancers occasionally show acoustic enhancement.

COMPUTED TOMOGRAPHY (CT)

When is CT used as a primary means of evaluating the breast?

CT is occasionally used to evaluate chest wall involvement of breast cancer. It is also useful for showing recurrent lesions deep in the axilla.

NUCLEAR MEDICINE

How is nuclear medicine used to evaluate the breast?

Technetium 99m (Tc-99m) sestamibi scans may be helpful for evaluating dense, lumpy breasts, by showing uptake in many malignancies.

MAGNETIC RESONANCE IMAGING (MRI)

How is MRI used to evaluate the breast?

MRI can be used to:
1. Evaluate the extent of cancer (i.e., to look for multifocal disease)

2. Detect chest wall involvement of breast cancer
3. Differentiate between scar tissue and recurrent breast cancer in a lumpectomy bed
4. Detect invasive cancers, especially in dense, lumpy breasts
5. Evaluate implants for rupture

Which enhances more rapidly with contrast on MRI— malignant or benign lesions?

Malignant lesions enhance more rapidly. The critical period is the first 3 minutes after injection.

How sensitive and specific is MRI for the evaluation of breast malignancy?

For invasive cancers larger than 1 cm in diameter, MRI has a sensitivity of 88%– 100% and a specificity of 30%–90%.

Which type of cancer may not enhance on MRI?

Only 50% of ductal carcinoma *in situ* (DCIS) cases show enhancement.

Should MRI be used to evaluate the malignant character of microcalcifications?

No. Calcifications of this size are not detectable on MRI.

OBTAINING SAMPLES FOR CYTOLOGIC ANALYSIS

What are 4 ways to obtain samples of suspicious lesions of the breast for cytologic analysis?

1. Core-needle biopsy
2. Needle localization and surgical biopsy
3. Fine needle aspiration
4. Surgical biopsy without localization (palpable masses)

If the lesion is not palpable, how can biopsy be obtained?

Mammographic, stereotactic, or ultrasonographic guidance can be used to localize the lesion. A core-needle biopsy or fine needle aspiration can then be performed. If the lesion is to be biopsied surgically, a needle is placed through the lesion. A wire is placed inside the needle and the needle is removed. The tissue around the wire is then removed at surgery ("needle" or "wire" localization).

What are the two guidance methods commonly used for performing core-needle biopsy?

Ultrasound and stereotactic guidance

What is stereotactic guidance?

Stereotactic guidance uses images obtained by obtaining two x-rays at a 30° angle to one another to localize the abnormality within the breast. The images may be obtained with either film or digital imaging.

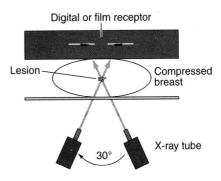

What are the sensitivity and specificity of:

    Core-needle biopsy?

    98% and 98%

    Surgical biopsy with localization?

    98% and 98%

What are the indications for:

    Core-needle biopsy?

    Suspicious (BIRADS 4) or malignant (BIRADS 5) lesion; probably benign (BIRADS 3) lesion, if the patient is excessively anxious about short-term follow-up or is unreliable

    Needle localization and surgical biopsy?

    Same as for core-needle biopsy

What are the advantages of core-needle biopsy over surgical biopsy?

Less invasive, lower complication rate, lower cost
If the lesion is malignant, the patient can chose mastectomy or lumpectomy before surgery has been performed. If it is invasive cancer, axillary dissection can be done during the initial surgery.

EVALUATING A MAMMOGRAM

FILM ANALYSIS

How are mammography films properly hung for reading?

The films are hung back-to-back with the chest wall toward the center. The MLO views are hung so that the axilla is at the top, and the CC views are hung so that the lateral aspect is at the top. Comparison views are hung directly above the views from the most recent examination. Note that the markers indicating the view and the technologist identification number are always placed closest to the axilla.

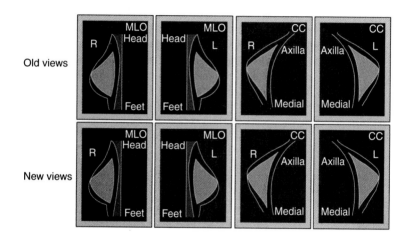

List 10 steps for evaluating a mammogram.

1. Check film quality. Is all of the breast tissue visualized?
2. Check the patient's name and age. Age may affect the differential for a lesion.
3. Determine the normal mammographic background pattern.
4. Check for symmetry. Be aware of any history of surgery.
5. Inspect the skin and subcutaneous fat. Look specifically for skin thickening.
6. Compare the nipples and subareolar regions.
7. Inspect every square centimeter of each breast.

8. Reinspect with a magnifying glass.
9. Specifically evaluate the axillary region.
10. Reevaluate any asymmetry to determine an explanation if one is not already evident.

What is a very important eleventh step?

Compare the current film with the patient's previous films!

How old should a comparison mammogram be?

The comparison mammogram should be at least 2 years older than the current mammogram. Some breast cancers grow slowly; therefore, a change may not be noticeable if the current film is compared with a film that was taken in the previous year.

What are the Breast Imaging Reporting and Dictation System (BIRADS) reporting codes and what follow-up is recommended for each code?

0: Additional evaluation (e.g., magnification or spot compression views, old films for comparison, additional projections, or ultrasound) needed

1: Breasts are symmetric and normal; annual screening recommended

2: Benign lesion (e.g., stable mass, simple cyst, calcified fibroadenoma, scattered benign calcifications, normal lymph node); annual screening recommended

3: Probably benign lesion (e.g., multiple rounded densities, round calcifications, circumscribed mass on a first mammogram); short-interval follow-up suggested (i.e., in 6 months)

4: Suspicious lesion (10%–30% chance of malignancy); biopsy recommended

5: Malignant lesion (spiculated lesion = 90% chance of malignancy); appropriate action (e.g., biopsy, excision) should be taken

MASSES

What are the 3 most important criteria for the analysis of masses detected on a mammogram?

1. Shape
2. Margins (judge the worst portion of the lesion)
3. Density

Using these criteria, describe the characteristics of a:

Benign mass

Shape: Round, oval, or macrolobulated (no more than 3 gentle lobulations)
Margins: Circumscribed
Density: Radiolucent or low-to-medium

Malignant mass

Shape: Irregular, microlobulated
Margins: Ill-defined or spiculated
Density: Medium-to-high

List 3 other typical characteristics of benign masses.

1. May have a halo (i.e., a low-density rim that surrounds the mass)
2. May contain fat (like a lymph node)
3. Lesion is stable or becomes smaller over time

List 2 other typical characteristics of malignant masses.

1. Architectural distortion
2. Enlargement over time

What are the 3 most common palpable masses?

Fibroadenoma (patients younger than 35 years)
Cyst (patients between the ages of 35 and 50 years)
Carcinoma (patients older than 50 years)

What are the differential diagnoses for:

A well-defined mammographic mass? (List 14)

1. Cyst
2. Fibroadenoma
3. Phylloides tumor
4. Carcinoma
5. Metastases
6. Papilloma
7. Hematoma
8. Hamartoma
9. Lipoma
10. Intramammary lymph node
11. Abscess
12. Oil cyst (fat necrosis)
13. Galactocele
14. Raised skin lesion

An ill-defined mammographic mass? (List 6)

1. Carcinoma
2. Abscess

3. Hematoma
4. Radial scar
5. Fibrocystic changes
6. Myoblastoma

A spiculated mammographic mass? (List 3)

1. Invasive carcinoma (99%)
2. Surgical scar
3. Radial scar

A circumscribed, fat-containing (radiolucent) mass? (List 5)

1. Lymph node
2. Lipoma
3. Hamartoma
4. Oil cyst (fat necrosis)
5. Galactocele

Are fat-containing masses always benign?

No. All *circumscribed* fat-containing masses are benign. However, an irregular or spiculated mass that contains fat may be malignant.

Which cancers may present as a circumscribed mass on mammogram?

Mucinous carcinoma, medullary carcinoma, and phylloides tumor typically present as well-defined masses, but they are uncommon breast cancers. Infiltrating ductal carcinoma only presents as a well-defined mass 6% of the time, but because it is the most common histologic type of breast cancer, it is statistically the most common cause of a malignant well-defined nodule.

List 7 mammographic signs of malignancy that are caused directly by a tumor.

1. Mass
2. Spiculated or ill-defined margin
3. Malignant calcifications (microcalcifications)
4. Focal asymmetric density
5. Neodensity
6. Architectural distortion
7. Single enlarged duct

List 6 mammographic signs of malignancy that occur indirectly as a result of a tumor.

1. Architectural distortion
2. Skin thickening
3. Nipple retraction
4. Lymphadenopathy (enlarged or dense lymph nodes)
5. Trabecular thickening (breast edema)
6. Asymmetry of breast tissue

CALCIFICATIONS

What 4 criteria are used to differentiate benign and malignant mammographic calcifications?	Distribution, size, shape, stability
What are the characteristics of calcifications in:	
Benign lesions?	Scattered, macro (> 2 mm in diameter), smooth, uniform

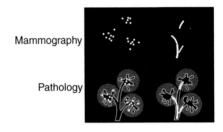

Malignant lesions?	Clustered, micro (< 0.5 mm in diameter), irregular, variable

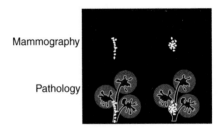

What are ductal casts?	Ductal casts, which occur when necrotic debris and secretions calcify within the duct, are another characteristic of malignant calcifications. The casts may be fine (sand-like) or granular ("broken needles," "crushed stone").
List 2 malignant lesions that are associated with calcifications.	DCIS and infiltrating ductal carcinoma (usually DCIS that has progressed to invasion)

List 8 benign mammographic findings and the typical calcification pattern of each.

1. Fibroadenoma: "Popcorn" calcifications

2. Fibrocystic changes: Scattered microcalcifications, usually round, but sometimes amorphous and indistinct
3. Oil cyst (fat necrosis): Ring-like calcifications with lucent centers
4. Plasma-cell mastitis ("secretory disease"): Needle-like calcifications oriented along ducts
5. Arteries: "Tram-track" lines (i.e., pairs of parallel lines)
6. Skin: Small, round calcifications with lucent centers located along the medial and lower edges of the breast, usually within sebaceous glands
7. Artifacts: Deodorant (aluminum hydroxide) and talcum powder most common culprits
8. Silicone: Foreign-body granulomas, may have very bizarre appearance

What is a "milk of calcium" lesion? Is it benign or malignant?

A "milk-of-calcium" lesion, a benign finding, results from cystic hyperplasia, which is a type of fibrocystic change. Lobules become cystically dilated and debris within the fluid calcifies. On a true lateral view [i.e., a mediolateral (ML), not an MLO, view], the dependent debris has a linear configuration ("teacups"). Calcifications are often difficult to visualize on the CC view, but may be round ("pearls"). (see figure on next page)

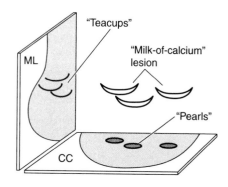

"Teacups"

"Milk-of-calcium" lesion

ML

"Pearls"

CC

SKIN THICKENING

What is the upper limit of normal for breast skin thickness?

3 mm (usually < 1.5 mm)

List 8 benign causes of a thickened skin pattern.

1. Inadequate compression
2. Irradiation or surgery
3. Acute mastitis
4. Cardiac failure
5. Renal failure
6. Hypoalbuminemia
7. Thrombophlebitis of the breast (Mondor's disease)
8. Thrombus in the subclavian vein or superior vena cava (SVC)

List 4 malignant causes of a thickened skin pattern.

1. Locally advanced primary cancer (focal thickening)
2. Recurrent carcinoma after lumpectomy and radiation therapy
3. Lymphatic obstruction owing to metastatic axillary nodes (including lymphoma)
4. Inflammatory breast cancer (diffuse thickening)

DUCTAL CHANGES

What causes a dilated duct?

Obstruction, such as that caused by DCIS, papilloma, ductal adenoma (a rare benign epithelial tumor), or debris (especially related to lactation and galactocele)

Duct ectasia (benign periductal fibrosis),

which is usually retroareolar and may be associated with a palpable mass and nipple retraction

What 3 options are available to the radiologist for further evaluation of a ductal lesion?

Ultrasound, spot compression view, magnification view

DISORDERS OF THE BREAST

BREAST CANCER

Incidence and epidemiology

What is the incidence of breast cancer in the United States?

One in ten American women develop breast cancer.

What are the risk factors?

Female sex (female:male > 100:1)
Age > 40 years
Family history of breast cancer, especially premenopausal or bilateral breast cancer in a first-degree relative (mother or sister)
Previous history of breast cancer, lobular carcinoma *in situ* (LCIS), or atypia
Early menarche and late menopause
Nulliparity or age > 35 years at first full-term pregnancy

What percentage of breast cancers occur in patients with no risk factors except gender and age?

75%

What is the overall death rate associated with breast cancer?

35%–50% of breast cancer patients eventually die from the disease.

Which 4 tumors commonly metastasize to the breast?

Lymphoma, leukemia, melanoma, lung cancer

Types of breast cancer

What are the histologic types of breast cancer?

Invasive ductal: 65%
Intraductal carcinoma (DCIS): 15%
Invasive lobular: 10%
Tubular carcinoma: 3%

Medullary carcinoma: 2%
Mucinous carcinoma: 2%
Phylloides tumor: 1%
Paget's disease: 1%
Inflammatory carcinoma: 1%

Ductal carcinoma

What are the characteristics of DCIS on physical examination?

The breast is usually normal, but thickening or a discrete mass may be palpable.

What is the risk of developing invasive ductal carcinoma with DCIS?

DCIS becomes invasive in approximately 30% of patients if left untreated.

What are the radiographic characteristics of invasive ductal carcinoma?

Usually presents as a spiculated, high-density mass on mammogram

Lobular carcinoma

What are the clinical characteristics of invasive lobular carcinoma?

Invasive lobular carcinoma often presents with thickening rather than a discrete palpable mass.

What are the radiographic characteristics of invasive lobular carcinoma?

A spiculated mass is the most common mammographic finding, but is seen much less often than in invasive ductal carcinoma. Invasive lobular carcinoma is often not as dense on mammography as other cancers, and the mammogram usually underestimates the amount of tumor present. Invasive lobular carcinoma is more commonly mammographically occult than invasive ductal carcinoma, a fact with medicolegal significance.

Inflammatory breast cancer

What is the histologic hallmark of inflammatory breast cancer?

Cancer in the dermal lymphatics

What is the clinical presentation of inflammatory breast cancer?

Red, swollen, painful breast

How is inflammatory breast cancer definitively diagnosed?	Biopsy should include a section of skin; therefore, fine needle aspiration is usually not sufficient to make the specific diagnosis.

Phylloides tumor

What is a phylloides tumor?	A phylloides tumor is a rare type of breast tumor that usually presents as a rapidly enlarging mass in an older woman (average patient age = 70 years). On histologic examination, a phylloides tumor appears similar to a fibroadenoma, but the stroma is more cellular and epithelium-lined branching clefts are typical.
What are the radiographic characteristics of a phylloides tumor?	Mammographically, a phylloides tumor presents as a round, circumscribed, solid mass that may resemble a fibroadenoma.
How can a phylloides tumor be differentiated from a fibroadenoma?	The patient's age usually helps differentiate the two entities (fibroadenomas are most common in young women).
What percentage of phylloides tumors are malignant?	15%–20%; cannot predict malignancy from histology
When malignant, what is the most common site of metastasis?	Lung (rather than the nodes)

Lymphoma of the breast

What are the radiographic characteristics of lymphoma of the breast?	Primary lymphoma presents as a mass with minimal spiculation. Secondary lymphoma of the breast presents as diffuse involvement with skin thickening.

Paget's disease

What is Paget's disease?	Thickening or erosion of the nipple associated with ductal cancer
What are the two theories of histogenesis associated with Paget's disease?	Migratory cells *De novo* appearance in nipple

Screening

Why are screening mammograms done?

Mortality is reduced if breast cancer is found at an early stage.

What are the American Cancer Society (ACS) guidelines for screening mammography?

Baseline mammogram between the ages of 35 and 39 years; yearly mammogram starting at age 40

What are the ACS guidelines for clinical breast examination and breast self-examination (BSE)?

Patients should receive a clinical breast examination from a health professional every 3 years between the ages of 20 and 39 years, and yearly starting at age 40. BSE should be performed monthly beginning at age 20 years.

What is the best time of the month for premenopausal women to perform a BSE or have a mammogram?

During days 5–10 of the menstrual cycle (i.e., during the postmenstrual week) because the breasts are least tender and lumpy at this time of the cycle.

How does hormone replacement therapy (HRT) affect the breast clinically and mammographically?

Clinically, approximately 25% of women starting HRT develop breast tenderness. Mammographically, about 30% have an increase in breast fibroglandular density, which is usually bilateral and symmetric but may be unilateral or focal.

Staging and prognosis

What system is used for pathologic staging?

TMN: Tumor, **M**etastases, **N**odal involvement

What are the stages?

0:   DCIS
I: Invasive tumor < 2 cm in diameter, no regional nodes, no distant metastases
II: Invasive tumor < 5 cm in diameter, not fixed to chest wall, +/− few regional nodes, no distant metastases
III: Invasive tumor any size, may be fixed to chest wall, + regional nodes, no distant metastases
IV: Distant metastases

What is the most important prognostic factor for patients with primary breast cancer?

Axillary node status

What is the most important prognostic factor for patients with stage N_0 disease?

Estrogen receptor (ER) status

Describe the three levels of axillary lymph nodes.

Level I: Lateral to the pectoralis minor muscle
Level II: At the pectoralis minor muscle
Level III: Medial to the pectoralis minor muscle

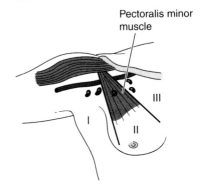

What is the 5-year survival rate after treatment (by stage at the time of diagnosis)?

Locally invasive: 90%
Regional spread: 68%
Distant spread: 17%
When the cancer is noninvasive, the 5-year survival rate approaches 100%, hence the benefit of early detection.

What is the risk of recurrence based on nodes and ER status?

Risk of Recurrence	*Nodes*	*ER Status*
Low	−	+
Intermediate	−	−
Intermediate	+	+
High	+	−

To where does breast cancer typically metastasize?

Ipsilateral lymph node (< 25% for screening-detected cancers, 50% for palpable cancers)
Bone—(most common site)
Lung
Pleura
Soft tissue
Liver
Brain

Treatment

Mastectomy

What are the 5 criteria for inoperability of breast cancer?	1. Extensive skin edema or arm edema 2. Fixation of the primary tumor to the chest wall 3. Primary tumor > 5 cm in diameter 4. Massive involvement or fixation of the axillary, supraclavicular, or internal mammary nodes 5. Distant metastases
Define the following types of mastectomies:	
Halstead radical mastectomy	Excision of all breast tissue, including the nipple, pectoralis major and minor muscles, and all axillary lymph nodes; rarely performed today
Modified radical mastectomy	Excision of all breast tissue, including the nipple and axillary lymph nodes, but preservation of the muscles
Total (simple) mastectomy	Excision of all breast tissue, including the nipple, but preservation of the muscles and nodes
Subcutaneous mastectomy	Excision of most breast tissue, but the nipple is left intact and the muscles and nodes are preserved
Partial mastectomy (lumpectomy)	Excision of some breast tissue. The nipple, the muscles and possibly the nodes are left intact
Why should women who have had a subcutaneous or partial mastectomy have mammograms?	Because breast tissue is still present and therefore the patient is still at risk for cancer
Is mammography useful for women who have had a radical, modified radical, or simple mastectomy?	No. There is no significant breast tissue remaining. If physical examination is inconclusive or suspicious, CT can be useful.

How does the survival rate after treatment with radical, modified, simple, and partial mastectomies vary?	There are no significant differences among the types of surgery in terms of survival rate.

Chemotherapy and radiation therapy

What are the National Cancer Institute chemotherapy recommendations for patients with the following status following surgical evaluation?

Premenopausal, + nodes, + or − ER status	Combination chemotherapy
Premenopausal, − nodes, + or − ER status	Consider chemotherapy, depending on the patient's situation
Postmenopausal, − nodes, + or − ER status	No further treatment indicated
Postmenopausal, + nodes, − ER status	Consider chemotherapy, depending on the patient's situation
Postmenopausal, + nodes, + ER status	Tamoxifen

What percentage of patients will respond to endocrine therapy:

When their ER status is positive?	57%
When their ER status is negative?	8%
What effect does radiation therapy have on the recurrence and survival rates?	Radiation therapy improves the local recurrence rate but not the distant recurrence rate or the survival rate.

BENIGN LESIONS

Lobular carcinoma *in situ* (LCIS)

What are the physical examination and mammographic characteristics of LCIS?	None. LCIS, an incidental finding on biopsy, is not detectable on physical examination and is mammographically occult.

How does LCIS differ from DCIS?

Unlike DCIS, which may progress to invasive ductal carcinoma, LCIS does not progress to invasive lobular carcinoma. Therefore, LCIS is not a true carcinoma, and is often now termed "lobular neoplasia." However, a biopsy showing LCIS is associated with a high risk of developing breast cancer.

In patients with a previous history of LCIS, what is the risk of developing invasive cancer?

Patients have a 30% risk of developing invasive carcinoma (most commonly invasive ductal carcinoma) in either breast (50/50) over 20 years.

Simple cyst

How does a simple breast cyst develop?

A cyst results from dilatation of the terminal ductule.

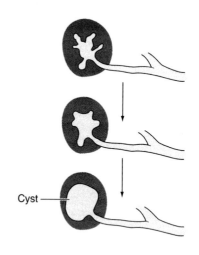

How are simple breast cysts diagnosed?

The mammographic appearance (i.e., of a well-defined nodule) is not pathognomonic; ultrasound is required for diagnosis.

What are the 3 ultrasound criteria for a simple cyst?

Anechoic, well-defined back wall, acoustic enhancement

When should a breast cyst be aspirated?

A cyst should be aspirated when it is tender, or when it is new or enlarging and the ultrasound criteria for a simple cyst are not met. In the latter situation, aspiration confirms that the mass is cystic and not solid.

Fibroadenoma

What are the clinical characteristics of a fibroadenoma?

Fibroadenomas are the most common palpable mass in patients younger than 35 years. They are nontender, rubbery, and freely moveable. Typically, fibroadenomas begin in adolescence and may grow to 2–3 centimeters in size. They may become very large during puberty, in which case they are called juvenile fibroadenomas.

How do fibroadenomas appear radiographically?

They are smooth and lobulated. Fibroadenomas may involute after menopause and develop pathognomonic "popcorn" calcifications ("ancient" fibroadenomas).

Papilloma

What is a papilloma?

A benign intraductal epithelial lesion, usually single and located in the retro-areolar area

What are the clinical characteristics of a papilloma?

Papillomas are the most common cause of a bloody discharge. They are typically nonpalpable.

How do papillomas appear radiographically?

They may infarct, undergo sclerosis, and then calcify.

Hematoma

What are the clinical characteristics of a hematoma?

Ill-defined palpable mass

How is a hematoma diagnosed?

Diagnosis depends on the proper clinical setting (i.e., a recent history of trauma, biopsy, or surgery).

Hamartoma

What is a hamartoma?

Normal tissue in an abnormal location

What are the characteristics of a hamartoma:

Clinically?

Usually not palpable because hamartomas

are composed of same tissue as the rest of the breast

Mammographically?

Hamartomas present as a mixed-density mass ("breast within a breast"). The appearance is pathognomonic if a capsule is seen.

Lipoma

What are the characteristics of a lipoma:

Clinically?

Often not palpable because lipomas are composed of the same tissue as the rest of breast

Mammographically?

Lipomas are entirely radiolucent. Demonstration of a capsule separates a true lipoma from simply a fatty component of the breast.

Abscess

How is an abscess diagnosed?

An abscess may be well-defined or ill-defined on mammography. Carcinoma may mimic this appearance; therefore, diagnosis requires the proper clinical setting (i.e., fever or erythema and tenderness at the site).

What follow-up is indicated for a patient with a suspected abscess?

If an abscess is thought to be present clinically, the patient should be re-examined in 2–4 weeks after antibiotic therapy to ensure that the mass resolves, because carcinoma can mimic an abscess.

Oil cyst (fat necrosis)

What are the clinical characteristics of an oil cyst?

An oil cyst presents clinically as a firm, nontender mass, usually following trauma or surgery.

How does an oil cyst appear radiographically?

An oil cyst appears as a circumscribed radiolucent mass on mammography. The mammogram is pathognomonic if a capsule (which often calcifies) is identified.

Galactocele

What is a galactocele?

A cystic structure containing inspissated milk

What are the clinical characteristics of a galactocele?

A galactocele is usually caused by the sudden cessation of nursing. It presents as a hard mass, which may or may not be tender.

How does a galactocele appear on a mammogram?

Mammography shows the galactocele to be fat density (i.e., radiolucent). The galactocele may contain a fat-fluid level and is not calcified.

Mondor's disease

What is Mondor's disease?

Superficial thrombophlebitis of the veins of the breast; the thoracoepigastric vein (on the lateral aspect of the breast) is most often involved

How does Mondor's disease present clinically?

Painful swelling of the breast

Radial scar (radial sclerosing lesion, sclerosing capillary proliferation, nonencapsulated sclerosing lesion)

What are the radiographic characteristics of a radial scar?

Radial scars typically appear as a small spiculated mass on mammogram, occasionally with microcalcifications. The lesion may have central lucency ("black star"), as opposed to the central density seen with invasive cancers ("white star").

With which condition can radial scar be confused?

Mammographically and histologically, radial scars can be confused with carcinoma; therefore, biopsy must be performed.

Are radial scars associated with cancer?

Yes, especially tubular carcinoma

Fibrosis and fibrocystic changes

In what age group does fibrosis or fibrocystic change occur?

Women between the ages of 35–50 years

How is fibrocystic change defined histologically?	Fibrosis with cyst formation
How does fibrocystic change appear radiographically?	Mammography may show more glandular tissue than expected for the patient's age and parity Microcalcifications, typically scattered, are common "Milk-of-calcium" areas may be seen with cystic hyperplasia
How does fibrocystic change appear on ultrasound?	Ultrasound shows macrocysts or microcysts (< 3 mm in diameter)

Lymph nodes

On mammography, what is the typical appearance of:

Normal axillary nodes?	< 1.5 cm in diameter if not fatty replaced; they may be considered normal at any size if fatty replaced Well-circumscribed Often demonstrate a fatty hilum (i.e., a notch of fat density)
Intramammary lymph nodes?	Typically located in the upper breast, in a band along the lateral aspect Demonstration of a fatty hilum is diagnostic
What are the causes of abnormal axillary nodes and how do the nodes appear radiographically?	Abnormal lymph nodes lose their fatty hilum and increase in density. Causes of abnormal axillary nodes include: **Primary lymphoma:** Node margins usually remain well-defined **Metastases from breast primary:** Node margins may become ill-defined; may contain microcalcifications **Metastases from non-breast primaries:** Node margins usually become ill-defined; usually no calcifications **Nonmalignancies** [e.g., sarcoidosis, rheumatoid arthritis (injected gold salts may look like microcalcifications), psoriasis, systemic lupus

erythematosus (SLE), scleroderma, granulomatous infections]

CONDITIONS ASSOCIATED WITH NIPPLE DISCHARGE

What are the most common causes of nipple discharge?	Benign intraductal papilloma (90% of cases), DCIS, intraductal debris, fibrocystic change
When is nipple discharge worrisome?	When it is bloody or serous (clear) When it is spontaneous When it is unilateral and affects a single duct
When is nipple discharge usually benign?	When it is green, milky, yellow, or brown When it is expressible only (i.e., not spontaneous) When it is bilateral and affects multiple ducts
What lesion may cause a milky discharge (galactorrhea) and headache or peripheral vision loss?	Pituitary adenoma (prolactinoma)
What test is useful for evaluating worrisome nipple discharge?	A galactogram (ductogram). A small catheter is placed in the duct of origin of the discharge and contrast is injected. Mammogram images are then obtained to look for an intraductal mass (papilloma or intraductal cancer).

IMPLANT RUPTURE

What are most breast implants made from currently?	A silastic bag filled with saline or silicone
What reaction does the breast have to implants?	It forms a fibrous capsule around the implant.

What are the two types of implant rupture?

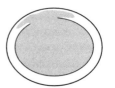

Intracapsular rupture
(implant shell only)

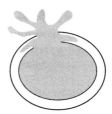

Extracapsular rupture
(implant shell and
fibrous capsule)

What might calcifications signify in patients with implants?

Leaking silicone can induce tissue calcifications of a variety of shapes and sizes.
An inflammatory response can cause capsular calcification.

MRI evaluation

What components of the implant are seen on the MRI scan?

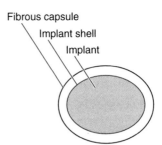

Fibrous capsule
Implant shell
Implant

Why is the ability to discern the components of the implant important?

It allows for evaluation of the contour of the silastic bag and the fibrous capsule.

On MRI, is silicone bright or dark?

Silicone has long T_1 and long T_2. Therefore, silicone (like water and saline) is dark on T_1 and bright on T_2.

What is the "linguine" sign?

Lines within the implant that may

represent the collapsed walls of an intracapsular rupture

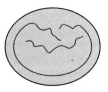

What are radiating folds?	Normal redundant folds in the silastic envelope, not to be confused with rupture

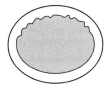

What do crenelated margins indicate?	Capsular contracture

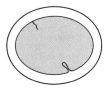

What can a focal bulge represent?	Herniation through the fibrous capsule (as below) or rupture

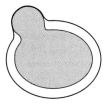

What is the "inverted teardrop" sign?	The "inverted teardrop" sign occurs when silicone enters a radial fold and then leaks between the implant and the capsule. It is a nonspecific sign that may be seen with extensive gel bleed or focal intracapsular rupture. [Silicone gel may traverse an

intact implant shell ("bleed"). This occurs to some extent with most implants, but may be extensive in some cases.]

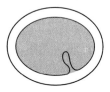

How sensitive and specific is MRI for evaluating implant rupture?

94% sensitivity and 97% specificity

Ultrasound evaluation

How do normal implants appear on ultrasound?

Implants are normally anechoic. Echogenic implants are abnormal.

What descriptors have been used to describe the ultrasound appearances of:

Extracapsular rupture?

"Snowstorm" appearance (i.e., extreme echogenicity with extensive shadowing)

Intracapsular rupture?

"Stepladder" appearance (similar to the "linguine" sign on MRI)

How sensitive and specific is ultrasound for evaluating implant rupture?

70% sensitivity and 70% specificity

10

Obstetric and Gynecologic Imaging

David Cressler Heasley, Jr.

ANATOMY

Identify the following structures on this sagittal section (see image on next page):

A = Fallopian tube
B = Uterine fundus
C = Round ligament of the uterus
D = Uterovesical pouch
E = Bladder
F = Symphysis pubis
G = Urethra
H = Vagina
I = Anus
J = Rectum
K = Posterior fornix of the vagina
L = Cul-de-sac or rectouterine pouch (pouch of Douglas)
M = Sigmoid colon
N = Sacrum
O = Uterine cervix
P = Uterine corpus
Q = Ovary

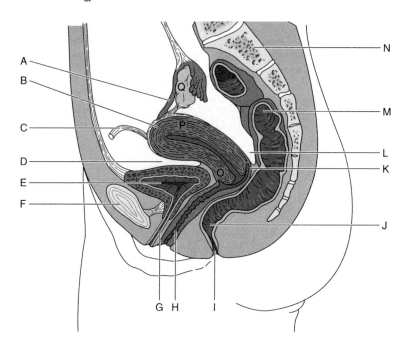

Through what structure is a culdocentesis (aspiration of ascites) performed?

The posterior fornix of the vagina

Identify the following structures on this coronal section (see image on next page):

A = Ureters
B = Uterine fundus
C = Uterine cornu
D = Uterine corpus
E = Uterine isthmus
F = Sigmoid colon
G = Bladder
H = Vagina
I = Uterine cervix
J = Parametria
K = Internal iliac vessels
L = Broad ligament
M = Common iliac vessels
N = Iliopsoas muscle

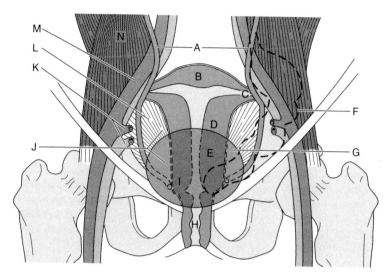

Describe the uterus in each of the following pictures.

A = Anteflexed
B = Retroverted
C = Retroflexed
D = Anteverted

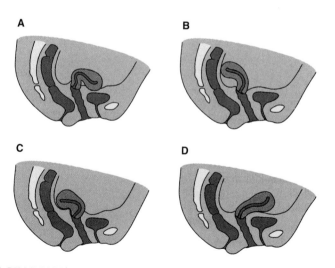

IMAGING MODALITIES

OBSTETRICS

What imaging modality is the mainstay of obstetric radiology?

Ultrasound, either transabdominal or transvaginal (endovaginal)

List 6 common indications for the use of ultrasound in pregnancy.	1. Confirmation of intrauterine pregnancy (IUP) 2. Evaluation of suspected ectopic pregnancy 3. Determination of fetal estimated gestational age (EGA) 4. Investigation of vaginal bleeding 5. Evaluation of fetal well-being 6. Evaluation of an abnormal α-fetoprotein (AFP) level
When is MRI used in pregnancy?	When a problem affecting the mother's health arises and ultrasound cannot provide the answer
When is computed tomography (CT) used in pregnancy?	Work-up of maternal trauma when a rapid diagnosis is essential
List 3 advantages that transvaginal (endovaginal) ultrasound offers over transabdominal ultrasound.	1. A full bladder is not required (indeed, it is not desired). 2. Pregnancy can be detected earlier, because the transducer is closer to the structures of interest and a higher frequency can be used. 3. Higher resolution images are possible because higher frequency transducers can be used.

GYNECOLOGY

Which modality is best for initial evaluation of suspected uterine or endometrial pathology?	Ultrasound
What are some indications for transvaginal ultrasound in terms of assessing a potential gynecologic disorder?	Abnormal vaginal bleeding (transvaginal ultrasound allows better visualization of the endometrium than transabdominal ultrasound) An adnexal mass
What structures may be missed by endovaginal ultrasound?	Any structure more than 8–10 cm away from the transducer (e.g., the ovaries, if they are positioned in the upper pelvis;

other structures normally located in the upper region of the pelvis)

What is a contraindication to endovaginal ultrasound?

Prepubertal condition

List 6 indications for using MRI to image the uterus.

1. Staging of cancers of the endometrium and uterine cervix
2. Differentiation of fibroids from adenomyosis
3. Preoperative assessment of fibroids if myomectomy is being considered
4. Clarification of pelvic mass origin (adnexal versus uterine) when ultrasound is equivocal
5. Clarification of septate and bicornuate uterine anomalies
6. Noninvasive monitoring of endometriosis

What are 5 advantages of MRI over CT for imaging the uterus?

1. Improved soft tissue contrast
2. Can distinguish the zonal anatomy of the uterus and cervix
3. Absence of ionizing radiation
4. Intravenous contrast not usually necessary
5. Multiplanar imaging capability

What are 5 disadvantages of MRI for imaging the uterus?

1. High cost (compared with ultrasound; only slightly higher than CT)
2. Long examination time
3. Contraindicated in patients with pacemakers or certain ferromagnetic implants
4. Poor visualization of calcification
5. Possible intolerance to the procedure (e.g., as a result of claustrophobia)

What pelvic structures do T_1-weighted MRI scans distinguish well?

Soft tissue (from fat), lymph nodes, hemorrhagic lesions

Name a strength of T_2-weighted MRI in terms of evaluating gynecologic disorders.

T_2-weighted MRI distinguishes the zonal anatomy of the uterus, which is useful for staging cervical and endometrial cancer and evaluating adenomyosis.

In T$_2$-weighted MRI scans, give the relative signal strengths of the following tissues:

Endometrium	High signal intensity
Junctional zone (inner myometrium)	Low signal intensity
Outer myometrium	Intermediate signal intensity

What is a hysterosalpingo-gram (HSG)?

A fluoroscopic image of the pelvis taken after injecting contrast material through the cervix and into the uterus and fallopian tubes; normally, contrast fills the endometrial cavity (U) and freely spills into the peritoneal cavity (P) through the patent fallopian tubes (T)

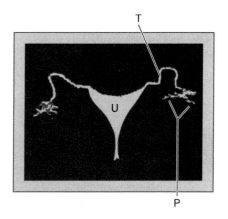

Name 2 common indications for obtaining an HSG.

1. As part of an infertility work-up (to evaluate tubal patency)
2. To evaluate uterine congenital anomalies

List 4 causes of infertility that can be revealed by an HSG.

1. Congenital anomalies
2. Submucosal leiomyomas
3. Asherman's syndrome (i.e., intrauterine synechiae, menstrual dysfunction, and infertility secondary to dilation and curettage)
4. Obstructed or adherent fallopian tubes

List 2 clinical precautions that should be taken with regard to an HSG.

1. Perform only on days 6–12 after the patient's last menstrual period (LMP).
2. Administer prophylactic doxycycline if tubal dilation is observed (to reduce the risk of infection and a tubo-ovarian abscess).

What risks are associated with an HSG?

Pain, infection, contrast allergy, and radiation-associated problems

What radiation dose does an ovary receive during an HSG?

100–600 mrad

Name 4 contraindications to performing a HSG.

1. Pregnancy
2. Active tubal or uterine infection
3. Active menstruation
4. Recent uterine surgery

OBSTETRICS

PREGNANCY IN THE FIRST TRIMESTER

List 7 features that one should attempt to identify by first-trimester ultrasound in a patient with a normal pregnancy.

1. Gestational sac
2. Yolk sac
3. Embryo
4. Cardiac activity
5. Crown-rump length (CRL)
6. Uterine anatomy
7. Placental location

How is the CRL defined?

The CRL is the distance from the top of the embryo's head to the bottom of the torso.

At which point in development can endovaginal ultrasound detect the following:

IUP (i.e., a gestational sac)

When the β-human chorionic gonadotropin (β-hCG) level exceeds 1000 mIU/ml

Fetal yolk sac

When the mean gestational sac diameter is greater than 8 mm

Embryo or fetal pole

When the mean gestational sac diameter is greater than 16 mm

Cardiac activity	When the fetal pole (embryo) is greater than 4 mm
At what point in development can transabdominal ultrasound detect the following?	
IUP	When the β-hCG is greater than 3600 mIU/ml
Fetal yolk sac	When the mean gestational sac diameter is greater than 20 mm
Embryo or fetal pole	When the mean gestational sac diameter is greater than 25 mm
What findings definitively confirm the diagnosis of an early IUP?	Cardiac activity and the presence of a yolk sac
What other sign may be seen in early pregnancy?	The "double decidual sac" sign (i.e., visualization of two echogenic rings)
What 3 structures make up the "double decidual sac" sign?	1. Decidua parietalis 2. Decidua capsularis 3. Decidua basalis

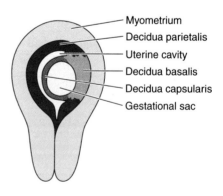

What does the "double decidual sac" sign indicate?	IUP
What is gestational age?	The time since the first day of the LMP— not from the moment of conception

Give the gestational age of the following:

Gestational sac less than 8 mm without a visible embryo or yolk sac	5.0 weeks
Gestational sac of 8–16 mm with a visible yolk sac but no visible embryo	5.5 weeks
Heart beat with or without visible embryo	6.0 weeks

Tell how the EGA is best assessed sonographically at the following times:

6–13 weeks	CRL (in mm)
14–26 weeks	Biparietal diameter at the level of the thalami (in mm)
27–40 weeks	Femur length (in mm) or a combination of multiple measurements (e.g., biparietal diameter, humerus length, head circumference, and abdominal circumference)

Name 4 causes of vaginal bleeding in the first trimester.

1. Miscarriage (approximately 15% of all recognized pregnancies)
2. Small subchorionic hemorrhage (approximately 15% of all pregnancies)
3. Ectopic pregnancy
4. Molar pregnancy

What are 4 causes of a positive β-hCG test in the absence of a visualized IUP?

1. Early IUP
2. Ectopic pregnancy
3. Spontaneous abortion
4. Molar pregnancy

What would you expect to find in terms of the β-hCG level in each of the following situations?

Early IUP	Doubles approximately every 48 hours
Ectopic pregnancy	Increases, but does not double every 48 hours

Spontaneous abortion   Falls to 0 mIU/ml

Molar pregnancy   Increases dramatically

What are 3 clinical symp-   Pelvic pain, vaginal bleeding, and pelvic
toms of ectopic pregnancy?   mass

List 5 sonographic findings   1. No intrauterine gestational sac
suggestive of ectopic preg-   2. Complex or solid adnexal mass
nancy.   (representing the ectopic gestation),
                                     possibly with fetal heart activity
                                  3. Blood in the cul-de-sac (if the ectopic
                                     pregnancy has ruptured)
                                  4. Tubal ring (i.e., an echogenic ring in
                                     the ovary or fallopian tube)
                                  5. Single layer of decidua in the
                                     endometrium (decidual reaction)

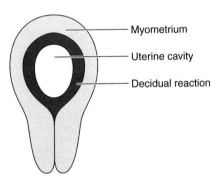

Myometrium

Uterine cavity

Decidual reaction

Name the 5 most common   1. Fallopian tube (95%–97% of cases)
sites of ectopic pregnancy   2. Uterine cornu (2%–5% of cases)
(from most to least common). 3. Ovary (1% of cases)
                                  4. Cervix (< 0.1% of cases)
                                  5. Abdomen (< 0.1% of cases)

Can ectopic pregnancy and   Yes; this phenomenon occurs in about 1
IUP coexist?   out of every 7000 pregnancies.

What is the appearance of   A molar pregnancy appears as a "cluster
molar pregnancy on ultra-   of grapes" (i.e., an echogenic mass in the
sound?   uterine cavity with small cystic spaces).
                                  Bilateral theca lutein ovarian cysts are
                                  often seen secondary to stimulation from
                                  an elevated β-hCG level.

What condition may mimic   Missed abortion
a molar gestation?

What is a missed abortion?

Death of the fetus, but fetal tissue is retained *in utero;* now known as embryonic demise

List 4 sonographic findings that are suggestive of impending abortion.

1. Angular or collapsed gestational sac
2. Absence of visible cardiac activity at the appropriate EGA
3. Irregular trophoblastic rim
4. Discrepant gestational sac or embryo size

PREGNANCY IN THE SECOND AND THIRD TRIMESTERS

Why is examination of the fetus by ultrasound in the second trimester particularly useful?

Organs are fully formed

Anatomy is easier to visualize

Dates (i.e., gestational ages) are as accurate as in the first trimester if examined before the 24th week of pregnancy

Abortion may be an option at the beginning of the second trimester, but not in the third trimester

Is examination of the fetus by ultrasound technically easier during the second trimester or at full term?

During the second trimester, because:

The amniotic fluid-to-body bulk ratio is higher than in the third trimester

It may still be possible to image the entire fetus

The bones are less calcified and therefore cause less shadowing

In each of the following areas, name the specific features that should be routinely examined during the second-trimester using ultrasound:

Head, neck, and spine

Biparietal diameter, atria of the lateral ventricles, cerebellum, cisterna magna, and spine

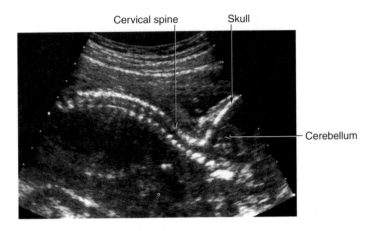

<table>
<tr><td>**Chest**</td><td>The heart (all four chambers), the great vessels, and the heart rate; also check that no abdominal contents are in the thoracic area</td></tr>
</table>

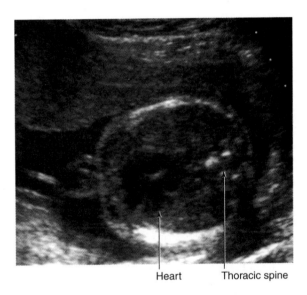

<table>
<tr><td>**Abdomen**</td><td>Abdominal circumference, stomach, umbilical cord insertion, kidneys, and bladder</td></tr>
</table>

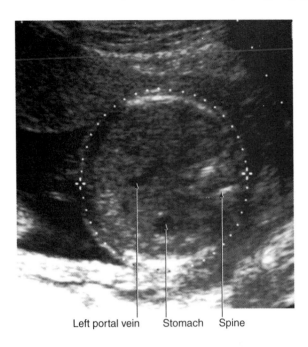

Left portal vein   Stomach   Spine

Extremities   Femur length; also, ensure that all four
                                   extremities are present

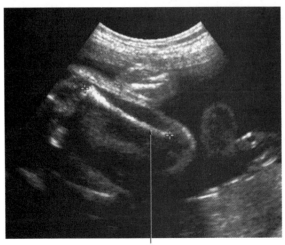

Femur

What other factors should be evaluated using ultrasound during the second trimester?

Amniotic fluid volume
Placental location (rule out placenta previa)
Cervical length and competence
Umbilical cord and vessels

How do you check for spina bifida?

Scan the entire spine in the transverse plane from the base of the skull to the rump, looking for orientation of the posterior elements and any mass or disruption of the skin

Name 2 reasons why it is important to examine the umbilical cord.

1. To confirm the presence of two arteries and one vein (a two-vessel cord is found in 1% of fetuses and is associated with other congenital anomalies)
2. To confirm normal insertion, which excludes gastroschisis and omphalocele

Where is the biparietal distance measured?

From the outer table to the inner table of the skull (at the level of the thalami)

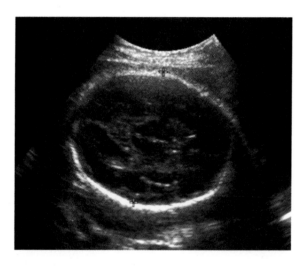

Where is the abdominal circumference measured?

In the plane of the umbilical vein and the portal vein

What is the normal ratio of head circumference to abdominal circumference at 12 weeks?

Approximately 1.3

What is the normal ratio of head circumference to abdominal circumference after 36 weeks?

Approximately 1.0

List 6 conditions in which the ratio of head circumference to abdominal circumference is abnormal.

1. Maternal diabetes
2. Asymmetric intrauterine growth retardation (IUGR)
3. Abdominal masses or ascites
4. Diaphragmatic hernia
5. Hydrocephalus
6. Microcephaly or anencephaly

What is the biophysical profile (BPP)?

An *in utero* APGAR score (maximum score = 10)

Parameter	*Points*
Nonstress test (reactive)	2
Fetal body movements (3 or more)	2
Fetal breathing movement (30 seconds or more)	2
Fetal tone (1 episode of flexion and extension)	2
Amniotic fluid volume (at least one 2 cm × 2 cm pocket)	2

What BPP score indicates severe fetal compromise?

A score of 4 or less necessitates delivery

MULTIPLE GESTATIONS

What percentage of pregnancies result in twin births?

About 1.2% (1 in 85)

What percentage of pregnancies result in triplet births?

About 0.014% (1 in 85^2, or 1 in 7225)

What percentage of twins are dizygotic?

70%

What percentage of twins are monozygotic (identical)?

30%

What are the various types of monozygotic twins?

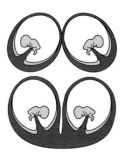

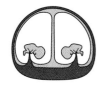

Dichorionic diamniotic (30%)

Monochorionic diamniotic (69%)

Monochorionic monoamniotic (1%)

What fetal syndrome can be seen in monochorionic diamniotic twins?

Twin-twin transfusion syndrome as a result of vessel anastomoses in the common placenta

How can monochorionic monoamniotic twins be identified by ultrasound?

The absence of an intertwin membrane with cord entanglement is the only definitive sonographic sign.

What is the "twin peak" sign in dichorionic diam-niotic twin pregnancies?

Extension of placental or myometrial tissue into the intertwin membrane (this is an early sign)

COMPLICATIONS OF PREGNANCY

What is the differential for an increased AFP level?

GE MINER CO
Gastroschisis
Esophageal atresia
Multiple gestations
Incorrect menstrual dates (most common)
Neural tube defects

Error (laboratory)
Renal disease (polycystic kidney disease, obstruction, dysplasia, congenital nephrosis)
Chorioangioma
Omphalocele

What are 6 causes of a decreased AFP level?

1. Trisomy 18
2. Trisomy 21
3. Absence of fetal tissue (molar pregnancy or lack of pregnancy)
4. Fetal demise
5. Misdated pregnancy
6. Normal pregnancy

What is the significance of the following intrauterine tissues?

Chorioamnionic membrane

If seen after 16–17 weeks, it may be secondary to separation

Intertwin membrane

Twins

Bands

Amniotic band syndrome

Synechiae (usually much thicker than bands)

Amniotic sheet

Fetal anomalies

Central nervous system (CNS) anomalies

Name 3 defects of neural tube closure.

1. Anencephaly (most common)
2. Spina bifida
3. Encephalocele

List 3 spinal sonographic findings that may be associated with neural tube defects.

1. Lordosis or kyphosis
2. Splaying of the posterior ossification centers
3. Cystic sac adjacent to the spine

Name 3 cranial sonographic findings that may be associated with neural tube defects.

1. "Banana" sign (banana-shaped cerebellum, instead of the usual "3" shape)
2. Ventriculomegaly
3. "Lemon" sign (enfolding of the frontal bones of the skull); resolves before 24 weeks' gestation

Name 4 causes of fetal ventriculomegaly.	**ABCD** **A**queductal stenosis **B**leed with secondary hydrocephalus **C**hiari II malformation **D**andy-Walker syndrome
What 3 features of Chiari II malformation are apparent on obstetric ultrasound?	1. Small posterior fossa (banana-shaped) 2. Lateral ventriculomegaly with a normal fourth ventricle (obstruction at the level of the aqueduct of Sylvius) 3. Myelomeningocele
What is a Dandy-Walker malformation?	Congenital absence of the cerebellar vermis and cystic enlargement of the fourth ventricle (resulting from malformation of the foramina of Luschka and Magendie); may be accompanied by hydrocephalus
What is the Dandy-Walker variant?	Partial absence of the cerebellar vermis; accompanied by enlargement of the fourth ventricle and hydrocephalus in 20% of cases
Which is highly associated with chromosomal and structural abnormalities— the Dandy-Walker malformation or its variant?	Both
What is holoprosencephaly?	Cerebral malformations resulting from incomplete division of the forebrain into the cerebral hemispheres
Name the 3 forms of holoprosencephaly.	Alobar, semilobar, and lobar
What distinguishes these types?	**Alobar holoprosencephaly** is most severe; no division occurs. **Lobar holoprosencephaly** is characterized by a near-total division. **Semilobar holoprosencephaly** is characterized by partial division (i.e., more than alobar holoprosencephaly, but less than lobar holoprosencephaly).

Which one of these forms can be difficult to detect sonographically?

Lobar

What sonographic findings are associated with holoprosencephaly?

1. Fusion of the thalami (seen in lobar and semilobar holoprosencephaly)
2. Presence of a dorsal sac (i.e., a fluid-filled intracranial space with mono-ventricle)
3. Absence of the falx and septum pellucidum
4. Midline facial abnormalities
5. Abnormalities of the cardiovascular and gastrointestinal systems, abnormal hands, and spina bifida

What is the differential diagnosis of a cystic mass at the back of the head or neck of the fetus?

Encephalocele or meningocele (skull not intact)
Cystic hygroma (skull intact)
Teratoma (usually solid but may be cystic)

What is the significance of an encephalocele or meningocele?

Possibly an isolated fetal defect with a 1%–3% chance of recurrence in subsequent pregnancies
Possibly associated with other defects

What is the classic ultrasound appearance of a cystic hygroma?

Posterior large nuchal fluid collection with a midline septation

What is the possible significance of a cystic hygroma?

High association with chromosomal abnormalities (especially Turner's syndrome), structural abnormalities, and fetal hydrops; if fetal hydrops is present, the prognosis for the fetus is very poor

Where are fetal teratomas located most often, and what is their appearance on ultrasound?

Sacral (most commonly); either complex or solid

What are the 2 important clinical considerations when a teratoma is discovered?

1. If the tumor is very exophytic, a cesarean delivery may be necessary.
2. There is a high likelihood of malignant degeneration if the tumor is not removed within 4 months of the baby's birth.

Chest anomalies

What percentage of fetal cardiac anomalies can be detected on a four-chamber view?	As many as 85%
What are these anomalies?	Ventricular septal defect (VSD), endocardial cushion defect, hypoplastic left heart, and tricuspid atresia
What other views may be obtained to evaluate the possibility of fetal cardiac anomalies?	Views of the ventricular outflow tract (right and left) are necessary to diagnose transposition of the great vessels or truncus arteriosus.
Name 7 intrathoracic masses seen in the fetus.	1. Bronchopulmonary sequestration 2. Bronchogenic cyst 3. Cystic adenomatoid malformation 4. Chest wall hamartoma 5. Diaphragmatic hernia 6. Diaphragmatic eventration 7. Neuroblastoma
Can these masses be differentiated using ultrasound?	It is difficult to differentiate intrathoracic masses from one another using ultrasound, but specific identification is not really important. It is more important to merely detect the mass.
What complication may occur if an intrathoracic mass is present?	Pulmonary hypoplasia of the compressed lung or lungs. With bilateral hypoplasia, the newborn may not survive.

Gastrointestinal anomalies

What is the "double bubble" sign?	Two dilated fluid-filled structures in the abdomen
List 4 causes of the "double bubble" sign in the fetus.	**LADS** **L**add's bands **A**nnular pancreas **D**uodenal atresia **S**tenosis of the duodenum (high-grade duodenal obstruction is most common)
What 2 masses may be seen near the umbilical cord insertion?	Gastroschisis and omphalocele

Name 4 features that characterize fetal gastroschisis.

1. Defect to the right of the midline
2. Lack of a covering membrane
3. Loops of bowel that are freely floating in amniotic fluid (often seen)
4. Gastrointestinal complications (e.g., atresia, malrotation, obstruction); very rarely seen

When is an omphalocoele normal?

A physiologic omphalocoele may be present until 12 weeks' gestation

List 4 features that characterize fetal omphalocele.

1. Midline defect, with the umbilicus inserting into the apex
2. Membranous covering (amnion and peritoneum)
3. Extra-abdominal location of the liver and sometimes, the small bowel as well
4. Commonly associated with other defects (e.g., cardiovascular, genitourinary, chromosomal)

What are the components of the lethal condition known as the "pentalogy of Cantrell?"

1. Omphalocele
2. Sternal cleft
3. Cardiac exstrophy
4. Cardiovascular malformations
5. Anterior diaphragmatic hernia

With what syndrome is the pentalogy of Cantrell associated?

Trisomy 21 (approximately 30% of cases)

Genitourinary anomalies

At what week does the fetal kidney begin making significant urine?

About week 16

What organ is the most common origin of cystic abdominal masses in the fetus?

Kidney (> 50%)

What steps are involved in evaluating a mass in the fetal abdomen?

1. Identify the organ of origin if possible.
2. Characterize the abnormality (i.e., hydronephrosis versus polycystic kidney disease).
3. Check the contralateral kidney (more than 50% of anomalies are bilateral).

4. Check the fetal bladder.
5. Assess the amniotic fluid volume.
6. Check for posterior urethral valves, especially in male fetuses.

Amniotic fluid anomalies

Where is amniotic fluid produced?

Before 16 weeks' gestation: Via transport of the maternal blood across the amnion

After 16 weeks' gestation: In the fetal kidneys (urine)

Where is amniotic fluid resorbed?

In the fetal gastrointestinal tract after the fluid has been swallowed; it is returned to the maternal circulation via the placenta

Why is abnormal amniotic fluid volume an indicator of congenital abnormalities?

Lack of fetal urination results in oligo-hydramnios
Lack of swallowing or upper gastro-intestinal obstruction by the fetus may lead to polyhydramnios

What is the normal volume of amniotic fluid at birth?

About 1 L

List 4 methods for estimating amniotic fluid volume.

1. Subjective assessment (via ultrasound)
2. Amniotic fluid index (a summation of the measurements of the largest fluid pockets in each of the four quadrants of the abdomen) [normal = 5–20 cm]
3. Measurement of the vertical depth of the largest pocket, as assessed using ultrasound
4. Dye dilution with para-amino hippurate

Give 3 definitions of oligo-hydramnios.

1. Amniotic fluid index less than 5
2. Largest fluid pocket less than 1–2 cm
3. Fluid volume at term less than 500 cm^3

List 5 causes of oligohy-dramnios.

DRIPP
Demise of fetus
Renal anomalies bilaterally
IUGR (most common)
Premature rupture of membranes
Postmaturity

List 4 renal anomalies associated with oligohydramnios.

1. Posterior urethral valves (males)
2. Infantile polycystic kidney disease
3. Renal agenesis
4. Renal dysgenesis (multicystic kidney disease)

Give 3 definitions of polyhydramnios.

1. Amniotic fluid index more than 20–24
2. Largest fluid pocket greater than 8 cm
3. Fluid volume at term 1500–2000 cm^3

List 5 causes of polyhydramnios.

TARDI
Twin-twin transfusion syndrome
Anomalies (CNS and gastro-
    intestinal in 20% of cases)
Rh incompatibility (hydrops fetalis)
Diabetes
Idiopathic (60%)

Placental anomalies

Name 3 common causes of vaginal bleeding in the third trimester.

1. Placenta previa (painless)
2. Abruptio placentae (painful)
3. Vaginal or cervical trauma

What is placenta previa?

Location of the placenta such that it partially or completely covers the internal cervical os or is within 2 cm of the os

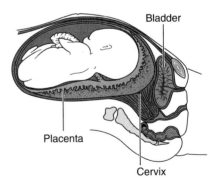

What is the clinical presentation of placenta previa?

Painless vaginal bleeding in the late second or third trimesters

What is the greatest danger associated with assessment of suspected placenta previa?

Catastrophic hemorrhage, which may result from even minor trauma to a placenta previa (through digital examination or instrumentation)

How should placenta previa be evaluated sonographically?

Translabial ultrasound is used in most centers. Endovaginal ultrasound is theoretically safe because there is no need for the probe to touch the cervix.

What is abruptio placentae?

Premature disengagement of the placenta from the uterus

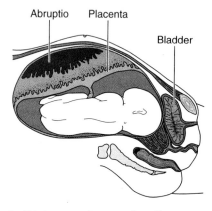

Abruptio   Placenta

Bladder

List 2 ultrasound findings suggestive of abruptio placentae.

1. Distinct visualization of a collection between the placenta and the uterus
2. Thickened placenta (> 4–5 cm) as a result of fresh bleeding

List 5 other causes of thickened placenta.

1. Maternal diabetes
2. TORCH infections
   Toxoplasmosis
   Other (e.g., enterovirus)
   Rubella
   Cytomegalovirus (CMV)
   HIV and **H**erpes simplex
3. Oligohydramnios
4. Fetal hydrops
5. Placental tumor

m

GYNECOLOGY

DISORDERS OF THE UTERUS

Endometrial thickening

Identify the following phases of menstruation according to the ultrasonographic appearance of the endometrium:

A = Late menstrual phase ("single line")
B = Early proliferative (follicular) phase ("three line")—the endometrium is thickened but hypoechoic
C = Late proliferative (periovulatory)

phase ("thickened three line")—the endometrium is thickened and becoming echogenic at the base

D = Late secretory (luteal) phase—the endometrium is diffusely hyper-echoic and thickened

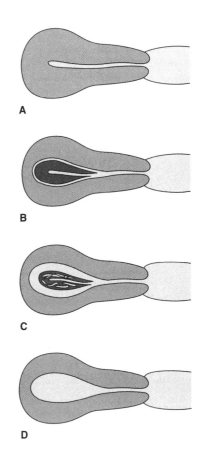

A

B

C

D

What is the upper limit of normal endometrial thickness for a premenopausal woman?	20 mm
How should a premenopausal woman with a thick endometrium be managed clinically?	Reevaluate the endometrium at the end of the menstrual cycle; if it is still thick, the problem is acyclic and may represent endometrial cancer. Biopsy may be indicated for these patients.

What is the upper limit for endometrial thickness for a postmenopausal woman?

5 mm

What is the differential diagnosis of postmenopausal endometrial thickening?

Endometrial carcinoma, endometrial hyperplasia, and polyp

What are indications for a sonohysterogram (transvaginal imaging performed after placing fluid in the endometrial canal)?

Mildly thickened postmenopausal endometrium or thickened acyclic premenopausal endometrium (to rule out polyps, hyperplasia, and carcinoma)
Leiomyomas of unclear location
Infertility (to rule out interuterine adhesions or submucosal leiomyomas or polyps)

How can a sonohysterogram be useful in making treatment decisions?

A sonohysterogram may be used to help determine the best treatment; for example, by differentiating between diffuse and focal thickening or polyps with broad bases as opposed to stalks.

What therapy is indicated for a postmenopausal woman with endometrial thickening?

Curettage and biopsy

What is the differential diagnosis of vaginal bleeding in a woman who is not pregnant?

CEEASE
Cervical cancer
Endometrial cancer or polyp
Endometrial hyperplasia
Adenomyosis
Submucosal fibroids
Ectopic pregnancy

m

Endometriosis

What is endometriosis?

Ectopic endometrium outside the uterus

Where are deposits from endometriosis typically found?

Peritoneal surfaces (e.g., cul-de-sac, orifices of the fallopian tubes, bowel)

What is the clinical presentation of endometriosis?

Premenstrual abdominal pain
Dysmenorrhea
Chronic pelvic pain
Dyspareunia

Which imaging modality is best for diagnosing endometriosis?	No imaging technique is particularly useful. Most lesions are too small to image radiographically. They usually have the appearance of small, focal nodules or a sheet-like coating on pelvic structures. Laparoscopy is the gold standard for the diagnosis of endometriosis, but MRI is occasionally used.
What role does MRI play in the diagnosis and treatment of endometriosis?	Noninvasive assessment of patients who are not candidates for operative assessment (not very sensitive) Noninvasive monitoring of endometriomas
What is a "chocolate cyst?"	An endometrioma (i.e., a large focal collection resulting from endometriosis)
What is the appearance of endometriomas on MRI?	High signal intensity on both T_1-weighted and T_2-weighted images High signal intensity on a fat-suppression sequence (not fat) Profound decrease in signal on gradient-recalled echo (GRE) sequences owing to the paramagnetic effect of old blood
What is the appearance of an endometrioma on ultrasound?	A complex cystic mass; swirling echoes or septations may be seen

Adenomyosis

What is adenomyosis?	Invasion of the myometrium by the basal layer of endometrium; also known as "internal endometriosis"
What is the clinical presentation of adenomyosis?	Noncyclical dysmenorrhea and metrorrhagia and uterine enlargement; sometimes patients are asymptomatic
What is the best imaging modality for diagnosing adenomyosis?	T_2-weighted MRI
What is the appearance of adenomyosis on MRI?	Focal or diffuse thickening of the junctional zone to more than 12 mm High-intensity foci in the junctional zone

on T_1-weighted images and low or
high signal intensity on T_2-weighted
images, indicative of blood products
("salt and pepper" appearance)
Boundary of adenomyosis and
myometrium may be lobulated or
spiculated

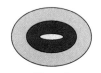

Normal

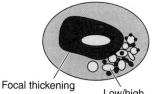

Focal thickening

Low/high
signal intensity

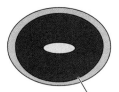

Diffuse thickening

What is the appearance of adenomyosis on ultrasound?	Nonspecific (i.e., heterogeneous echo-texture and uterine enlargement that is usually indistinguishable from diffuse fibroid change)
What is the clinical treatment for adenomyosis?	Hysterectomy

Uterine fibroids (leiomyomas)

What clinical symptoms are associated with leiomyomas?	Abdominal pain; dysfunctional, cyclical uterine bleeding; and infertility (especially common with submucosal fibroids); sometimes patients are asymptomatic

How common are leiomyomas?

Found in 20%–30% of women older than 30 years

List the types of leiomyomas, based on their location in the uterus.

There are 4 types of uterine leiomyomas: submucosal, intramural, subserosal (some are pedunculated), and cervical (these are rare). Extrauterine leiomyomas rarely occur as well.

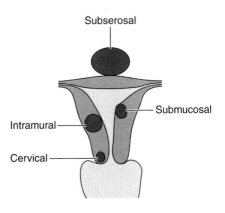

What is the appearance of leiomyomas on ultrasound?

They are usually hypoechoic with a whorled heterogeneous echotexture, but they may be calcified. An affected patient may present with discrete masses, a distorted uterus, or a diffusely enlarged uterus. Some degenerated fibroids may be partially cystic; many have calcification.

What is the appearance of leiomyomas on MRI?

Distinct, round masses
Uniformly low signal intensity on both T_1- and T_2-weighted images

How can leiomyomas and leiomyosarcomas be differentiated on MRI?

Central degeneration (high T_2-weighted signal) and rapid size change may be suggestive of sarcoma. Usually these masses cannot be distinguished definitively on MRI.

What is the appearance of a fibroid on CT?

A mass with the same density as the uterus, or an irregularly enhancing mass
Possible calcification
Irregular uterine contour

What is the clinical treatment for women with leiomyomas?	Myomectomy, hysterectomy, or in some centers, uterine artery embolization

Developmental (müllerian duct) disorders

List 4 types of congenital müllerian duct anomalies.

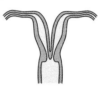

Uterus didelphys
(two uteri
and cervices)

Bicornuate uterus
(incomplete fusion)

Septate uterus
(failure of resorption
of the septum)

Unicornuate uterus

What genital tract anomalies can be seen following *in utero* diethylstilbestrol (DES) exposure?	Hypoplastic, "T"-shaped uterus with irregular cavity Cervical stenosis or incompetence Increased risk of clear cell cancer of the vagina
What is the clinical presentation of müllerian duct anomalies?	Menstrual disorders, infertility, or problems late in pregnancy (e.g., dystocia or premature labor) may be seen, or the patient may be asymptomatic.
How common are müllerian duct anomalies?	They affect approximately 1 in 200 women.
How are müllerian duct anomalies best imaged initially?	HSG
Describe what is shown on each of the following HSGs:	A = Normal uterus B = Unicornuate uterus C = Bicornuate uterus D = Uterus didelphys

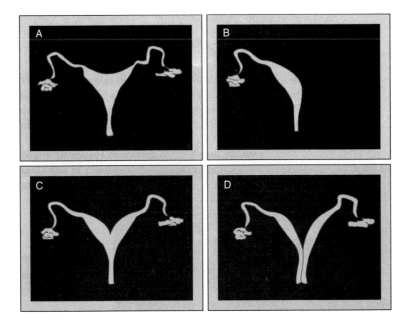

When should ultrasound be used in the work-up of müllerian duct anomalies?

Ultrasound is indicated when uterine obstruction is suspected [e.g., vaginal agenesis, bicornuate uterus (may have obstruction of one horn)]. Ultrasound may be able to distinguish the anomaly and should be the first imaging procedure ordered when these conditions are suspected.

When should MRI be used in the work-up of müllerian duct anomalies?

MRI should be used for distinguishing a bicornuate uterus from a septate uterus when ultrasound is equivocal. Although MRI is highly accurate, routine use is probably not justified.

Why is it important to distinguish a bicornuate uterus from a septate uterus?

These conditions are treated with different surgical approaches (laparotomy and hysteroscopy, respectively).

What additional area should sometimes be imaged in patients with a müllerian duct anomaly?

Urinary tract imaging should be performed if ultrasound is abnormal because kidney and ureter malformations are associated with approximately 50% of müllerian duct anomalies.

DISORDERS OF THE OVARIES AND ADNEXA

What imaging modality should be used for initial evaluation of the ovaries and adnexa?

Ultrasound

What is the appearance of the ovaries on T$_2$-weighted MRI?

Adnexal structures that contain multiple follicles of high signal intensity

How is the approximate volume of an ovary calculated?

$0.5 \times$ length $\times$ width $\times$ depth (an ellipsoid)

What is the volume of a normal ovary?

Premenopausal: Less than or equal to 18 cm^3 (i.e., less than or equal to $0.5 \times 3 \times 3 \times 4$ cm^3)

Postmenopausal: Less than or equal to 8 cm^3 (i.e., less than or equal to $0.5 \times 2 \times 2 \times 4$ cm^3)

What changes does an ovary normally undergo during the menstrual cycle?

Follicular phase (approximately days 1–14): Development of a graafian follicle

Ovulation (approximately day 14): Rupture of the follicle and release of the ovum

Luteal phase (approximately days 15–28): Formation of the corpus luteum

What size is a mature graafian follicle?

15–30 mm

What signs on ultrasound may signal impending ovulation?

Irregularity of the follicle wall and decreased echogenicity around the follicle

Is free fluid in the cul-de-sac pathologic during ovulation?

No, it may be normal (especially during ovulation)

Name 4 structures that may mimic the ovary on ultrasound.

1. Bowel loops
2. Cervix that contains multiple Nabothian cysts
3. Lymph nodes
4. Blood vessel

Ovarian cysts

What is the appearance of a hemorrhagic cyst on ultrasound?	A "ground-glass," fenestrated, or lace-like pattern within the cyst; no discrete solid components
What findings are suggestive of a neoplasm on ultrasound?	Solid components, especially if color Doppler ultrasound shows vascular flow within these areas

What is the differential diagnosis of a complex adnexal mass?

CHEETAH

m

Cystadenoma or **C**ystadenocarcinoma (typically solid vascularized components)

Hemorrhagic cyst (usually fenestrated with no discrete solid components)

Endometrioma (typically diffuse low-level echos)

Ectopic pregnancy

Teratoma or dermoid cyst (typically echogenic shadowing component—"dermoid plug")

Abscess (from nearby intestine, as in diverticulitis or a tubo-ovarian abscess)

Hematoma

What is the appearance of a unilocular ovarian cyst on ultrasound?	No internal echoes, smooth walls, good transmission of sound waves through the cyst to underlying structures
Are simple, unilocular cysts a cause for concern in postmenopausal women?	No.
What follow-up should be provided for premenopausal women with unilocular cysts or probable hemorrhagic cysts that are larger than 3 cm in diameter?	Repeat sonogram in 4–6 weeks
What is the most common cause of ovarian enlargement in young women?	Functional cysts (frequently 4–10 cm in diameter)
Name 3 other common causes of ovarian enlargement.	1. Ovarian torsion 2. Polycystic ovary syndrome 3. Ovarian mass

Functional cysts

What is a functional cyst?	A physiologic, hormonally active cyst that has not yet involuted
What are the 3 types of functional cyst?	1. Follicular cyst (small, unilateral, usually asymptomatic) 2. Corpus luteum cyst (large, unilateral) 3. Theca lutein cyst (large, multiple and bilateral, associated with excess β-hCG)
How can these 3 types be distinguished using ultrasound?	They cannot be distinguished from one another using ultrasound.
How should functional cysts be managed clinically?	The patient should return for a repeat sonogram during a different menstrual phase or after hormonal therapy; most functional cysts resolve spontaneously.
What are 3 potential complications of functional cysts?	Hemorrhage, rupture, and torsion
What is the typical clinical picture of ovarian torsion?	Extreme sudden pelvic pain, especially in a child or adolescent
What 3 findings are suggestive of ovarian torsion on ultrasound?	1. Unilateral ovarian enlargement 2. Multiple peripheral cortical follicles 3. Fluid in the cul-de-sac Note that the absence of blood flow on Doppler is not diagnostic.

Polycystic ovary syndrome

What are other terms for polycystic ovary syndrome?	Chronic anovulatory syndrome and Stein-Leventhal syndrome
What is the clinical triad of polycystic ovary syndrome?	Oligomenorrhea, hirsutism, and obesity
What is the appearance of the ovaries in polycystic ovary syndrome on ultrasound?	Bilateral enlargement Increased echogenicity of the fibrous central stroma Multiple peripheral follicles (none ever mature)

A. Normal

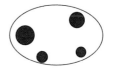

B. Polycystic ovary syndrome

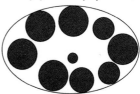

How often do the ovaries appear normal in polycystic ovary syndrome?	In about 25% of cases

Disorders of the fallopian tubes

Are the fallopian tubes normally visible on endovaginal ultrasound?	Not unless they contain or are surrounded by fluid (however, the broad ligament is often visible)
Which is the best modality for imaging the fallopian tubes?	HSG
What is hydrosalpinx?	Obstruction of the fallopian tube leading to fluid accumulation and tubal dilation
What is the usual cause of hydrosalpinx?	Scarring secondary to pelvic inflammatory disease (PID)
What are the imaging features of hydrosalpinx?	Fluid accumulation and tubal dilation Convoluted appearance Polypoid nodules protruding into the lumen (these nodules represent infolding of the wall)
What are the possible sonographic findings of PID?	Thickened, ill-defined endometrium as a result of endometritis Pus in the cul-de-sac Hydrosalpinx or pyosalpinx

Ill-defined ovarian masses as a result of ovarian abscesses

Normal

What are the 4 possibilities if fluid is noted in the cul-de-sac?	1. Normal finding (if ovulating) 2. Ascites 3. Blood (as a result of trauma, endometriosis, postoperative status, ruptured ectopic pregnancy, or ruptured ovarian cyst) 4. Pus (as a result of PID)

GYNECOLOGIC CANCERS

What is the most common gynecologic malignancy in women?	Cervical cancer

Cervical cancer

Name 3 risk factors for cervical cancer.	1. Human papillomavirus infection 2. Multiple sexual partners 3. Early age at time of first intercourse
What imaging modality is best for screening for cervical cancer?	Imaging is not effective for this purpose. A Papanicolaou (pap) smear is the screening method of choice.
What imaging modality is best for staging cervical cancer?	T_2-weighted MRI; using the sagittal plane is key
Why is T_2-weighted MRI so useful?	It distinguishes cancer (a high-intensity signal) from the surrounding connective tissue (which has a lower signal intensity), and it can detect invasion of the stroma, parametrium, or bladder as well as lymph node involvement (sagittal and axial images are particularly useful).
What is the typical sequence of spread of cervical cancer?	Local invasion, nodal spread, and hematogenous dissemination
What characterizes stage IIIb disease?	Extension to the pelvic side wall

What is the significance of tumor extension to the parametrium (stage IIb cancer)?

This development affects treatment; usual treatment of stage IIb cancer is radiation therapy rather than surgery.

What complication may be seen when pelvic side wall extension is present?

Hydronephrosis as a result of ureteral obstruction

What distinguishes stage IVa disease from stage IVb disease?

Stage IVa disease involves only the adjacent organs (e.g., the bladder and rectum) and stage IVb involves spread to distant organs (i.e., metastases).

What are the 3 most common sites of nodal spread in cervical cancer (from most to least common)?

Obturator, common iliac, and para-aortic nodes

Name 4 common locations of distant metastasis.

Liver, lungs, brain, and bone

When is a pelvic exenteration performed?

In patients with recurrent cervical cancer when radiotherapy has failed

What are the 3 types of pelvic exenteration?

1. Total: The bladder, rectum, anus, uterus, vagina, and adnexa are removed.
2. Anterior: The rectum and anus are left intact and the ureters are diverted.
3. Posterior: The bladder is left intact and a colostomy is created.

Endometrial cancer

What is the classic presentation of endometrial cancer?

Postmenopausal vaginal bleeding is characteristic. However, most cases of postmenopausal bleeding are not caused by endometrial cancer.

List 4 risk factors for endometrial cancer.

NOEL
Nulliparity
Obesity
Estrogen stimulation (unopposed)
Late menopause

m

What imaging modality is best for diagnosis of endometrial cancer?

No imaging technique is particularly useful. Diagnosis is made on the basis of examination of biopsy tissue.

What MRI scans are most helpful in staging endo- metrial cancer?	Sagittal T_2-weighted images Sagittal T_1-weighted images with gadolinium contrast
What MRI findings are significant in endometrial cancer?	1. Maximal endometrial thickness greater than 5 mm in postmenopausal women or 14 mm in premenopausal women (measured from junctional zone to junctional zone) 2. Invasion of the junctional zone and myometrium 3. Extension into adjacent organs
What is the risk when deep invasion (i.e., invasion of more than 50% of the myo- metrium) has occurred?	Nodal metastasis
What treatment is indicated for women with more than 50% myometrial invasion (stage IC cancer)?	Hysterectomy and lymph node dissection
What differentiates stage III endometrial cancer from stage II disease?	Extrauterine extension

Vaginal cancer

What are the 4 most com- mon sites of nodal spread in vaginal cancer (from most to least common)?	Inguinal, external iliac, obturator, and para-aortic nodes
How is nodal spread from cancer of the upper third of the vagina different from that of cancer of the lower two thirds of the vagina?	It resembles cervical cancer in its predilection for spread to the obturator, common iliac, and para-aortic nodes. The inguinal nodes are not usually involved.

Ovarian neoplasms

What is the clinical presen- tation of an ovarian neo- plasm?	Increased abdominal girth; pressure symptoms Chronic abdominal pain from enlarge- ment and adhesions Menstrual irregularity Acute pain from torsion or hemorrhage

What is the peak decade of life for discovery of ovarian cancer?	Sixth decade
Which ovarian neoplasms are most often found in younger women?	Dermoid cysts and dysgerminomas
List 3 risk factors for ovarian cancer.	1. First-degree relative with ovarian cancer 2. Nulliparity 3. Breast cancer
What radiologic findings suggest malignancy of an adnexal mass (premeno-pausal or postmenopausal)?	Solid mass or a cyst with any solid components Cyst greater than 5 cm with vascularized septations
Name the 4 tissue types of ovarian tumors (from most common to least common)	1. Epithelial: 70% 2. Germ cell: 15% 3. Sex chord or stromal: 5%–10% 4. Metastatic (extraovarian): 5%–10%
What are the common benign epithelial neoplasms?	Serous and mucinous cystadenoma
What are the most common malignant epithelial neo-plasms?	Serous and mucinous cystadenocar-cinoma
Give the typical ultrasound pattern associated with:	
Epithelial neoplasms (cystadenoma/adenocar-cinoma, endometrioid tumors, clear cell cancer)	Cystic (malignant forms may have solid elements)
Teratomas	Typically focal echogenic shadowing; "dermoid plug" Occasionally not distinguishable from a functional or hemorrhagic cyst
Tumors of germ cell, sex chord, or stromal origin (i.e., Sertoli-Leydig cell tumors, thecomas, fibromas)	Solid and cystic or entirely solid

How often are epithelial tumors found bilaterally?	Serous cystadenocarcinoma (50%) Endometrioid tumors (50%) Mucinous cystadenocarcinoma (25%) Dermoid cysts (10%)
What is Krukenberg's tumor?	A gastric or colon cancer metastatic to the ovary
What is Meigs' syndrome?	Pleural effusion and ascites from fibroma (or other ovarian cancer)
What is pseudomyxoma peritonei ("jelly belly")?	Rupture of a mucin-producing adenoma or adenocarcinoma of the ovary, appendix, colon, or rectum that results in peritoneal seeding
What disease stage is represented by pseudomyxoma peritonei?	Stage III (intraperitoneal metastasis)
What distinguishes stage II from stage I ovarian cancer?	Involvement of both ovaries, not just one
What is the most common stage of ovarian cancer at the time of discovery?	Stage IV disease (extra-peritoneal metastases) is seen in 65% of patients.
What are common findings of ovarian cancer spread on CT?	Ovarian mass with solid components Ascites (as a result of peritoneal spread) Peritoneal masses (e.g., subcapsular liver fluid collections) Omental caking (i.e., thickened omentum with increased soft tissue attenuation) Lymphadenopathy
What is the most common site of nodal spread in ovarian cancer?	The most common site of nodal spread in ovarian cancer is to the para-aortic nodes at the level of the renal veins, where the ovarian veins drain into the inferior vena cava (IVC) or left renal vein. Note that this is also the embryologic location of origin of the ovaries before they descend to the pelvis.

Dermoid cysts

What is a dermoid cyst?	An ovarian teratoma containing tissues derived from only ectoderm (hair, teeth, fat)

How common are dermoid cysts?	Dermoid cysts account for 5%–10% of all ovarian neoplasms; they are the most common childhood ovarian neoplasm.
What is the clinical presentation of dermoid cysts?	Patients may experience pain, torsion, or mass effect, or they may be asymptomatic.

What are the findings associated with dermoid cysts on the following radiographic studies?

Plain film	Radiopaque densities suggestive of teeth or fat density
Ultrasound	Echogenic, highly attenuated (shadowing) mass; "dermoid plug" of fat in patients with complex masses
CT	Fat-fluid level; fragments of bone or teeth
MRI	"Dermoid plugs" within a cystic mass Floating debris on fat-suppression sequences

How are dermoid cysts definitively distinguished from endometriomas?	If a mass shows fat suppression on MRI, it is a dermoid cyst. Endometriomas do not show fat suppression.
What complications are associated with dermoid cysts?	Torsion and hemorrhage
What is the clinical therapy for dermoid cysts?	Surgical removal

11   Pediatric Imaging

Matthew L. Cohen
Brent K. Milner

GENERAL CONSIDERATIONS

In what way is pediatric radiology different from adult radiology?	Patient age is far more critical when determining a differential diagnosis in a child.
What category of disease must be remembered when constructing a pediatric differential diagnosis?	Congenital anomalies
Describe how development influences interpretation of pediatric images.	Anatomy develops throughout the pediatric period (e.g., the thymus involutes with time, certain structures are not ossified in infancy).

HINTS FOR MANAGEMENT OF THE PEDIATRIC PATIENT

What examination is a useful adjunct to any radiologic study?	A focused physical examination (perform it yourself)
Under what circumstances can a child be left alone in a room?	Never; a parent, technician, resident, or radiologist should always be with a pediatric patient, even one who is restrained.
How should parents be handled?	Parents may be handled in various ways. A child is often more cooperative with the parents in the room, and one or both parents may be just the thing a child needs. A parent may provide an extra set of hands. Be sure to explain what is happening, and always respect parental wishes and concerns. Remember that *an*

anxious parent leads to an anxious child.

How much clothing should be removed?	Generally, remove as much as possible. Warmth is a consideration in the very young child, and modesty is an issue in the older child.
What is a child most afraid of in the radiology department?	The "unknown"
How does a child manifest anxiety?	Nonverbally (most often) Fearfulness without speaking Crying Calling for parents
At what age is separation anxiety most likely to present a problem?	6 months to 3 years
What can be done to allay a child's fears?	Ask what the child fears—often, it is unrelated to radiology.
What can be done to put a child at ease?	Use stuffed animals, toys, and/or colorful decorations. Keep the room lighted. Keep the technician in the room (ensure no hidden surprises). Loosen restraining devices while films are being processed.
How can rapport with a child be easily established?	Be warm, sympathetic, and reassuring. Use the child's correct name or nickname. Bribe the child with stickers and quick reunion with parents. Demonstrate equipment noises and motions before beginning the examination.
What is a good strategy for dealing with the uncooperative child?	Let the child operate the machines and explore them before trying to use them for examination.
How should the angry child be dealt with?	Firmly (e.g., "Let's get on with this and get it over with")

What is the most common cause of poor pediatric films?

Poor immobilization

Which is less traumatic, being held down by several people or immobilization?

Immobilization, which also exposes personnel to less radiation

What hazards are associated with immobilization?

Cutting of circulation to extremities, airway compromise, strangulation, and skin abrasion

How do you get a child to cooperate with respiration?

Infant younger than 6 months: Occlude the nose between the thumb and forefinger at end inspiration.

Older infant: Induce crying by making a loud noise or pinching the infant on the heel.

Toddler or young child: Have the child blow soap bubbles for deep inspiration. Teach the child to close her mouth and nose for breath holding.

How can a child be encouraged to face a particular direction?

Via strategic placement of a toy or noise maker

When should sedation be used?

Use it as a last resort, and then only after consulting the primary physician. Try reassurance and rapport first.

What drugs are useful for sedation?

Chloral hydrate or Conway's formula (meperidine, promethazine, and chlorpromazine cocktail)

POSITIONING OF LINES AND TUBES

Trace the flow of blood through the fetal circulation.

Umbilical vein → left portal vein → ductus venosus → hepatic vein → inferior vena cava (IVC) → heart → pulmonary artery → ductus arteriosus → aorta → common iliac arteries → internal iliac arteries → umbilical arteries

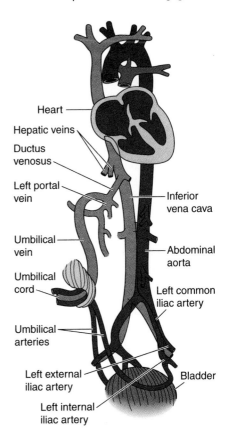

What is the ideal position for:

The tip of an umbilical vein catheter?

Inferior right atrium, so that it does not enter the renal vein and cause thrombosis

The tip of an umbilical artery catheter?

Just below the renal arteries (below L2), to prevent any emboli that might form from entering the renal arteries (which could cause hypertension)

A feeding tube?

In the third or fourth portion of the duodenum, to prevent reflux into the stomach (which could lead to vomiting and aspiration)

An endotracheal tube?

Midway between the vocal cords and carina—if it is too low, it could enter a main stem bronchus, and if it is too high, it could fall out

DISORDERS OF THE RESPIRATORY SYSTEM

LUNG PARENCHYMA AND PLEURA

Conditions in newborns

What chest findings in newborns suggest the need for medical (as opposed to surgical) treatment?

Diffuse findings suggest diffuse conditions such as pneumonia, respiratory distress syndrome (RDS), and congestive heart failure (CHF), which are usually treated medically.

What chest findings in newborns suggest the need for surgical (as opposed to medical) treatment?

Unilateral findings may suggest conditions that are better treated surgically (e.g., pneumothorax, chylothorax, pleural effusion).

What major radiographic patterns are seen in the lungs of neonates?

Opaque hemithorax, lobar opacity, and bubbly hemithorax

What are 5 causes of opaque hemithorax in newborns?

1. Pleural effusion
2. Chylothorax
3. Atelectasis
4. Pulmonary agenesis
5. Hypoplastic lung

What other lesions cause a similar appearance if they are fluid-filled (before they fill with air)?

Diaphragmatic hernia, congenital lobar emphysema, and cystic adenomatoid malformation

What is the best radiologic procedure for differentiating fluid from other solid lesions in an opaque hemithorax?

Ultrasound

What are 7 causes of pleural effusion in infants?

1. Trauma during delivery
2. CHF
3. Hypervolemia
4. Esophageal rupture
5. Idiopathic
6. Erythroblastosis fetalis
7. Turner's syndrome (XO)

What is the most common cause of large pleural effusions in newborns?	Chylothorax
Do infants with chylothorax present immediately after birth?	50% develop symptoms in the first day, and 70% develop symptoms by the end of the first week. Note that lymph in the pleural space becomes chylous only after milk or formula is ingested.
Are infants with chylothorax usually full-term infants who were born following a normal labor and delivery?	Yes.
What treatment is appropriate for chylothorax?	Most infants respond to thoracentesis. Ultrasound or computed tomography (CT)-guided drainage and parenteral nutrition may be necessary.
What is the prognosis for neonates with chylothorax?	Excellent
What is the most common cause of pneumothorax in neonates?	Barotrauma resulting from ventilation
What are 5 causes of lobar opacity in neonates?	**I HEAR** **m** **I**nfection (group B streptococci, Gram-negative rods) **H**emorrhage **E**dema [transient tachypnea of the newborn (TTN), severe coarctation, hypoplastic left heart, total anomalous pulmonary venous return (TAPVR) with obstruction, hypervolemia/hyperviscosity] **A**spiration (amniotic fluid, meconium) **R**DS
What is a radiologic pattern typical of pulmonary edema?	Enlarged, indistinct pulmonary vessels with perihilar haziness, often with infiltrates

Concerning the differential diagnosis of a pulmonary edema pattern and *normal* heart size:

What are 3 conditions associated with *no improvement* in 24–72 hours?

1. Hypoplastic left heart
2. TAPVR with obstruction
3. Pulmonary lymphangiectasia

What are 4 conditions associated *with improvement* in 24–72 hours?

1. TTN
2. Aspiration of amniotic fluid
3. Intracranial hemorrhage
4. Hyperviscosity/hypervolemia

Concerning the differential diagnosis of a pulmonary edema pattern and *cardiomegaly*:

What are 3 conditions associated with *no improvement* in 24–72 hours?

1. Hypoplastic left heart (heart may be normal or enlarged)
2. Severe coarctation (often associated with a left-to-right shunt)
3. Myocardiopathy

What are 2 conditions associated *with improvement* in 24–72 hours?

1. Asphyxiated myocardium
2. Maternal diabetes

What 4 conditions most commonly cause respiratory distress in newborns?

1. RDS, especially in premature infants (most common)
2. TTN, especially in infants born by cesarean section
3. Meconium aspiration (patchy infiltrates and hyperinflated lungs)
4. Pneumonia (segmental infiltrate or diffuse infiltrates)

What helps distinguish patchy infiltrates in newborns?

The size of the lung volumes—whether they are small or large

What are 3 causes of patchy infiltrates and small lung volumes?

1. RDS
2. Pulmonary hypoplasia
3. Hypoventilation

What are 5 causes of patchy infiltrates and large lung volumes?

I HEAR
Infection (pneumonia)
Hemorrhage
Edema (including TTN and, rarely, nephrotic syndrome)
Aspiration (especially of meconium)
RDS (in a patient on ventilator therapy)

What is RDS?	RDS, also known as hyaline membrane disease, affects premature neonates. These infants do not have sufficient surfactant production because the cells that line the alveoli are immature. This lack of surfactant causes poor compliance of alveoli.
What amniotic fluid indicator is useful for identification of infants with RDS?	The lecithin:sphingomyelin ratio (decreased)
When does RDS usually manifest clinically?	In the first few hours of life
What radiographic findings occur in premature infants with mild RDS?	Diffuse granular pattern Small lung volumes Peripherally extending air bronchograms
What is TTN?	TTN is a condition caused by retained fluid within the lung that was not squeezed out during birth (wet lungs). The edema pattern rapidly clears in 24–48 hours. TTN often affects infants who were delivered by cesarean section.
What is the frequency of meconium aspiration?	10% of newborns have meconium staining of amniotic fluid, and 10% of these infants experience respiratory distress. Therefore, meconium aspiration occurs in less than 1% of deliveries.
What radiographic findings are characteristic of meconium aspiration?	Patchy, bilateral, asymmetric areas of opacity Hyperinflation of the lungs with flattened diaphragmatic domes Pneumothorax or pneumomediastinum (25% of cases) Slow clearing of radiologic findings despite clinical improvement
What are the common agents in neonatal pneumonia?	Group B streptococci and Gram-negative rods
What is the typical radiologic appearance of neonatal pneumonia?	Diffuse infiltrates, but the appearance varies—it may mimic edema or hemorrhage.

What 4 conditions lead to a bubbly-appearing hemithorax in newborns?	1. Pulmonary interstitial emphysema (PIE) 2. Cystic adenomatoid malformation 3. Bronchopulmonary dysplasia (BPD) [may be asymmetric and is usually not present until 2–4 weeks] 4. Diaphragmatic hernia
What is PIE?	PIE is a complication of performing artificial ventilation in lungs that have low compliance. Air passes into the interstitium and lymphatics and causes a streaky appearance. PIE may progress to pneumothorax.
What other 2 complications occur as a result of ventilator therapy?	BPD and pneumothorax

Conditions in older infants, children, and adolescents

What causes parenchymal opacity in older children?	Pneumonia, congenital anomalies, and tumor (rare)
What 4 radiographic findings are typical of viral pneumonia?	1. Hyperinflation 2. Peribronchial thickening (an interstitial process) 3. Bilateral infiltrates (not lobar) 4. Shifting atelectasis The overall pattern is diffuse obstructive airways disease that resembles asthma.
What is respiratory syncytial virus (RSV) infection?	A viral infection of the bronchioles
What are the "3 Ws" of RSV?	**3 Ws** **W**heezing **W**inter Ne**W**born
What are 5 radiologic characteristics typical of RSV?	1. Bronchiolitis 2. Bronchiolitis plus interstitial edema 3. Subsegmental atelectasis 4. Patchy perihilar atelectasis (from mucous plugging) plus bronchiolitis 5. Hazy lungs (rare) plus bronchiolitis
What is a common pattern in RSV?	Collapse of the right upper lobe (RUL)

What 3 radiographic findings are typical of bacterial pneumonia?

Focal infiltrates, air bronchograms (alveolar process), and pleural fluid

What is the most common pathogen in bacterial pneumonia (patients of all ages)?

Streptococcus pneumoniae

What is "round" pneumonia?

A pattern seen commonly in children where pneumonia appears as a mass

What 9 conditions should be considered in the differential diagnosis of recurrent pneumonia?

1. Cystic fibrosis (CF)
2. Atopic asthma (pulmonary shadows are usually atelectasis)
3. Gastroesophageal reflux disease (GERD)
4. Tracheoesophageal fistula
5. Chronic granulomatous disease or other immune deficiency
6. BPD
7. Bronchiectasis
8. Foreign body
9. Sequestration

What radiographic findings characterize early CF?

Hyperinflation and recurrent RUL atelectasis may occur; the appearance is often normal in early infancy.

What 7 radiographic findings characterize advanced CF?

1. Increased linear perihilar markings
2. Peribronchial cuffing
3. Bronchial mucous plugging
4. Bronchiectasis
5. Atelectasis caused by mucous plugging
6. Patchy pneumonias
7. Hilar enlargement (adenopathy and pulmonary artery hypertension)

What are 6 complications of advanced CF?

1. Scarring
2. Bronchiectasis
3. Lobar atelectasis (common)
4. Pulmonary hypertension with cor pulmonale (frequent, owing to hypoxemia)
5. Pneumothorax due to rupture of bleb or bullae
6. Hemoptysis as a result of enlarged bronchial collaterals (uncommon)

What is the most useful radiologic method for following pulmonary hypertension with cor pulmonale in a patient with CF?	Comparison films to follow the heart and the hilum are most helpful. The heart is enlarged in cor pulmonale; however, a normal-sized heart may actually represent cor pulmonale, because the heart is usually small in patients with CF as a result of hyperinflation of the lungs.
What is a noninfectious cause of pneumonitis?	Chemical pneumonitis
What materials can typically cause chemical pneumonitis?	Hydrofluorocarbons such as gasoline, kerosene, lighter fluid, and aerosols
How soon do radiographic changes appear after aspiration of chemicals?	6–12 hours (clearance in weeks to months)
Where is chemical pneumonitis usually seen?	Dependent portions of the lungs
What are 3 radiographic findings in chemical pneumonitis?	Hyperemia, pulmonary edema, and infiltrates
What is the delayed complication of chemical pneumonitis?	Pneumatocele
What are common congenital causes of opacity or density on plain film?	Hernia, sequestration, and bronchogenic cyst
Where is Bochdalek's hernia located?	Think "**BochdaLek = B**ack and to the **L**eft" (posteriorly, and most are left-sided)—these hernias often contain the upper pole of the kidney and retroperitoneal fat, but may contain bowel
Where is the Morgagni's hernia located?	Think "**MorgAgni = M**edially and **A**nteriorly," in the cardiophrenic angle (i.e., where the right side of the heart rests on the diaphragm)—these hernias often contain bowel or fat
Which hernia is a more common congenitally, Bochdalek's or Morgagni's?	Bochdalek's

What is sequestration of the lung?	A congenital mass of pulmonary tissue with no normal connection with the bronchial tree or pulmonary artery
Name the 2 types of sequestration of the lung.	Intralobar (more common) and extralobar
What is the typical location of sequestration?	Usually the posterior basilar segments of the lower lobe (left more often than right)
What arteries supply the sequestered lung?	Anomalous arteries off the aorta
What veins drain the sequestered lung?	Pulmonary veins (intrapulmonary sequestration) Systemic veins and the IVC (extrapulmonary sequestration)
What are the symptoms of sequestration?	**Intralobar** sequestration is frequently **asymptomatic** until adolescence, when superimposed infection may occur. Recurrent **pneumonia** at a young age is common in patients with **extralobar** sequestration.

AIRWAYS

What symptom is indicative of an airway obstruction in children?	Stridor
What causes stridor?	Tracheobronchitis (croup) Epiglottitis Retropharyngeal abscess or mass Vascular ring Granuloma or stricture (postintubation) Papilloma of larynx or trachea Foreign body
Where does the obstruction occur in patients with:	
Inspiratory stridor?	Above the thoracic inlet
Expiratory stridor?	Below the thoracic inlet; with severe narrowing, both inspiratory and expiratory stridor may occur

Compare croup and epiglottitis in terms of the:

Nature of the disease

Croup: Self-limited
Epiglottitis: Acute and emergent

Age of typical occurrence

Croup: 6 months–3 years
Epiglottitis: 3–6 years

Shape of the airway

Croup: "Steeple" sign (subglottic edema)
Epiglottitis: "Thumb" sign more so than "steeple" sign (epiglottic, glottic edema)

Type of pathogen

Croup: Viral
Epiglottitis: Bacterial

What is the "steeple" sign?

Narrowing of the trachea gives a pointed appearance to the subglottic airway on a frontal plain film in patients with croup.

What is the "thumb" sign?

The enlarged epiglottis looks like a thumb on a lateral plain film in patients with epiglottitis.

Where is an aspirated foreign body most likely to be found?

In the right main stem bronchus

How can a nonradiopaque foreign body be identified?

1. **Fluoroscopy:** The mediastinum moves away from the side of obstruction on expiration as a result of air trapping.
2. **Lateral decubitus film:** Normally, the dependent side hypoaerates, but it stays hyperaerated with a foreign body.

On a chest film, how can it be determined whether a coin is in the trachea or the esophagus?

If on a lateral projection, the coin is parallel to the projection (slim appearance), then it is in the esophagus. If the coin is perpendicular to the projection (round), then it is usually in the trachea.

MEDIASTINUM

What structures are normally located in the anterior mediastinum?

Thymus and lymph nodes

What structures are normally located in the middle mediastinum?	Heart, lymph nodes, and trachea
What are the "5 birds" of the posterior mediastinum?	1. Azy-"goose" (azygos vein) 2. Hemiazy-"goose" (hemiazygos vein) 3. Va-"goose" [vagus nerve (cranial nerve X)] 4. Esopha-"goose" (esophagus) 5. Thoracic "duck" (thoracic duct)
What are the causes of an anterior mediastinal mass?	**4 Ts + C** *m* **T**hymus (normal gland, hyperplastic gland, or thymic tumor) **T**hyroid (extension from neck) **T**eratoma (germ cell tumor) **T**errible lymphoma **C**ystic hygroma (extends from neck)
What causes a middle mediastinal mass?	Lymphadenopathy [e.g., lymphoma, tuberculosis (TB)] Cyst (e.g., bronchogenic cyst, neurenteric cyst)

What are 4 causes of a posterior mediastinal mass?	1. Neurogenic tumor (most common)
	  Neuroblastoma (patients younger than 2 years)
	  Ganglioneuroblastoma (patients younger than 10 years)
	  Ganglioneuroma (patients between the ages of 6 and 15 years)
	  Neurofibroma or schwannoma (patients older than 20 years)
	2. Neurenteric cyst
	3. Extramedullary hematopoiesis
	4. Sequestration

What is the "sail" sign?	A normal thymus that is shaped like a sail; especially visible in small children

DISORDERS OF THE CARDIOVASCULAR SYSTEM

When taking a systematic approach to cardiac disease, what factors are important to evaluate?	Heart size and chamber enlargement Pulmonary vascular pattern Situs abnormalities (site of the aortic arch; abdominal visceral situs)

Is heart size as determined on a chest radiograph (CXR) reliable?

In small children, size may depend on the respiratory phase.

What is a good clue to full inspiration on CXR in children?

Straightening of the trachea on a frontal projection. If the trachea is buckled, the film probably depicts expiration.

What structure complicates evaluation of the heart size and aortic arch in young infants?

The thymus, which usually obscures part of the heart and aortic arch

What terms can be used to describe the pulmonary vascular pattern?

Normal, increased/decreased, and symmetric/asymmetric

What is situs?

Situs refers to the position of asymmetric parts of the anatomy—the lungs, aorta, spleen, liver, and stomach—in relation to the midline.

Define the following types of situs:

    Situs solitus

Normal positioning

    Situs inversus

"Mirror image" positioning (i.e., aortic arch, heart, and liver are on the right side)

    Situs ambiguous

Bilateral right-sidedness (eparterial bronchi, trilobar lungs), asplenia, horizontal liver, and midline stomach

What is the best indicator of situs?

Positions of the aortic arch and liver/stomach (look for stomach bubble)

How can a CXR be used to evaluate congenital heart disease (CHD)?

A CXR can be used as a screening tool and may also indicate whether the patient is in CHF

What other modalities are useful for evaluating CHD?

Echocardiography, angiography, and magnetic resonance imaging (MRI) may be useful for making specific diagnoses.

What is the most common congenital cardiac anomaly?

Bicuspid aortic valve occurs most often, but is not the most common symptomatic lesion. The resultant condition presents in adulthood.

What are the 8 most common congenital cardiac anomalies of childhood (in order of frequency)?

1. Ventricular septal defect (VSD) [isolated (29%); one component of CHD (> 50%)]
2. Atrial septal defect (ASD) [11%]
3. Pulmonic stenosis (9%)
4. Patent ductus arteriosus (PDA) [8%]
5. Tetralogy of Fallot (6%)
6. Aortic stenosis (5%)
7. Coarctation of the aorta (5%)
8. Transposition of the great vessels (4%)

What clinical observation helps categorize children with CHD?

Color—cyanotic (bluish) or acyanotic (normal color)

ACYANOTIC CHD

What are common causes of acyanotic CHD?

Left-to-right shunt lesions such as VSD, ASD, and PDA (no deoxygenated blood on the systemic side)

What is the most common congenital heart lesion associated with increased pulmonary arterial flow?

VSD

Ventricular septal defect (VSD)

See also Chapter 4, "Cardiac Imaging"

What is the most common type of VSD?

A defect in the membranous portion of the septum high in the septum, toward the tricuspid valve, is most common. A muscular septal defect (lower in the septum) is the next most frequently occurring type. A supracristal VSD occurs below the aortic valve.

In what fraction of patients does spontaneous closure of a VSD occur?

One third

Patent ductus arteriosus (PDA)

What is PDA?

PDA occurs when the ductus arteriosus, the communication between the aorta and the pulmonary artery, does not close after birth. Aortic pressures are higher in diastole and systole, resulting in a continuous left-to-right shunt.

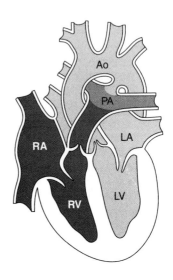

What is the appearance of PDA on CXR?	Cardiomegaly Increased size of the main pulmonary artery with increased pulmonary vascularity Normal-to-large aortic arch
What 4 lesions are associated with PDA?	**Left**-sided congenital lesions: 1. Aortic valvular stenosis 2. Coarctation 3. Interrupted aorta 4. Hypoplastic left heart syndrome

Atrial septal defect (ASD)

See also Chapter 4, "Cardiac Imaging"

What is the most common type of ASD?	Ostium secundum defect
Is ASD found more often in girls or boys?	Girls
What is the endocardial cushion?	A structure that partially forms the ventricular septum, the septal leaflets of the mitral and tricuspid valves, and the atrial septum

What angiographic signs are seen in an endocardial cushion defect?	Gooseneck deformity of the aortic outflow tract Abnormally oriented scalloped mitral valve Mitral regurgitation Left-to-right shunting (to right atrium and right ventricle)
With what syndrome is endocardial cushion defect associated?	Down syndrome

CYANOTIC CONGENITAL HEART DISEASE (CHD)

What is the physiologic basis of the cyanosis in CHD?	Right-to-left shunting with an admixture of deoxygenated blood
What are 5 causes of cyanotic CHD?	**5 Ts** (remember 1–5) **T**runcus arteriosus (1: one common trunk) **T**ransposition of great vessels (2: two-vessel switch) **T**ricuspid atresia (3: tricuspid valve) **T**etralogy of Fallot (4: tetralogy) **T**APVR (5: five words)
What are the changes in pulmonary blood flow associated with each of these 5 causes?	Truncus arteriosus: Increased flow Transposition of the great vessels: Variable flow Tricuspid atresia: Decreased flow (increased in 10%–15% of patients) Tetralogy of Fallot: Decreased flow TAPVR: Increased flow
What are the 2 most common cyanotic congenital heart lesions in neonates and infants?	**Tetralogy of Fallot** (most common cause of cyanosis in infants) and **transposition of the great vessels** (most common cause of cyanosis in neonates)

Tetralogy of Fallot

What are the hallmarks of tetralogy of Fallot?	Right ventricular outflow obstruction (infundibular and pulmonic stenosis) Large, subaortic VSD Overriding aorta Right ventricular hypertrophy

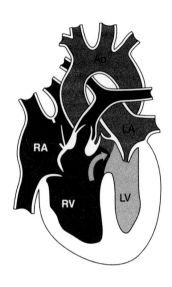

What characteristic of tetralogy of Fallot determines the severity of the symptoms?	The degree of right ventricular outflow obstruction
What is the classic appearance of tetralogy of Fallot on CXR?	"Boot-shaped" heart (right-sided enlargement, upturning of left apex) Diminished pulmonary vascularity Right-sided aortic arch (common)
What treatment is appropriate for tetralogy of Fallot?	Medical: Prostaglandins to maintain PDA temporarily Surgical: Blalock-Taussig shunt (palliative) and other surgical shunts; total correction
What is the Blalock-Taussig shunt?	Creation of a conduit from the subclavian artery to the pulmonary artery with a Gortex graft to increase pulmonary blood flow

Transposition of the great vessels

What is transposition of the great vessels?	Reversal of the great vessels so that the right ventricle empties into the aorta and the left ventricle empties into the pulmonary artery

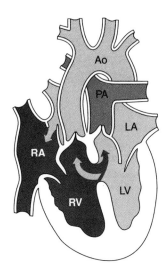

What flow pattern results from transposition of the great vessels?

Two completely separate circuits of blood flow—one oxygen saturated and one oxygen unsaturated—occur in parallel. This condition is fatal unless a communication (e.g., PDA, VSD, ASD) exists.

What is the typical appearance of transposition of the great vessels on CXR?

Enlarged heart and narrow mediastinum, with "egg-on-a-side" pattern

What treatment is appropriate for transposition of the great vessels?

Medical: Prostaglandins to keep the duct open (temporary)
Surgical: Rashkind atrial septostomy to increase mixing (temporary) or Jatene arterial switch procedure (definitive)

Tricuspid atresia

What is tricuspid atresia?

Failure of development of the tricuspid valve and the inflow portion of the right ventricle

How can children survive tricuspid atresia?

An interatrial shunt (often a stretched foramen ovale) and a VSD reroute blood flow into the right ventricular outflow tract and compensate for complete atresia of a tricuspid valve.

What treatment is appropriate for tricuspid atresia?

The **Fontan** procedure (connection of the right atrium to the main pulmonary artery or without a valve) is definitive. The Glenn procedure [anastomosis of the superior vena cava (SVC) to the right pulmonary artery] is also performed.

What is Ebstein's anomaly?

Downward displacement of the tricuspid valve ring into the right ventricle, in which tricuspid regurgitation leads to right atrial enlargement and decreased functional right ventricular output

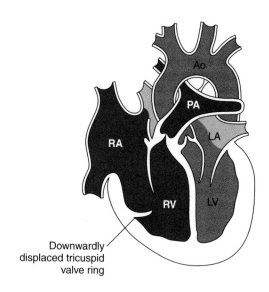

Downwardly displaced tricuspid valve ring

What is the appearance of Ebstein's anomaly on CXR?

Enlarged heart (usual in neonates; may be massive in older children or adults)
Diminished pulmonary vascularity
Resemblance to pericardial effusion

Total anomalous pulmonary venous return

Describe the 3 types of TAPVR.

In all three types, the pulmonary veins ultimately drain into the right atrium.
A = Supracardiac (drainage to the left brachiocephalic vein)
B = Intracardiac (drainage to the coronary sinus)
C = Infracardiac (drainage below the

diaphragm through the esophageal hiatus to the portal vein, which is often obstructed, leading to severe CHF)

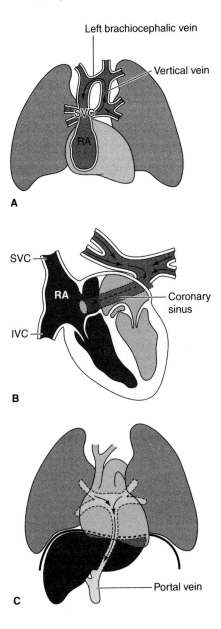

Left brachiocephalic vein

Vertical vein

SVC

RA

A

SVC

RA

IVC

Coronary sinus

B

Portal vein

C

What is the characteristic appearance of the supra-cardiac type of TAPVR on CXR?

"Snowman" pattern

How is partial anomalous pulmonary venous return (PAPVR) different from TAPVR?

Although both TAPVR and PAPVR are left-to-right shunts at the atrial level, patients with PAPVR are acyanotic. PAPVR is associated with other acyanotic lesions, notably ASD; 15% of patients with ASD have PAPVR.

What is the appearance of PAPVR on CXR?

Scimitar syndrome—the name is derived from the fact that the anomalous right pulmonary vein at the border of the right side of the heart looks like a Turkish sword. The syndrome is characterized by a hypoplastic right lung, dextroposition of the heart, and partial anomalous pulmonary venous drainage.

What is hypoplastic left heart syndrome?

Underdevelopment of the aorta, aortic valve, left ventricle, and mitral valve

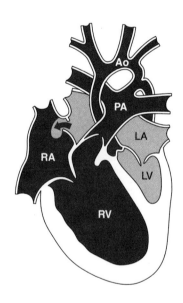

When does hypoplastic left heart syndrome become manifest?

Affected infants present in the first week of life with metabolic acidosis, shock, hypovolemia, cardiomegaly, and pulmonary edema. Lack of forward flow is the problem. The condition often causes death in the first week.

What is the typical appearance of hypoplastic left heart syndrome on CXR?

Cardiomegaly, CHF, and pulmonary overcirculation

What 2 other causes of congenital cardiomegaly in newborns both result in right atrial enlargement?

Pulmonary atresia and Ebstein's anomaly

AORTIC ARCH ANOMALIES

Right aortic arch

What is the significance of a right aortic arch?

A right aortic arch is associated with **cyanotic heart disease** in almost all cases.

Which way is the trachea deviated in a right aortic arch?

Leftward or midline, with no aortic knob visible on the left

What are the 5 most common lesions associated with a right aortic arch?

1. Truncus arteriosus (30%–35%)
2. Tetralogy of Fallot (30%)
3. Pulmonary atresia with VSD (30%)
4. Double-outlet right ventricle (20%)
5. Tricuspid atresia (3%–5%)

Coarctation of the aorta

What is coarctation of the aorta?

Coarctation is a focal narrowing of the aorta at the isthmus between the arch and the descending aorta

What are the 2 forms of coarctation of the aorta?

Pre- and postductus arteriosus

What bony change may be seen with coarctation of the aorta?

Rib notching develops when collateral flow occurs from the subclavian arteries through the internal mammary arteries and the intercostal arteries to the aorta below the level of the obstruction. This increased flow leads to the enlargement of the subcostal groove because of the tortuosity of the intercostal arteries.

What are the radiographic findings in coarctation of the aorta?

An indentation in the aorta is apparent on the posterior—anterior (PA) film (the "3" sign)

Rib notching (from intercostal artery collaterals)

What other studies may show the coarctation?	MRI (may show deformity of the arch, dilated internal mammary arteries, and collateral circulation) Angiography Transesophageal echocardiography (TEE)
What chromosomal syndrome has a high incidence of coarctation of the aorta?	Turner's syndrome (45, XO)

Vascular rings

What are vascular rings?	Embryologic anomalies of the aortic arch or its branches that encircle the trachea; symptoms are caused by tracheobronchial compression
What aortic lesions form vascular rings?	Double aortic arch and right aortic arch with aberrant left subclavian artery or left ligamentum arteriosum
What is the appearance of a double aortic arch on CXR?	Bilateral aortic arch shadows, with the right higher than the left, and anterior tracheal impression
What is the appearance of a double aortic arch on barium swallow?	Anterior esophageal and posterior tracheal impressions
What is a pulmonary sling?	Passage of the left pulmonary artery between the esophagus and the trachea

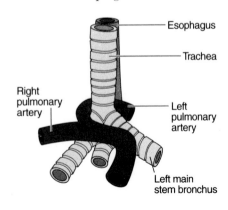

Esophagus

Trachea

Right pulmonary artery

Left pulmonary artery

Left main stem bronchus

What is the appearance of a pulmonary sling on barium swallow?	Anterior indentation on esophagus at about the level of the carina
Is the pulmonary sling a vascular ring?	No, the pulmonary artery does not encircle the bronchus or esophagus. However, affected patients may have respiratory problems as a result of hypoplasia of the trachea and carinal region.

DISORDERS OF THE GASTROINTESTINAL SYSTEM

OBSTRUCTIVE DISEASE

What is the radiographic *sine qua non* of mechanical obstruction?	Disproportionate dilatation of one segment of bowel compared with a distal segment; there is a **transition point** between the dilated and normal bowel segments
How is paralytic ileus characterized?	Paralytic ileus is characterized by gas, fluid, or both in all parts of the gastro-intestinal tract; generalized dilatation; late-onset pain; and absent bowel sounds.
List 7 common causes of bowel obstruction in neo-nates.	1. Esophageal atresia and tracheo-esophageal fistula 2. Hypertrophic pyloric stenosis 3. Duodenal atresia 4. Midgut volvulus 5. Jejunoileal atresia 6. Meconium plug 7. Hirschsprung's disease
What is the most common gastrointestinal disease of infancy?	Hypertrophic pyloric stenosis
What are 6 common causes of small bowel obstruction in children?	**AAIIMM** **A**dhesions **A**ppendicitis **I**ntussusception (most common cause) **I**nguinal hernia **M**alrotation (duodenal) with volvulus **M**eckel's diverticulum

Esophageal atresia and tracheoesophageal fistula

List the 3 most frequently occurring types of esophageal atresia and tracheoesophageal fistula.

A = Esophageal atresia with distal fistula
B = Esophageal atresia without fistula
C = Tracheoesophageal fistula without esophageal atresia (H-type)

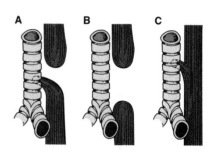

What is the most common type of esophageal atresia and tracheoesophageal fistula?

Esophageal atresia with distal fistula (80%)

What is the clinical/radiographic appearance of esophageal atresia and tracheoesophageal fistula?

Inability to pass a nasogastric tube and absence of air in the gastrointestinal tract

With what syndrome is tracheoesophageal fistula associated?

VACTERL syndrome
Vertebral anomalies
Anal atresia
Cardiovascular anomalies
Tracheo**E**sophageal fistula
Renal anomalies
Limb (especially radial) anomalies

Hypertrophic pyloric stenosis

Who tends to be affected?

Boys (boy:girl ratio is 4:1)
Whites (white:black ratio is 2:1)

When does this disease become manifest?

Between the second and sixth weeks of life (peaks at third week)

How do patients with hypertrophic pyloric stenosis present?

With projectile nonbilious vomiting (the vomitus hits the wall behind you if it is truly projectile)

What is involved in the imaging work-up?	Palpable "olive" (hypertrophied pylorus): Surgery (no need for imaging) Nonpalpable "olive" (hypertrophied pylorus): Ultrasound
What findings on ultrasound are diagnostic?	The presence of a hypoechoic ring, a pyloric ring greater than 4 mm in transverse view, and a pyloric channel greater than 14 mm in longitudinal view are diagnostic.
What study may yield a definitive diagnosis if the ultrasound findings are equivocal?	A barium study
What is the "string" sign in hypertrophic pyloric stenosis?	The "string" is the narrow lumen of the pylorus in hypertrophic pyloric stenosis, visible on an upper gastrointestinal series.

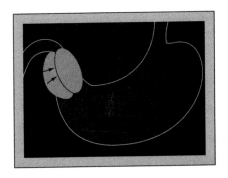

What treatment is appropriate for hypertrophic pyloric stenosis?	Pyloromyotomy

Duodenal obstruction

What does the "double bubble" appearance on a pediatric abdominal film represent?	Stomach and proximal duodenum dilatation
What causes the "double bubble"?	Obstruction at the duodenum, which may be caused by duodenal atresia, annular pancreas, choledochal cyst, or malrotation with midgut volvulus

With what syndrome is duodenal atresia associated?

Down syndrome

What is malrotation?

Normally, the bowel rotates a total of 270° counterclockwise, causing the transverse portion of the duodenum to cross to the left of the spine and relocating the cecum to the right lower quadrant. In malrotation, the bowel rotates less than 270°, the duodenal-jejunal junction does not reach its expected location to the left of the spine at the level of the duodenal bulb, and the colon may be on the left.

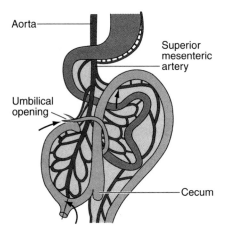

Aorta

Superior mesenteric artery

Umbilical opening

Cecum

What radiologic study determines the diagnosis of malrotation?

Finding the ligament of Treitz in an abnormal position on an upper gastrointestinal series confirms the diagnosis. (Normally, the ligament, demarcated by the junction of the fourth portion of the duodenum and the proximal jejunum, is located to the left of the spine, at or above the level of the pylorus.)

What appearance does the proximal bowel have in a malrotation with midgut volvulus?

Corkscrew appearance

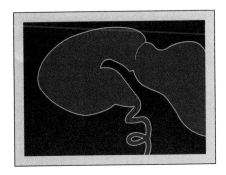

What problems does malrotation cause?

The body tries to "tack down" the abnormally positioned bowel with peritoneal fibrous bands known as "Ladd's bands." **Ladd's bands** can cause bowel obstruction and bilious vomiting. **Midgut volvulus** (twisting of the mesentery) leads to obstruction and vascular compromise or infarction of the gut.

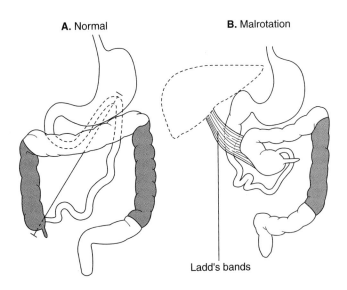

A. Normal   **B.** Malrotation

Ladd's bands

What diseases are associated with malrotation or may predispose to it?

Omphalocele, gastroschisis, and congenital diaphragmatic hernia

List 4 major differences between omphalocele and gastroschisis.	*Omphalocele*	*Gastroschisis*
	Defect at the midline (umbilicus)	Defect lateral to the midline (right)
	Viscera covered with amnion and peritoneum	Viscera not covered
	Abnormal rotation (Ladd's bands or midgut volvulus)	Malrotation
	Associated with severe anomalies	Less likely to have associated anomalies

Can omphalocele and gastroschisis be diagnosed by ultrasound *in utero*?

Yes.

Intussusception

What is intussusception?

Telescoping of one portion of the bowel into another

On the following figure depicting intussusception, what are the components *A* and *B* called?

A = Intussuscipiens
B = Intussusceptum

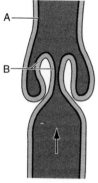

In what part of the bowel does intussusception almost always occur?

Ileocolic (terminal ileum invaginates into the colon)

What is the most common cause (lead point) of intussusception in children?

Idiopathic condition resulting from hypertrophied Peyer's patches

What 7 other lesions can serve as lead points in intussusception?	1. Meckel's diverticulum 2. Tumor 3. Duplication 4. Lymphoma 5. Mesenteric lymphadenopathy 6. CF 7. Hemorrhage
What is a Meckel's diverticulum?	A congenital remnant from foregut development
What is the "rule of 2s" in Meckel's diverticulum?	Occurs in **2**% of the population Located **2** feet from the ileocecal valve Presents at age **2**
What radiologic technique is used for the diagnosis of Meckel's diverticulum?	Technetium 99m-tagged red blood cell (RBC) scan
What radiologic finding is diagnostic?	"Hot" ectopic gastric mucosa in the diverticulum (pertechnate uptake)
What radiologic study is used for evaluation of intussusception?	Air or barium enema, which is used both to confirm or exclude the diagnosis and reduce the intussusception (i.e., it is diagnostic as well as therapeutic)

Distal bowel obstruction

What are 7 causes of distal obstruction?	1. Jejunal or ileal atresia owing to intrauterine vascular event 2. Meconium plug syndrome (barium enema shows cast of meconium in colon; 10% of patients have Hirschsprung's disease) 3. Small left colon (associated with maternal diabetes) 4. Meconium ileus (almost always associated with CF) 5. Hirschsprung's disease 6. Intussusception (patients 5–9 months of age; "coiled spring" appearance on radiograph) 7. Necrotizing enterocolitis (seen in premature infants)
What is the radiologic triad of a meconium ileus?	1. "Soap bubble" appearance in the right lower quadrant (RLQ)

2. Variation in caliber of distended loops
3. Paucity of air-fluid levels

What is the most common cause of meconium ileus?

CF

Describe Hirschsprung's disease.

Hirschsprung's disease is characterized by an aganglionic distal segment of colon. A transition zone is present between the dilated normal section of bowel and the diseased bowel. The sigmoid colon is larger than rectum, and evacuation is disordered.

What radiographic findings are seen in necrotizing enterocolitis?

Pneumatosis and pneumoperitoneum on CXR; gas in the portal venous system (late)

Match the findings on barium enema with the diagnosis.

A = Meconium plug syndrome
B = Hirschsprung's disease
C = Microcolon
D = Small left colon

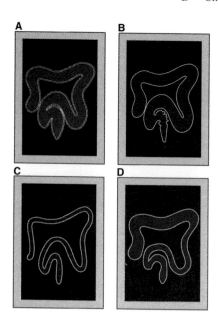

What is a microcolon?

An unused colon

What is the differential diagnosis of a microcolon?

Meconium ileus (the smallest of all microcolons)

Distal ileal atresia or stenosis
Hirschsprung's disease (if total)
Colonic atresia (distal to atresia)
Megacystis-microcolon-hypoperistalsis
    syndrome

NONOBSTRUCTIVE DISEASE

Polyposes

What are the 5 colonic polyposis syndromes seen in children?	1. Familial polyposis (polyps at puberty) 2. Juvenile polyps 3. Juvenile gastrointestinal polyposis (familial) 4. Gardner's syndrome (polyposis accompanied by osteomas, soft tissue fibromas, and sebaceous cysts) 5. Peutz-Jeghers syndrome (polyps primarily in jejunum)
Of these 5 syndromes, which have adenomatous polyps?	Familial polyposis and Gardner's syndrome
Why is this important?	The incidence of **malignancy** is greatly increased with **adenomatous polyps.**

Pneumatosis and pneumoperitoneum

What is pneumatosis?	Air seen in the bowel wall but not free in the peritoneum
What are 8 causes of pneumatosis?	1. Necrotizing enterocolitis (usually in neonates) 2. CF 3. Vascular injury 4. Sepsis 5. Hirschsprung's disease (with enterocolitis) 6. Toxic megacolon 7. Collagen vascular disease 8. Steroid therapy
What treatment is appropriate for pneumatosis caused by steroid therapy or CF?	In these cases, pneumatosis is a benign condition and requires no treatment. **In neonates,** however, **no pneumatosis is benign**—it signals necrotizing enterocolitis and the prognosis is poor.

What is pneumoperitoneum?	Free air in the peritoneum
What are 3 causes of pneumoperitoneum in neonates?	1. Necrotizing enterocolitis with perforation 2. Spontaneous gastric perforation 3. Air leak in chest and downward dissection
What are 4 radiographic signs of pneumoperitoneum?	1. "Double wall" or "Rigler's" sign on lateral view (air on both sides of the bowel wall) 2. Football-shaped lucency in midabdomen 3. Air outlining the falciform ligament 4. Hyperlucency of the entire abdomen

BILIARY DISEASE

Why are hepatobiliary scans performed for neonates with liver dysfunction?	To distinguish between biliary atresia and neonatal hepatitis
Why is it important to differentiate neonatal hepatitis from biliary atresia?	Surgery is indicated for biliary atresia but not for hepatitis
How are biliary atresia and neonatal hepatitis distinguished diagnostically?	**Biliary atresia:** Ultrasound may demonstrate dilated biliary ducts. A hepatobiliary scan indicates no bowel activity at 24 hours' post-injection. (Normally, bowel activity occurs within 24 hours.) **Hepatitis:** A hepatobiliary scan shows poor uptake of radionuclide (i.e., the liver is not as dark as usual) and poor excretion (although tracer should be seen eventually in the bowel). If biliary atresia has been present for a long time, there may be liver dysfunction and poor liver uptake, making it difficult to distinguish biliary atresia from hepatitis.
Is a hepatobiliary scan the "gold standard" for diagnosis of biliary atresia?	No. When a hepatobiliary scan suggests biliary atresia, an intraoperative cholangiogram is performed before any repair is attempted.

Why must a hepatobiliary scan be performed promptly?

Biliary atresia must be corrected by the Kasai procedure before permanent liver damage ensues. The procedure should be performed within 2–3 months of birth.

What routine premedication is appropriate for a neonate who is being evaluated for liver dysfunction?

Phenobarbital (usually 5 mg daily for 5–7 days) increases the activity of liver secretory enzymes.

What are 2 causes of biliary obstruction in a neonate or infant, aside from biliary atresia?

Choledochal cyst and enteric duplication

What are 4 types of choledochal cysts?

Type I: Dilatation of the extrahepatic ducts (80% of cases)
Type II: Eccentric diverticulum
Type III (choledochocele): Focal dilatation near the sphincter that extends into the duodenal wall
Type IV: Multiple dilatations

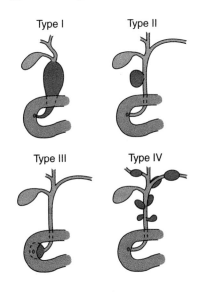

Patients with choledochal cysts are at increased risk for what condition?

Carcinoma of the bile ducts (cholangiocarcinoma)

Do children develop gallstones?

Yes.

What are the 2 major categories of gallstones?	Nonhemolytic and hemolytic

What are the causes of:

Nonhemolytic gallstones? (List 4)	1. Idiopathic (most common) 2. CF 3. Pancreatitis 4. Sepsis
Hemolytic gallstones? (List 3)	1. Sickle cell disease 2. Thalassemia 3. Spherocytosis

DISORDERS OF THE GENITOURINARY SYSTEM

How should an abdominal mass in a neonate be evaluated?	Supine and upright or decubitus abdominal films should be obtained. If the films show obstruction, an upper gastrointestinal series or a barium enema should be performed. If the films are negative, an ultrasound should be performed to identify the organ of origin or confirm hydronephrosis. A CT may be indicated in the case of a solid mass.
Name 16 causes of abdominal mass in neonates.	**Renal causes** 1. Hydronephrosis (most common) 2. Multicystic dysplastic kidney 3. Infantile polycystic kidney disease 4. Mesoblastic nephroma **Genital causes** 5. Ovarian cyst (result of stimulation by maternal hormones) 6. Hydrometrocolpos **Gastrointestinal causes** 7. Enteric duplication or mesenteric cyst 8. Dilated bowel proximal to obstruction or atresia 9. Volvulus 10. Meconium ileus **Retroperitoneal causes** 11. Adrenal hemorrhage 12. Teratoma 13. Neuroblastoma **Hepatobiliary causes** 14. Hepatoblastoma

15. Hemangioma or hemangio-
    endothelioma
16. Choledochal cyst

**What is the initial diag-
nostic test in the evaluation
of an abdominal mass in an
older infant or child?**

As with neonates, ultrasound is most
likely to be helpful, but CT or MRI may
be needed ultimately.

**Name 10 causes of abdom-
inal mass in older infants
and children.**

Renal causes
1. Wilms' tumor (20% of cases)
2. Hydronephrosis (20% of cases)

Retroperitoneal causes
3. Neuroblastoma (20% of cases);
   displaces kidney
4. Pancreatic pseudocyst

Gastrointestinal causes
5. Appendiceal abscess
6. Hepatobiliary mass
7. Enteric duplication or mesenteric
   cyst

Genital causes
8. Ovarian cyst
9. Hydrometrocolpos
10. Ovarian teratoma or dermoid cyst

**What is the most frequently
occurring primary neo-
plasm of the kidney in
young infants?**

Mesoblastic nephroma

HYDRONEPHROSIS AND OTHER BENIGN CONDITIONS

What is hydronephrosis?

Dilatation of the renal collecting system

**What are the causes of
hydronephrosis?**

PURE P
Posterior urethral valves
Ureteropelvic obstruction
Reflux
Ectopic ureterocele
Prune belly syndrome

m

**How is the level of obstruc-
tion identified?**

Dilated ureters signify obstruction distal
to ureters, and a dilated bladder signifies
obstruction distal to bladder. In chronic
obstruction, the bladder may become
trabeculated and thick walled.

If necessary, how can the function of a kidney be demonstrated in obstruction?	By use of a furosemide renogram (see Chapter 2, "Imaging Techniques")
What is the most common cause of unilateral hydronephrosis in children?	Ureteropelvic junction (UPJ) obstruction

Ureteropelvic junction obstruction

What is a congenital UPJ obstruction?	An intrinsic abnormality of the proximal ureter that causes a functional obstruction
What is the radiographic appearance of a congenital UPJ junction obstruction?	Hydronephrosis without a hydroureter and without a mass or stone
How often is a UPJ junction obstruction bilateral?	20% of the time
With what congenital anomaly may a congenital UPJ junction obstruction be associated?	Horseshoe kidney
What are 6 complications of horseshoe kidney aside from increased UPJ junction obstruction?	1. Increased incidence of Wilms' tumor 2. Higher incidence of adenocarcinoma 3. Greater susceptibility to trauma 4. Increased incidence of renovascular hypertension 5. Increased vesicoureteral reflux 6. Increased stone formation

Vesicoureteral reflux

What is vesicoureteral reflux?	Reflux of urine from the bladder into the ureter caused by an abnormal course of the ureter in the bladder wall
What are the grades of vesicoureteral reflux?	**I:** Reflux limited to the lower ureter **II:** Reflux extended to the renal pelvis **III:** Reflux with mild hydronephrosis and hydroureter **IV:** Reflux with moderate hydronephrosis and hydroureter **V:** Reflux with severe hydronephrosis

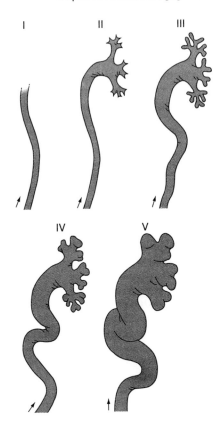

How may vesicoureteral reflux be manifest?

In girls, by recurrent urinary tract infections (UTIs)

In boys, just one UTI should arouse suspicion

What is involved in the work-up of UTI in children?

Voiding cystourethrography (VCUG), with ultrasound in older children and adolescents

Should boys and girls be studied at the same stage of disease?

No—boys should be studied after their **first UTI,** whereas girls should be studied after their second UTI or first episode of pyelonephritis.

How is VCUG used in the work-up of a UTI?

VCUG, which is the first test, demonstrates reflux and voiding abnormalities. If the VCUG is normal, obtain an ultrasound, and if the ultrasound is normal, no additional testing is necessary. If either the VCUG or the ultrasound is abnormal, an intravenous pyelogram (IVP) is necessary.

Why is it important to diagnose intrarenal reflux?

Because the condition may lead to renal scarring and possible hypertension

What treatment is appropriate for vesicoureteral reflux?

Prophylaxis with antibiotics while the urinary tract matures (vesicoureteral reflux may disappear)
Surgery for grades IV and V (hydronephrosis) with scarring

What test is used for follow-up in a patient with vesicoureteral reflux? Why?

A nuclear cystogram, because it exposes the patient to 1/100 of the radiation dose compared to VCUG

What congenital anomaly predisposes to vesicoureteral reflux?

Ureteral duplication, where two ureters drain one kidney, leads to vesicoureteral reflux. The ureters may join each other or both insert into the bladder.

What are the complications of ureteral duplication?

The upper pole moiety is associated with an invagination of the bladder wall (ectopic ureterocele) and is obstructed. The lower pole moiety (orthotopic) refluxes.

What is the "drooping lily" sign in ureteral duplication?

On a VCUG, reflux into the lower pole ureter is seen, but the calyces are displaced inferiorly (drooping) by the dilated, obstructed upper pole.

What are 3 clinical features of prune belly syndrome?

Hypoplasia of the abdominal musculature, undescended testes, and bulging flanks

What are 9 radiographic findings of prune belly syndrome?

1. Flaring of the lower ribs
2. Lung hypoplasia
3. Renal agenesis
4. Hydronephrosis
5. Ureteral atresia
6. Bladder diverticula
7. Vesicoureteral reflux
8. Urethral valves
9. Distended bladder

What is the most common cause of urethral obstruction in boys?	Posterior urethral valves
In which patients should the diagnosis of urethral obstruction be considered?	In male infants or children with voiding difficulties and upper urinary tract dilatation
What are the findings of urethral obstruction on ultrasound?	Hydronephrosis; ureterectasis; a thick-walled, distended, keyhole-shaped bladder
What is the imaging method of choice in urethral obstruction?	VCUG
What is the "spinnaker sail" sign?	A dilated posterior urethra seen on VCUG in patients with urethral valves
What treatment is appropriate for patients with urethral valves?	Surgical obliteration of the valves

MALIGNANT CONDITIONS

What are the 2 most common malignant tumors in children (in order of frequency)?	**Wilms' tumor** (10% of all childhood malignant tumors) and **neuroblastoma**
How often is Wilms' tumor bilateral?	In 4%–10% of cases
What is the most common presentation of Wilms' tumor?	Abdominal mass

Compare Wilms' tumor with neuroblastoma in terms of:

	Wilms' Tumor	*Neuroblastoma*
Abdominal radiograph findings	Bulging flank	Calcification (66% of cases)
IVP findings	Large kidney	Inferoanterior displacement of kidney
Possible CXR findings	Lung metastases	Paravertebral mass

Possible findings on bone radiography	None	Bony metastases
Findings on CT	Low-density mass	Suprarenal mass (75% are calcified)
Findings on nuclear bone scan	Rarely any	Tumor uptake on bone scan (75% of cases)
Ultrasound	Solid or cystic mass	Solid calcified suprarenal mass
Relationship to adjacent vasculature	Possible invasion of the renal vein	Usual encasement of vessels

ADRENAL CONDITIONS

List 2 causes of a supra-renal mass.

Neuroblastoma and adrenal hemorrhage

What ultrasound findings determine the diagnosis?

An echogenic, vascular mass is a neuro-blastoma. An anechoic, nonvascular mass is an adrenal hemorrhage.

How is adrenal hemorrhage manifested in neonates?

Patients may be asymptomatic or exhibit anemia and jaundice (as a result of re-sorption of the hematoma).

If adrenal hemorrhage is suspected, what radiologic study should be per-formed—ultrasound or CT?

Ultrasound, which shows a suprarenal anechoic mass with extrinsic renal com-pression. Follow-up is appropriate to ensure that the mass does not grow.

What is the prognosis for patients with adrenal hem-orrhage?

Excellent

What are 7 conditions in the differential diagnosis of adrenal calcifications?

1. Neonatal adrenal hemorrhage
2. Neuroblastoma
3. Pheochromocytoma
4. Adrenal carcinoma
5. Adrenal cyst
6. Addison's disease
7. Granulomatous disease (tuberculosis or histoplasmosis)

TRAUMATIC DISORDERS
OF THE MUSCULOSKELETAL SYSTEM

What accounts for more deaths in children than all diseases combined?	Trauma, which most commonly occurs as a result of abuse (nonaccidental trauma) and birth injuries
How are the bones different in children than in adults?	Children are still growing. Immature bones have open growth plates and cartilaginous epiphysis, with a thick, tough periosteum. Because of incomplete mineralization, these bones are more elastic.
At what age is ossification of the axis (C2) complete?	The subdental synchondrosis closes between 3 and 6 years of age, fusing the ossification center of the dens with the body of the C2 vertebra.
What are the 6 ossification centers of the pediatric elbow?	1. Medial epicondyle 2. Lateral epicondyle 3. Capitellum 4. Trochlea 5. Radial head 6. Olecranon of the ulna
What is the sequence of ossification of the elbow?	Come Rub My Tree Of Love Capitellum—1 year Radial head—5 years Medial epicondyle—7 years Trochlea—10 years Olecranon—10 years Lateral epicondyle—11 years

CHILD ABUSE

What are common sites of injury in children who have been abused?	The head is the most common site. Other common sites include the ribs (costochondral and costovertebral junctions), metaphyses, and long bones (spiral fractures). Note that the upper limbs are twice as likely to be affected as the lower limbs.
What are 4 radiographic signs of abuse?	1. Healing fractures of differing ages 2. Multiple fractures (e.g., multiple rib fractures if the child is otherwise healthy) 3. Fractures in unusual locations 4. Metaphyseal fractures

What 7 radiographic views should be obtained if abuse is suspected?	1. Two views of the skull 2. Lateral thoracic and lumbar spine 3. Frontal views of both upper extremities 4. Both hands 5. Pelvis 6. Both lower extremities 7. Both feet
What is a bucket-handle fracture?	This transverse fracture through a long bone metaphysis, which appears to result from avulsion caused by severe shaking, is pathognomonic for abuse.
What is the responsibility of a physician in a case of suspected abuse?	The physician is legally required to report cases of suspected abuse to a department of social services.

BIRTH INJURIES

What birth injuries are most common?	Skeletal injuries occur most often—fortunately, they are the least severe. A fractured clavicle is the most common type of skeletal injury.
What is the frequency of birth injuries?	2–7 cases per 1000 births
What are 3 fetal characteristics that lead to birth injury?	High birth weight, shoulder dystocia, and breech presentation

FRACTURES

Are fractures less common in children or adults?	Fractures are less common in children because children have more elastic bones. Bending and bowing injuries and partial fractures occur more readily than complete fractures in children.
Which occurs more often in children, ligamentous injuries or joint injuries to the physis?	Injuries to the physis rather than a ligament are more likely, because of the weakness of the open epiphyseal plate.
How do fractures heal differently in children as compared with adults?	The healing process, which involves an active remodeling process that corrects most traumatic deformities, is more rapid in children.

When do the radiographic changes of bone healing typically occur in children?	Periosteal new bone formation: 7–10 days Obliteration of the fracture line: 14–21 days Hard callus formation: 14–28 days Remodeling of bone: 12 months
What are the 5 common types of bone injuries in children?	1. Elastic deformation 2. Bowing deformation 3. Torus fracture 4. Greenstick fracture 5. Salter-Harris fracture
What is the difference between elastic and bowing deformation?	An elastic deformation is a momentary, impermanent bending injury to bone, whereas a bowing deformation causes a bone deformity that may or may not be completely corrected by remodeling.
What is a torus fracture (also called a buckle fracture)?	A type of fracture that involves buckling of one cortex
What is a greenstick fracture?	An incomplete transverse fracture that is common in elementary school-age children, with fracture in one cortex and periosteal rupture on the convex side of injury and an intact periosteum on the concave surface
What are Salter-Harris fractures?	Salter-Harris fractures involve the epiphyseal plate.
How common are these fractures in children?	Salter-Harris fractures, which occur primarily in children between the ages of 10 and 15 years, make up approximately one-third of all skeletal injuries in children.
How are Salter-Harris fractures classified?	**Type I:** Fracture through the physeal plate **Type II:** Fracture through the metaphysis and physis **Type III:** Fracture through the epiphysis and physis **Type IV:** Fracture through the metaphysis, physis, and epiphysis **Type V:** Crush injury of the physis

I   II   III

IV   V

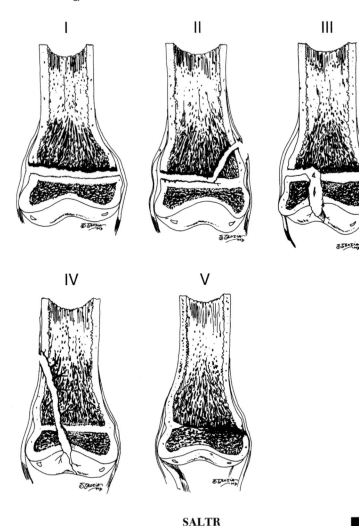

SALTR
Separated (type I)
Above (type II)
Lower (type III)
Through (type IV)
Ruined (type V)

m

HEAD TRAUMA

What is a ping-pong ball fracture?	A depression of the parietal bone that resembles a crunched ping-pong ball
What is the cause of a ping-pong ball fracture?	Forceps delivery

What are 2 common deformities of the head that develop in the immediate postnatal period?	**Caput succedaneum,** which is soft tissue swelling in the subcutaneous fat **Cephalohematoma,** which is a collection of blood trapped between the periosteum and the bony margin
How can caput succadeneum and cephalohematoma be distinguished radiographically?	Caput succadeneum crosses suture lines, whereas cephalohematoma does not.
What can be seen in a few months on a follow-up radiograph?	Normal-appearing head (condition resolves) or residual calcification (possible resemblance to a destructive bony lesion)

UPPER EXTREMITY TRAUMA

Shoulder trauma

What is the most common long bone fracture in children?	A clavicle fracture, usually through the distal clavicle physis, is much more common than shoulder dislocation or acromioclavicular joint separation in children (as opposed to adults).
What is pseudoarthrosis of the clavicle?	A rare congenital defect, which almost invariably occurs on the right side, that is manifest as a nonpainful palpable bony defect
What are the radiographic features of pseudoarthrosis of the clavicle?	A small gap in the middle third of the clavicle that exhibits no healing reaction at 2-week follow-up
What is "Little League" shoulder?	Activity-related pain of the dominant shoulder secondary to microtrauma from overuse
What are the radiographic features of "Little League" shoulder?	A widened, irregular, proximal humeral physis

Elbow trauma

What are 2 important radiographic lines in the elbow?	1. **Anterior humeral line,** which normally passes through the middle portion of the capitellum 2. **Radiocapitellar line** (line through the center of the radius), which normally

should pass through the capitellum on all views of the elbow

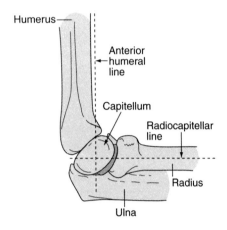

What is nursemaid's elbow?	Nursemaid's elbow, a common condition in toddlers, is **dislocation of the radial head** in toddlers without disruption of the annular ligament as a result of direct traction on the arm. Nursemaid's elbow may be difficult to see on radiographs because of incomplete ossification of the radial head, but one clue may be mal-alignment of the radiocapitellar line.
What are the most common distal humerus fractures in children?	Supracondylar fracture (60% of cases), followed by lateral and medial epi-condylar fractures
What is "Little League" elbow?	Medial epicondylitis
What are the radiographic features of "Little League" elbow?	Widened, irregular medial distal humeral physis and possible medial epicondyle avulsion

Hand and wrist trauma

What is epiphysiolysis of the distal radius?	This condition, which is analogous to "Little League" shoulder and elbow, is activity-related pain of the wrists due to overuse. It is commonly seen in gymnasts. Radiographs show widening and irregularity of the distal radial physis.

What is an extraoctave fracture?	Salter-Harris type I or II injury of the base of the fifth digit proximal phalanx

PELVIC TRAUMA

What is the most common pelvic fracture in children?	Avulsion fractures from ligamentous and tendonous stresses
What are the usual sites of pelvic avulsion fractures and the involved muscle attachments?	Anterior superior iliac spine: Sartorius Anterior inferior iliac spine: Rectus femoris Inferior pubic rami: Adductors, gracilis Lesser trochanter of the femur (as a result of stress on the iliopsoas tendon)

LOWER EXTREMITY TRAUMA

What is osteochondritis dissecans?	This articular injury, which most commonly affects the knee, usually involves unilateral separation of fragments of articular cartilage and subchondral bone. The condition is thought to result from chronic trauma.
How is osteochondritis dissecans manifested?	Knee pain
Who is most likely to develop this condition?	Children and young adults
How do tibial tubercle avulsion fractures occur?	Forceful quadriceps contraction, which is most common in adolescents
What is toddler's fracture?	This stress fracture of the lower extremity, usually occurring secondary to falls in children learning to walk, commonly leads to injuries such as spiral shaft fracture of the tibia and calcaneal and cuboid fractures.

SPINE TRAUMA

What is meant by pseudo-subluxation of the cervical spine?	As the prefix "pseudo" suggests, true injury to the cervical spine is uncommon in children. However, between 15% and 25% of children younger than 8 years have physiologic anterior displacement of

either the C2 or C3 vertebra as a result of normal ligamentous laxity.

What is an os odontoideum?
A congenital abnormality of fusion of the dens to the body at vertebra C2, which may be confused with a dens fracture

NONTRAUMATIC DISORDERS OF THE MUSCULOSKELETAL SYSTEM

SKULL DISORDERS

Which suture line closes prematurely in each of the 5 types of craniosynostosis [dolichocephaly (scaphocephaly), brachycephaly, turricephaly, oxycephaly, plagiocephaly]?
Dolichocephaly (scaphocephaly): Sagittal suture
Brachycephaly: Coronal sutures
Turricephaly: Complex fusion
Oxycephaly (small): All sutures
Plagiocephaly (oblique): Coronal or Lambdoidal suture

Which type of craniosynostosis is the most common?
Dolichocephaly

What is positional plagiocephaly?
Flattening of the back of the head, which results from the current practice of putting infants to sleep on their backs to prevent sudden infant death syndrome

What are 3 conditions in the differential diagnosis of primary craniosynostosis?
Idiopathic disease, Crouzon's disease, and Apert's syndrome

What are 5 causes of secondary craniosynostosis (secondary to abnormal brain development or bone growth)?
1. Cerebral degeneration
2. Anemia
3. Healing rickets
4. Mucopolysaccharidosis
5. Hyperthyroidism

What modality is most useful for the diagnosis of craniosynostosis?
CT. In addition to allowing diagnosis, CT with three-dimensional reconstruction can be used for surgical planning.

What are 7 causes of widened cranial sutures?
1. Prematurity
2. Increased intracranial pressure (ICP)
3. Rickets
4. Hypophosphatasia
5. Hypothyroidism
6. Osteogenesis imperfecta
7. Cleidocranial dysplasia

UPPER EXTREMITY DISORDERS

What is Sprengel's deformity?	Congenital elevation of the scapula is often associated with other anomalies such as cervical fusion, scoliosis, and cardiac and renal conditions. The involved scapula is typically smaller than normal.
What is radioulnar synostosis?	Congenital bony fusion of the proximal radius and ulna
What is Madelung's deformity?	Ulnar and palmar bowing of the distal radius with ulnar minus variant and triangularization of the distal radioulnar joint on radiography
What is radial club hand?	This radial deficiency of variable degree may involve absence of one thumb, shortening of the index finger, radial deviation of the hand, and a prominent distal ulna. This deficiency is associated with other conditions, including cardiovascular, genitourinary, and gastrointestinal problems.
What is ulnar club hand?	This ulnar deficiency, with extremely variable expression, may involve the absence of the small finger, ulnar deviation of the hand and wrist, shortening of the forearm with ulnar bowing, and even humeral shortening. This condition, which is much less common than radial club hand, is not associated with other anomalies.
What is cleft hand?	Central deficiency of formation of the hand, which is usually bilateral and associated with other cleft deformities
What is polydactyly?	This developmental anomaly is characterized by duplication of one or more digits. Postaxial or ulnar-sided polydactyly is more common in individuals of African origin and may indicate a serious abnormality in whites.

What is syndactyly?

This fusion of digits may be incomplete (not reaching the distal phalanx) or complete. The simple form involves webbed skin between the digits, and the complex form involves bony fusion.

What is macrodactyly?

This condition, characterized by enlargement of a digit, is a rare congenital malformation associated with neurofibromatosis, arteriovenous malformations (AVMs), and lymphangioma.

HIP DISORDERS

Name the common conditions of the hip that occur in children by age group.

Neonates, infants, and toddlers:
  Developmental dysplasia of the hip (DDH), which is also known as congenital dysplasia or dislocation of the hip
Children: Legg-Calvé-Perthes disease
Adolescents: Slipped capital femoral epiphysis (SCFE)

Developmental dysplasia of the hip (DDH)

What is DDH?

DDH is recurrent subluxation or dislocation of the hip secondary to acetabular dysplasia, abnormal ligamentous laxity, or both. The two components of acetabular dysplasia are increased acetabular angle and a shallow acetabular fossa. Chronic dislocation of the femoral head leads to exacerbated growth deformity of the acetabular fossa.

Which children are more likely to be affected?

Occurs much more commonly in firstborns and in female infants, possibly because of estrogen effects on ligamentous laxity

Which side of the body is most often involved?

DDH occurs in the **left** hip most frequently (70%). It is bilateral in only 5% of cases.

What clinical findings are characteristic of DDH?

Shortened leg with decreased range of abduction when flexed
Positive Ortolani's and Barlow's signs
Abnormal gait (older children)
Asymmetry of thigh folds

When are radiographs of the hip *not* useful in the diagnosis of DDH?

Radiographs are unreliable in children younger than 6–12 months because of a lack of skeletal ossification.

What radiographic view is best for evaluation of DDH?

Anterior-posterior (AP) radiography of the pelvis is most useful. Frogleg views are not helpful, because the hip is likely to be reduced in this position.

What are 8 radiographic features of DDH?

1. Shallow acetabulum
2. Increased acetabular angle
3. Small capital femoral epiphysis
4. Delayed ossification of the femoral head
5. Acetabular sclerosis
6. Loss of Shenton's curve
7. Femoral head lateral to Perkin's line
8. Femoral head superior to Hilgenreiner's line

What is Hilgenreiner's line?

A horizontal line through the triradiate cartilage of the acetabulum on an AP view of the pelvis

What is Perkin's line?

A vertical line that is perpendicular to Hilgenreiner's line from the lateral margin of the ossified acetabular roof and is normally tangential to the lateral margin of the ossification center of the femoral head

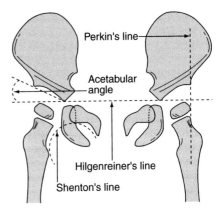

What is Putti's triad?

Superolateral displacement of femoral head
Acetabular angle greater than 35°
Small femoral epiphysis

What is the best imaging modality for the diagnosis of DDH?

Ultrasound, which should be performed in the first 6–12 months of life, while the epiphysis is not calcified and therefore cannot be seen on plain radiographs

How does DDH appear on ultrasound?

Decreased femoral head coverage by the acetabulum (< 50%)
Dynamic instability, as evidenced by displacement of the femoral head by the examiner during the study

Legg-Calvé-Perthes disease

What is Legg-Calvé-Perthes disease?

Idiopathic avascular necrosis of the femoral head

In what children is Legg-Calvé-Perthes disease suspected?

Children who are 3–8 years to age and have hip or knee pain or a limp

Are boys or girls more commonly affected?

Boys (boy:girl ratio is 5:1)

What is involved in the radiologic workup of Legg-Calvé-Perthes disease?

Plain films (frogleg view), bone scan, MRI

What are the findings on:

Plain film radiography?

Subchondral fractures (frogleg view)
Increased width of radiologic joint space

Bone scan?

Decreased activity in the femoral capital epiphysis

MRI?

A high signal on T_2-weighted images in the marrow

Which shows evidence of avascular necrosis first— plain film radiography or MRI?

MRI

What factor is a good prognostic indicator in Legg-Calvé-Perthes disease?	Age at onset, because if the onset of Legg-Calvé-Perthes disease occurs before 6 years of age, then the restoration of a spherical femoral head is more likely; otherwise, degenerative osteoarthritis is probable.

Other than Legg-Calvé-Perthes disease, what conditions can cause:

Unilateral avascular necrosis of the hip? (List 3)	1. Fracture of the femoral neck 2. Following surgery for DDH 3. Slipped capital femoral epiphysis (SCFE)
Bilateral avascular necrosis of the hip? (List 5)	1. Multiple epiphyseal dysplasia 2. Spondyloepiphyseal dysplasia 3. Gaucher's disease 4. Hypothyroidism 5. Sickle cell disease

Slipped capital femoral epiphysis (SCFE)

In which patients should SCFE be suspected?	Every adolescent who complains of hip or knee pain
Are boys or girls more often afflicted with SCFE?	**Boys** (ages 12–15 years) are affected twice as often as girls (ages 10–13 years).
What are the risk factors associated with SCFE?	Obesity, repetitive athletic stress, and endocrine disorders (hypothyroidism, hypopituitarism)
What are 4 signs of SCFE?	1. Osteoporosis (seen 7–10 days after slippage) 2. Widening of the physis 3. Disordered trabecula of the metaphysis 4. Incongruity of the head or neck of the femur at the physis
What radiographic view is best for the diagnosis of SCFE?	The frogleg view is essential, and minimal slippage is seen best.
When is diagnosis of SCFE most difficult?	When the slippage occurs bilaterally and symmetry is present

What is the prognosis for children with SCFE?	Good if the diagnosis is made before appreciable slippage occurs, because a favorable result can be obtained with surgical pinning, but poor if the diagnosis is made late
What is pistol grip deformity?	Flattening of the femoral neck, which occurs if SCFE is not diagnosed early, with the formation of an inferior notch at the femoral head

LOWER EXTREMITY DISORDERS

Knee disorders

What is Osgood-Schlatter disease?	Recurrent patellar tendonitis leading to a painful tibial tuberosity
Is Osgood-Schlatter disease more common in boys or girls?	The condition is most common in pre-adolescent boys (the boy:girl ratio is 5:1)
What are 4 radiologic findings of Osgood-Schlatter disease?	1. Soft tissue swelling about the patellar tendon 2. Thickened patellar tendon 3. Loss of the infrapatellar fat pad 4. Irregularity of the tibial tuberosity

Foot disorders

What is congenital vertical talus?	"Rocker bottom"-appearing foot as a result of fixed equinus contracture of the hindfoot with a pronated valgus heel, profound dorsiflexion, and abduction of the midfoot and forefoot
What are 3 radiographic features of vertical talus?	1. Sequential lateral neutral and plantar flexed weight-bearing films, which demonstrate the fixed nature of the deformity 2. Concave talar neck 3. Dislocation or subluxation at the calcaneocuboid joint
What are the 4 distinct components of talipes equinovarus (clubfoot)?	Hindfoot varus, equinus heel, metatarsus adductus (adduction and varus deformity of forefoot), and talonavicular subluxation
What is the major abnormality in clubfoot?	Deformity of the talus, which is smaller and deviated plantar and medially

How often does clubfoot occur?	A relatively common abnormality, with a frequency of up to 1/1000
Are girls or boys more commonly affected?	Boys (boy:girl ratio is 2:1)
What is the usefulness of radiographs in clubfoot and other deformities of the talus?	To assess the bones of the hindfoot so that the orthopedist may plan surgery in an attempt to place the foot in a nearly corrected position
What radiographs are required in clubfoot?	AP and lateral weight-bearing films
What are the radiographic characteristics of clubfoot?	Talocalcaneal angle ($< 20°$ on AP view; $< 35°$ on lateral view) Medial displacement of the first metatarsal relative to the long axis of talus Medial subluxation of the navicula in relation to the talus (frequently not appreciated because ossification has yet to occur at the time of diagnosis)
How often is clubfoot bilateral?	50% of the time
When is surgery required in clubfoot?	For a "true" deformity (as opposed to "postural" clubfoot, which arises from intrauterine malposition and is treated with conservative management)
What is tarsal coalition?	Congenital fusion of the tarsal bones, with complete or partial bony coalition or cartilaginous or fibrous fusion, that may manifest as chronic foot pain
What are the 2 most common types of tarsal coalition?	Calcaneonavicular (most common) and talocalcaneal
What are 2 radiographic features of tarsal coalition?	1. Calcaneonavicular bridge (oblique films) 2. Talocalcaneal joint obliteration (Harris axial film of the subtalar joint)
What is the best imaging modality for the diagnosis of tarsal coalition?	CT

Spine disorders

What spinal abnormality is commonly associated with Down syndrome?	Instability or subluxation at the atlanto-axial joint (C1–C2), which may occur in as many as 20% of patients with trisomy 21
What is Klippel-Feil syndrome?	The congenital fusion of two or more vertebrae in the cervical spine, which is most common from vertebrae C2 to C7 and may be single or multilevel
What are the clinical signs and symptoms of Klippel-Feil syndrome?	The clinical triad of short neck, low posterior headline, and limited range of motion of the neck is found in 50% of patients. Deafness is common, and there is an association with scoliosis.
What is scoliosis?	An "S"-shaped spine, usually convex to the right in the thoracic region, with a leftward compensation in the lumbar spine when it is idiopathic
What are 4 causes of scoliosis?	Congenital, neuromuscular, compensatory, and iatrogenic conditions
Does a spinal curve of 20° have the same significance in a 6-year-old child as it does in an 18-year-old young adult?	No, because the child has not yet undergone the growth spurt that will change the degree of curvature
At what degree of curvature does respiratory compromise occur?	Usually around 70°
What treatment is appropriate for severe scoliosis?	Bracing and fusion
What complications occur as a result of scoliosis?	Degenerative changes, with chronic pain and possible respiratory compromise
What are 3 causes of vertebra plana (flattened vertebral bodies)?	1. Eosinophilic granuloma (often one body only) 2. Leukemia (usually demineralized with multiple collapsed bodies) 3. Osteogenesis imperfecta (also demineralized with multiple collapsed bodies)

What is Scheuermann's disease?	Thoracic kyphosis, with or without pain, that is characterized by anterior wedging of at least 3 consecutive vertebrae and the presence of Schmorl's nodes
What film best reveals the deformity in Scheuermann's disease?	Lateral spine film
What are 5 entities in the differential diagnosis of the scalloping of the posterior margin of vertebral bodies?	1. Neurofibromatosis 2. Osteogenesis imperfecta 3. Marfan's syndrome 4. Achondroplasia (short pedicles) 5. Acromegaly
When posterior scalloping occurs only at one level, what else must be considered?	Spinal cord tumor or spinal dysraphism
Where can scalloping be normal?	Lumbar spine
What 5 conditions lead to an increased interpediculate space (distance between the pedicles) on an AP film?	1. Fracture 2. Dysraphic states (malformation of neural arch of spine—spina bifida) 3. Intramedullary tumor 4. Syringomyelia 5. AVM
In what condition is the interpedicular space decreased?	Achondroplasia

INFECTION

Osteomyelitis

What part of the bone is most commonly affected in osteomyelitis?	The **metaphysis**
What is the most common route of spread?	Hematogenous
What is the most common pathogen?	*Staphylococcus aureus*

What are the early plain film radiographic findings in osteomyelitis?

None. MRI or nuclear bone scan is more sensitive. Changes occur after thrombosis of the vasculature develops (usually not until 7–10 days). Common late radiographic findings include periosteal reaction and soft tissue swelling.

What are 3 other causes of periosteal reaction other than osteomyelitis?

1. Histiocytosis X
2. Periosteal hematoma
3. Primary or secondary malignant lesion

When should osteomyelitis be suspected in infants?

If pain occurs on passive movement ("pseudoparalysis")

TORCH infections

What are the so-called TORCH infections?

TORCH
Toxoplasmosis
Other (HIV, syphilis)
Rubella
Cytomegalovirus (CMV)
Herpes simplex virus (HSV)

m

What is the mode of transmission of the TORCH infections?

These infections either cross the placenta or are acquired at birth.

What are some radiographic findings associated with TORCH infections?

Irregularity of the metaphyses of the long bones ("celery stalking"—alternating radiodense and lucent lines), especially in rubella
Cerebral destruction (cerebral calcification, microcephaly)
Intracranial calcifications (especially in toxoplasmosis)
Curvilinear, paraventricular calcifications (especially in CMV infection)
Massive calcification of a small, atrophic brain (especially in HSV infection)

What changes result from syphilis in newborns?

Skeletal involvement occurs in 65% of patients:
Long bones show lucent bands of fragmentation and destruction (nonspecific)
Wimberger's sign (i.e., bilateral metaphyseal destruction in the upper middle tibias)

Well-marginated, lytic lesions in the skull
and flat bones
Diaphyseal periostitis in luetic diaphysitis
(solid periosteal reaction)
Deformity or chronic deformity of the
upper two thirds of the tibia

BONE TUMORS

What is Ewing's sarcoma?

A malignant tumor from undifferentiated
mesenchymal bone cells

Individuals in what age range are affected?

Adolescents; mean age is 11 years

What percentage of all primary bone tumors are represented?

10%

In what bones is Ewing's sarcoma distributed?

These tumors occur most often in the
bone shaft—70% in the diaphysis of the
lower extremity, and 25% in the flat
bones (scapula, sacrum). At the time of
presentation, 30% of patients have
metastases to the lung, other bones, and
lymph nodes.

What are the symptoms of Ewing's sarcoma?

Pain, swelling, leukocytosis, increased
erythrocyte sedimentation rate (ESR),
and occasionally fever

What are 5 radiographic findings in Ewing's sarcoma?

1. "Moth-eaten" appearance
2. Distribution in the long bones and flat
   bones
3. Lytic lesions with poorly defined
   margins and permeative pattern
4. "Onion skin" periosteum (nonspecific
   but suggestive finding)
5. Large soft tissue component

Is CT helpful in Ewing's sarcoma?

Yes, because it shows the soft tissue
masses better than plain films

What treatment is appropriate in Ewing's sarcoma?

This type of sarcoma is very radio-
sensitive, so patients should be sent to a
radiation oncologist. Chemotherapy is
used as adjunct therapy.

What is osteosarcoma?

Tumor originating in bone, usually in the metaphysis of the long bones, especially around the knee

Among the pediatric population, who is most commonly affected by osteosarcoma?

Males between the ages of 10 and 25 years

What are the radiographic findings in osteosarcoma?

Lytic, sclerotic, aggressive, eccentric
Usually does not cross the growth plate
"Moth-eaten" appearance with "sunburst" periosteal reaction or a Codman's triangle
Possible pathologic fracture (at presentation)

What diagnostic modalities are most useful in osteosarcoma?

MRI and CT are used to determine precise anatomic location and soft tissue extension, and plain film accurately shows the extent of the tumor.

Osteosarcoma typically metastasizes to what organs?

The lungs, where metastases may ossify, calcify, or cavitate
Other bones

What other tumors must be considered in the differential diagnosis of malignant bone lesions?

Neuroblastoma metastases, lymphoma, and leukemia

CONGENITAL ABNORMALITIES OF BONE FORMATION AND GROWTH

When and how should skeletal maturity be assessed?

Prenatally, by sonography
Neonatally, by looking at ossification centers (ossified humeral heads indicates at least 37 weeks' gestation) and by obtaining radiographs of the hands, feet, and knees

What film is routinely obtained to assess skeletal maturity (bone age)?

AP radiograph of the left hand and wrist

How is skeletal maturity determined?

The epiphyseal ossification of the bones of the hand, especially the metacarpals, is compared with an atlas of normal controls for each age.

Is skeletal maturity related to sexual maturity?

Yes. Skeletal maturity is more closely related to sexual maturity than to height.

What sex is more advanced in skeletal maturity for a given chronologic age?

Girls. In general, black children are more advanced in skeletal maturity than white children.

On what factors does ultimate height depend?

Present height and skeletal maturity (i.e., both short children with delayed bone age and tall children with advanced bone age will probably reach normal height)
Height of parents

Name the causes of retarded skeletal maturity.

Endocrine causes
Hypothyroidism (most extreme)
Adrenal cortical insufficiency (Addison's disease)
Adrenal cortical hyperactivity (Cushing's syndrome)
Exogenous steroids
Hypogonadism
Panhypopituitarism
Hyperpituitarism
Growth hormone deficiency
Chromosomal causes
Trisomy 18
Trisomy 21
Turner's syndrome (XO)
Klinefelter's syndrome (XXY, XXXXY)
Other causes
Malnutrition
Chronic disease
CHD
Maternal deprivation
Constitutional delay

Name the causes of accelerated skeletal age.

Endocrine causes
Hyperthyroidism
Idiopathic sexual precocity
Premature thelarche
Premature adrenarche
Hypothalamic tumors
Pineal tumors
Hypergonadism
Adrenogenital syndrome
Congenital causes
Pseudohypothyroid
Fibrous dysplasia

Other causes
Obesity

Neonatal short-limbed dwarfism

How are skeletal dysplasias categorized?

Usually by relative shortening of the proximal versus the distal long bones (e.g., humerus versus radius or femur versus tibia)

Describe the following types of skeletal dysplasia.

Rhizomelia

Shortening of the **proximal** limb relative to the distal limb

Mesomelia

Shortening of the **middle** limb

Acromelia

Shortening of the **distal** limb relative to the proximal limb

Micromelia

Shortening of **both** the proximal and distal limbs

What are the rhizomelic dwarfic states (affecting the proximal extremities)?

Achondroplasia (most common skeletal dysplasia) and thanatophoric dwarfism (usually lethal)

What is achondroplasia?

This rhizomelic growth deformity results from abnormal bone formation by enchondral ossification at growth plates but normal membranous ossification of flat bones. It is an autosomal dominant disorder.

What are 5 imaging features of achondroplasia?

1. Rhizomelia
2. Diminutive skull base with decreased foramen magnum with normal-sized calvaria
3. Shortened spinal pedicles distally
4. Spinal stenosis
5. Rounded iliac wings with decreased acetabular angle ("ping-pong paddle" pelvis)

What are the mesomelic dwarfic states (affecting the middle leg and forearm)?

Mesomelic dwarfism and Cornelia de Lange's syndrome

What are the acromelic (affecting distal extremities) dwarfic states?

Asphyxiating thoracic dystrophy
Chondroectodermal dysplasia
Acrodysostosis

What is chondroectodermal dysplasia (Ellis-Van Creveld syndrome)?

A condition characterized by acromelic limb shortening and polydactyly that is associated with ASDs (about 50% of cases)

Osteogenesis imperfecta

What is osteogenesis imperfecta?

A group of hereditary disorders of type I procollagen synthesis characterized by extremely fragile bones, resulting in multiple fractures

What is the characteristic clinical sign in osteogenesis imperfecta?

Blue sclerae

What are the most common types of osteogenesis imperfecta?

Tarda (develops later; less severe)—
    Frequency of 1:30,000; autosomal
    dominant
Congenita (develops at or before birth;
    lethal)—Frequency of 1:60,000;
    autosomal recessive

What are 3 radiographic characteristics of osteo-genesis imperfecta?

Demineralization, deformity, and fracture

Congenital tibia vara

What is congenital tibia vara (Blount's disease)?

A growth deformity of the medial proximal tibia secondary to abnormal enchondral ossification from stress and compression, which results in the bowing of the tibia

What children are most likely to be affected by congenital tibia vara?

Obese black children

What are 2 forms of con-genital tibia vara?

1. Infantile form (1–3 years of age)
2. Juvenile form (6–13 years)

What are 2 radiographic findings of congenital tibia vara?

1. Irregularity of the proximal medial tibia
2. Varus deformity (tibiofemoral angle > 15°)

Mucopolysaccharidoses

What are the mucopolysac-charidoses?

The mucopolysaccharidoses are a group of lysosomal storage diseases characterized by the accumulation of excess mucopolysaccharides [glycosaminoglycans (GAGs)]. Skeletal deformities occur secondary to the accrual of GAGs in the chondrocytes, resulting in abnormal ossification. Examples include Hurler's syndrome, Hunter's syndrome, Morquio's syndrome, Sanfilippo's syndrome, Maroteaux-Lamy syndrome, and other forms, depending on the site of the enzymatic defect.

What are 8 radiologic features of the mucopolysac-charidoses?

1. Osteopenia
2. Vertebral body deformities (hook-shaped vertebra L1 in Hurler's and Hunter's syndromes; platyspondylia in Morquio's syndrome; posterior vertebral body scalloping)
3. Scoliosis
4. Lordosis
5. "Mickey Mouse" ear iliac bones (widening and flaring of iliac wings)
6. Shortened limbs
7. Femoral epiphyseal dysplasia
8. Short, stubby phalanxes

Cleidocranial dysostosis

What is cleidocranial dysostosis?

An ossification disorder that affects both enchondral and membranous bone formation

What are 4 radiologic features of cleidocranial dysostosis?

1. Anomalous clavicles (absent, partial, or unfused)
2. Multiple epiphysis
3. Wormian bones (wide, serpiginous sutures in the skull)
4. Deficient midline ossification (failed closure of the fontanelles, neural arches, and symphysis pubis; delayed ossification of the mandible, sternum, and vertebral bodies)

What is the differential diagnosis of wormian bones?

COPD
Cleidocranial dysostosis
Osteogenesis imperfecta

Pyknodysostosis
Down syndrome

Osteopetrosis

What is osteopetrosis (marble bone disease of Albers-Schönberg)?

A rare inherited disorder of osteoclast functioning (the autosomal recessive form is usually lethal; the autosomal dominant form more benign)

What are the radiographic findings in osteopetrosis?

Short, block-like, radiodense bone
Widening of the epiphysis and metaphysis of the long bones, especially the distal femur (**Erlenmeyer flask deformity**)
Multiple fractures
Alternating sclerotic, osteopenic-appearing metaphyseal lines

METABOLIC DISORDERS

RICKETS AND RELATED DISEASES

What causes rickets?

Insufficiency of vitamin D, which leads to failure of normal bone mineralization

At what age is the diagnosis or rickets typically made?

Usually by 3–6 months, and almost always by 2 years

What are 4 common causes of rickets?

1. Nutritional (insufficient vitamin D in diet)
2. Malabsorption
3. Renal disease
4. Increased requirement for vitamin D

Do clinical findings precede the radiologic findings?

No.

What are the radiographic findings in rickets?

Demineralization, widening of the physis, deformity, and flared anterior ribs

What is hypophosphatasia?

A heritable metabolic disease characterized by decreased alkaline phosphatase activity, resulting in excess urinary loss of phosphate

What are 3 radiographic features of hypophosphatasia?

1. Severe osteoporosis
2. Marked widening of the physeal plates
3. Pathologic fractures

Mild cases may be indistinguishable
from other forms of rickets.

IDIOPATHIC OR INFLAMMATORY DISEASE

Caffey's disease

What is Caffey's disease?
Infantile cortical hyperostosis of unknown
cause

What is the age of onset of Caffey's disease?
9 weeks

What bones are most often affected?
Mandible and ribs (most frequently);
clavicle and humerus; tibia (most severely
affected)

What is the radiographic appearance of Caffey's disease?
Cortical thickening (actually a thick
periosteal reaction)

What is the differential diagnosis for symmetric periosteal reaction?
SCALP
Scurvy or **S**yphilis
Caffey's disease
Hypervitaminosis **A** or non-**A**ccidental
trauma
Leukemia
Physiologic or **P**rostaglandins

Histiocytosis X

What is histiocytosis X?
A disease of unknown cause that affects
the pediatric population in several ways

Describe the various types of histiocytosis X:

Eosinophilic granuloma
"Punched out" lytic skull lesion, with a
beveled edge
Vertebra plana
Lytic bone lesions in other bones

Letterer-Siwe disease
Acute, diffuse, and often fatal
Rash, adenopathy, hepatosplenomegaly,
diffuse lung involvement

Hand-Schüller-Christian disease
Chronic and diffuse
Classic triad is skull defects,
exophthalmos, and diabetes insipidus

Eosinophilic granuloma

For what bony lesion is eosinophilic granuloma notorious?

Spinal involvement and vertebral body collapse (also known as vertebra plana)

In what conditions might "floating teeth" be seen?

Periapical abscess
Eosinophilic granuloma
Primary mandibular tumors
Neuroblastoma
Lymphoma
Leukemia

Juvenile rheumatoid arthritis (JRA)

What is juvenile rheumatoid arthritis (JRA)?

JRA is a form of rheumatoid arthritis with onset before age 16 years. Monoarticular onset is characteristic of 20% of affected individuals. Up to 70% of patients with JRA are seronegative.

What is Still's disease?

JRA associated with lymphadenopathy, splenomegaly, and fever

What are 5 radiologic characteristics of JRA?

1. Soft tissue swelling
2. Periostitis
3. Overgrowth of epiphysis secondary to hyperemia
4. Premature physeal closure with growth retardation
5. Ankylosis (fusion) of spine articulation (especially cervical)

CENTRAL NERVOUS SYSTEM (CNS) DISORDERS

See also Chapter 12,
"Cranial and Spinal Imaging"

NEONATAL INTRACRANIAL HEMORRHAGE

What are the 2 most common predisposing factors for intracranial hemorrhage (the most common cause of neonatal death)?

Prematurity and hypoxia

What are 5 clinical signs of intracranial hemorrhage?

1. Obtundation
2. Hypotonia

   3. Falling hematocrit
   4. Metabolic acidosis
   5. Bloody CSF

What study is most useful in the radiologic work-up of intracranial hemorrhage?

Ultrasound is excellent for making an initial diagnosis and for following up.

What images are routinely obtained on the ultrasound?

Sagittal, parasagittal (angled with lateral ventricle), and coronal images

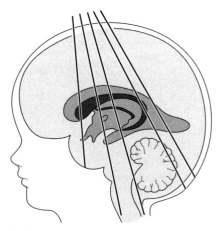

A. Planes of coronal sections

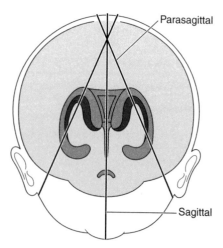

B. Planes of sagittal and parasagittal sections

What does hemorrhage look like on ultrasound?

Bright echoes in the brain or ventricles

What area in the brain is the most susceptible?

The subependymal germinal matrix just anterior to the caudothalamic groove

Select the letter that corresponds to the caudothalamic groove on this parasagittal section.

D

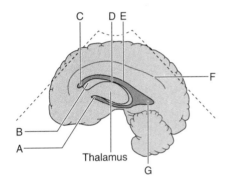

Thalamus

What are the grades of germinal matrix hemorrhage?

I: Hemorrhage confined to subependymal germinal matrix
II: Hemorrhage into nondilated ventricles
III: Hemorrhage into dilated ventricles
IV: Massive intraventricular and intracerebral hemorrhage

What is the prognosis associated with germinal matrix hemorrhage?

Grades I and II: Good
Grades III and IV: High frequency of death, neurologic morbidity, and hydrocephalus

HYDROCEPHALUS

What is the most common cause of an enlarged head before sutures close?

Hydrocephalus (i.e., enlargement of the ventricles)

What are the most common causes of hydrocephalus in neonates?

Aqueductal stenosis and Chiari malformation

What radiologic procedure is used to screen for increased hydrocephalus?	Ultrasound
What are 3 causes of unilateral ventricular obstruction?	Choroid plexus papilloma, meningioma, and intraventricular glioma

CONGENITAL DISORDERS

What are the 4 most common causes of a small skull?	Brain atrophy, craniosynostosis, poor brain growth, and shunt placement
What is the most common CNS anomaly?	Anencephaly
What is lissencephaly?	Absence of gyri, with a smooth cortical surface
What is pachygyria?	Broad, shallow gyri that are few in number
What is polymicrogyria?	Many tiny gyri
What are the phakomatoses?	A group of neurocutaneous disorders including neurofibromatosis, tuberous sclerosis, von Hippel-Lindau disease, Sturge-Weber syndrome, basal cell nevus syndrome, ataxia telangiectasia, and oculocutaneous melanosis
What is the most common neurocutaneous syndrome?	Neurofibromatosis (autosomal dominant), with type I disease (von Recklinghausen's disease) accounting for 90% of cases
What features are characteristic of type I neurofibromatosis?	Café-au-lait spots Plexiform neurofibromas Axillary or inguinal freckling (i.e., where the sun does not reach) Optic glioma Lisch nodules
What feature is diagnostic of type II NF?	Bilateral acoustic neuroma (diagnosed in adulthood)
What features are characteristics of Sturge-Weber syndrome?	Port-wine nevus (facial angioma) Mental retardation Seizures

Hemiparesis
Hemiatrophy
Cortical calcification

Describe the calcifications in Sturge-Weber syndrome.	Like a **tram track** that follows the convolutions of the cortex
What is the most common location of calcification in Sturge-Weber syndrome?	Parieto-occipital distribution

NEOPLASMS

What are the most common neoplasms of childhood?	Leukemia and CNS tumors

The age distribution of CNS tumors in children is tri-modal. What types of tumors are most common in:

Neonates?	Supratentorial tumors (astrocytomas, teratomas)
Young children (3–5 years)?	Infratentorial tumors (brain stem gliomas, cerebellar astrocytomas)
In older children (10–12 years)?	Supratentorial tumors
What is the most commonly used radiologic screening modality for CNS tumors?	CT (MRI is superior for posterior fossa imaging)
What are the 4 most common infratentorial neoplasms?	1. Juvenile pilocytic astrocytoma 2. Medulloblastoma 3. Ependymoma 4. Brain stem glioma
What are the common presenting symptoms of infratentorial masses?	Ataxia, headache, and increased ICP
Where do medulloblastomas arise?	Roof of the fourth ventricle (most commonly)
What is the radiographic appearance of medulloblastomas?	Hyperdense on unenhanced CT, with enhancement and a well-defined margin on enhanced CT

Where do ependymomas arise?

These heterogeneous, toothpaste-like lesions arise in the **ventricle** (where ependymal cells live). They fill the ventricle and may "squeeze out" through the foramina of Luschka or Magendie.

Where do juvenile pilocytic astrocytomas arise?

Cerebellar hemisphere (usually)

What is the appearance of a juvenile pilocytic astrocytoma?

A cyst with an enhancing mural nodule; some may be solid

What causes an enlarged sella turcica?

The most common causes are intrasellar tumor and parasellar tumor with extension into the sella. Other causes included increased ICP (the third ventricle bulges into sella), empty sella syndrome, Nelson's syndrome (pituitary gland hyperplasia after an adrenalectomy), and hypothyroidism.

What is the most common cause of a parasellar mass?

Craniopharyngiomas account for 50% of all parasellar masses and 10% of all intracranial neoplasms in children. To remember all of the causes of a parasellar mass, think "SATCHMO":
SATCHMO
Suprasellar germinoma
Adenoma (pituitary)
Tuberculosis (granulomatous disease)
Craniopharyngioma
Hypothalamic glioma
Meningioma
Oddball causes (e.g., epidermoid cyst, dermoid cyst, Rathke pouch cyst)

Where do craniopharyngiomas originate?

Rathke's pouch (they are remnants)

What treatment is appropriate for craniopharyngiomas?

Surgical removal

What is the most helpful modality for presurgical evaluation?

MRI

What do craniopharyngiomas look like?

Usually cystic with an unenhancing soft tissue nodule and calcification, although they can be solid

INFECTIOUS DISORDERS

What are common routes of entry for CNS infection in children?	Middle ear or paranasal sinus infection, which spreads to the adjacent epidural space Open skull fractures, which lead to abscess, empyemas (epidural or subdural) Hematogenous routes, which lead to spinal epidural abscess
What is the most common form of CNS infection?	Meningitis
What studies should be obtained in an unstable child who has suspected brain abscess?	Enhanced and unenhanced CT to look for intraparenchymal enhancing fluid collection

ORBITAL DISORDERS

What is the best way to evaluate the orbit radiologically?	CT or MRI
What symptoms are common in the presentation of intraocular lesions?	Leukocoria, periorbital inflammation, and strabismus
What are the causes of leukocoria?	The most common cause is retinoblastoma; other causes include congenital, inflammatory, and traumatic conditions.
List 11 masses of the orbit.	**Benign** 1. Dermoid cyst 2. Hemangioma 3. Inflammatory mass 4. Lymphangioma 5. Neurofibroma **Malignant** 6. Primary malignant tumor (i.e., retinoblastoma, rhabdomyosarcoma) 7. Metastatic malignant tumor (i.e., neuroblastoma) 8. Leukemia 9. Lymphoma 10. Optic nerve glioma 11. Sarcoma

What are the 2 most common benign orbital masses in children who are younger than 10 years (in order of frequency of occurrence)?	Capillary hemangioma, dermoid cyst
What is seen on CT of the orbit in capillary hemangioma?	Crescent-shaped mass within the lid, in the medial or lateral epicanthus, or retrobulbar area that exhibits well-defined homogenous enhancement after contrast administration
What is the most common malignant orbital mass?	Rhabdomyosarcoma (average age of diagnosis—7 years)
What features characterize the presentation of rhabdomyosarcoma?	Ptosis, swelling, redness, and unilateral exophthalmos
What is the best method for evaluation of rhabdomyosarcoma in the orbit?	CT
What is the most common location of rhabdomyosarcoma in the orbit?	Upper eyelid or medial epicanthal area
What is the most common malignant intraocular tumor?	Retinoblastoma
What is the most reliable sign of orbital abscess?	Presence of an air-fluid level within a mass
What is the most common cause of periorbital cellulitis?	Paranasal sinusitis

12

Cranial and Spinal Imaging

Erol Baskurt

ANATOMY

BRAIN ANATOMY

Identify the structures on the following computed tomography (CT) scans:

A = Frontal sinus
B = Orbit
C = Frontal lobe
D = Sphenoid sinus
E = Temporal lobe
F = External auditory canal
G = Mastoid air cells
H = Cerebellar tonsil
I = Foramen magnum

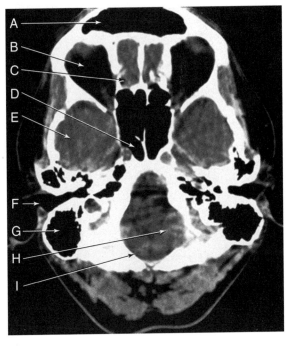

A = Frontal lobe
B = Sylvian fissure
C = Temporal lobe
D = Temporal horn of the lateral
    ventricle
E = Midbrain
F = Ambient cistern
G = Fourth ventricle
H = Cerebellar hemisphere

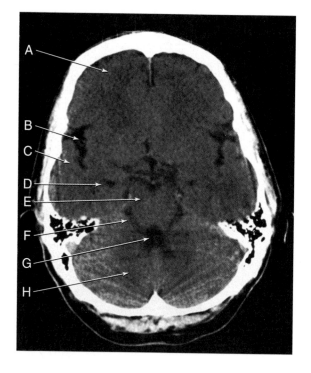

A = Falx
B = Frontal horn of the lateral ventricle
C = Caudate nucleus
D = Internal capsule (anterior limb)
E = Sylvian fissure
F = Basal ganglia
G = Third ventricle
H = Quadrigeminal plate cistern
I = Cerebellum

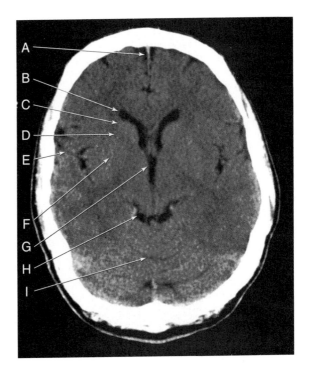

A = Interhemispheric fissure
B = Genu of the corpus callosum
C = Frontal horn of the lateral ventricle
D = Internal capsule
E = Thalamus
F = Pineal gland (calcified)
G = Cerebellar vermis
H = Straight sinus

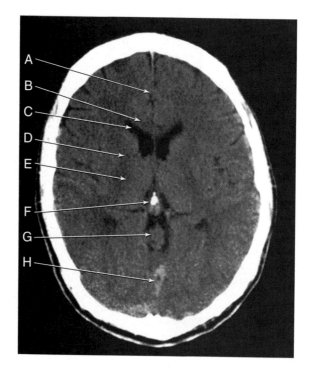

A = Falx cerebri
B = Frontal lobe
C = Parietal lobe
D = Body of the lateral ventricle
E = Occipital lobe

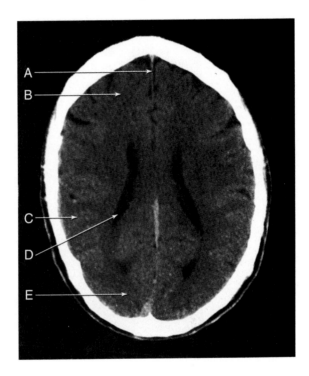

A = Falx cerebri
B = Sulcus
C = Gyrus
D = Central sulcus
E = Superior sagittal sinus

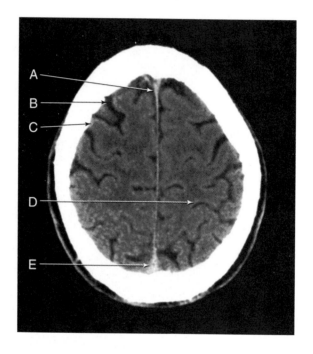

Identify the structures on the following axial magnetic resonance imaging (MRI) images:

A = Internal carotid artery
B = Medulla
C = Cerebellar hemisphere
D = Maxillary sinus
E = Sigmoid sinus
F = External auditory canal

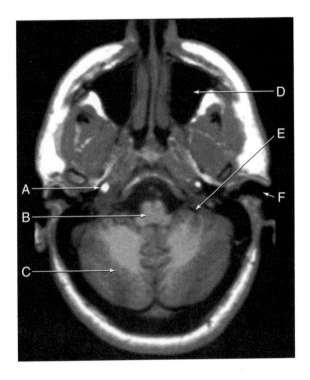

A = Sphenoid sinus
B = Internal carotid artery
C = Temporal lobe
D = Fourth ventricle
E = Basilar artery
F = Pons
G = Middle cerebellar peduncle
H = Cerebellum

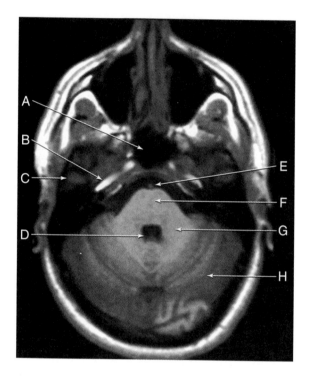

A = Orbit
B = Optic chiasm
C = Hippocampal formation
D = Cerebral peduncle
E = Tegmentum (midbrain)
F = Cerebral aqueduct
G = Tectum (midbrain)
H = Quadrigeminal cistern
I = Occipital lobe

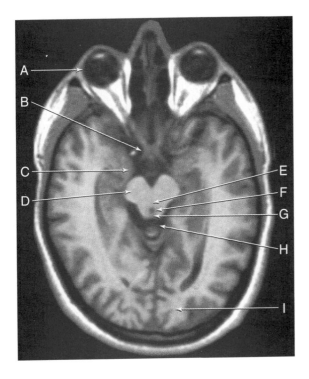

A = Caudate nucleus
B = Anterior limb of the internal capsule
C = Putamen
D = Fornix
E = Posterior limb of the internal
     capsule
F = Insula
G = Thalamus
H = Lateral ventricle (posterior horn)
I = Corpus callosum (splenium)

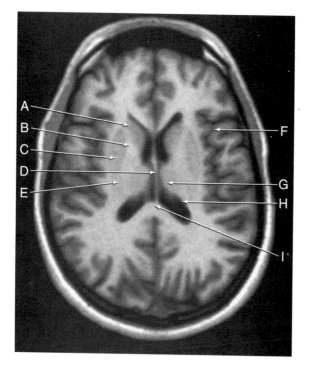

A = Lateral ventricle
B = Caudate nucleus
C = Septum pellucidum
D = Sylvian fissure
E = Corpus callosum (genu)
F = Gray matter
G = White matter

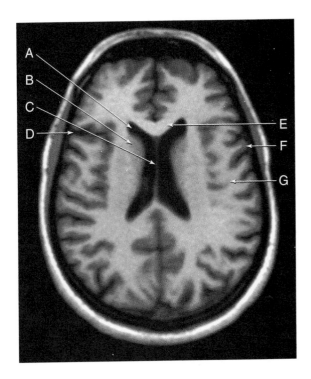

Identify the structures on the following coronal MRI images:

A = Intrahemispheric fissure
B = Corpus callosum
C = Lateral ventricle
D = Suprasellar cistern
E = Temporal lobe
F = Insular cortex
G = Sylvian fissure

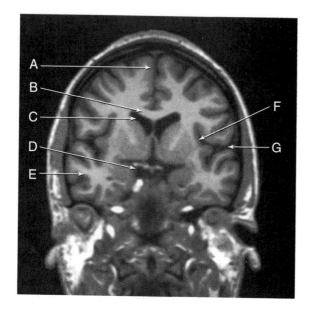

A = Superior sagittal sinus
B = Corpus callosum
C = Septum pellucidum
D = Lateral ventricle
E = Caudate nucleus
F = Internal capsule
G = Interventricular foramen of Monro
H = Third ventricle
I = Insular cortex

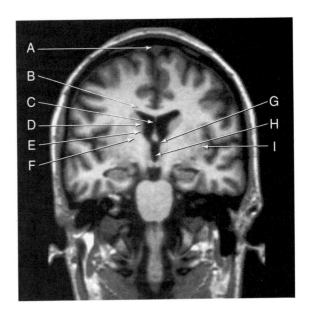

A = Corpus callosum (splenium)
B = Choroid plexus of the lateral ventricle
C = Hippocampal formation
D = Quadrigeminal cistern
E = Fourth ventricle
F = Cerebellar hemisphere
G = Tentorium cerebelli

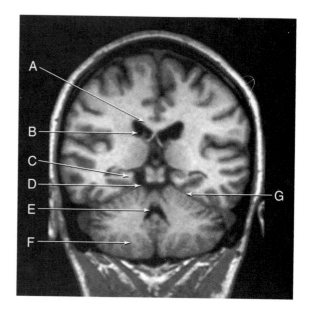

Identify the structures on the following sagittal MRI image:

A = Corpus callosum
B = Fornix
C = Thalamus
D = Optic chiasm
E = Pituitary gland
F = Pons
G = Dens (C2 vertebra)
H = Spinal cord
I = Pineal gland
J = Tectum (midbrain)
K = Cerebral aqueduct
L = Tegmentum (midbrain)
M = Fourth ventricle
N = Medulla

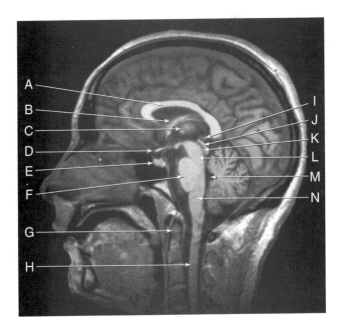

Identify the parts of the ventricular system on the following line drawing:

A = Frontal horn of the lateral ventricle
B = Body of the lateral ventricle
C = Occipital horn of lateral ventricle
D = Fourth ventricle
E = Foramen of Magendie (m = "middle")
F = Foramen of Luschka (l = "lateral")
G = Aqueduct of Sylvius

H = Temporal horn of the lateral
    ventricle
I = Third ventricle
J = Foramen of Monro

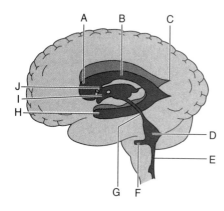

**Identify the branches of
the external carotid artery:**

A = Middle meningeal artery
B = Facial artery
C = Maxillary artery
D = Lingual artery
E = Superior thyroid artery
F = Ascending pharyngeal artery
G = Occipital artery
H = Posterior auricular artery
I = Superficial temporal artery

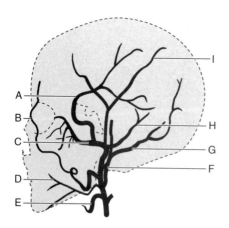

List the 3 parts of the extracranial internal carotid artery.

1. Cervical
2. Petrous
3. Cavernous

Name the branches of the intracranial internal carotid artery shown below:

A = Ophthalmic artery
B = Frontopolar artery
C = Callosomarginal artery
D = Anterior cerebral artery
E = Pericallosal artery
F = Temporal artery
G = Parietal artery
H = Anterior choroidal artery
I = Middle cerebral artery
J = Posterior communicating artery
K = Medial and lateral striates

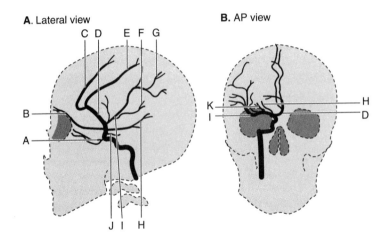

A. Lateral view

B. AP view

What constitutes the posterior circulation?

The flow supplied by the branches of the vertebral arteries.

Identify the branches of the vertebral artery:

A = Vertebral artery
B = Posterior inferior cerebellar artery
C = Basilar artery
D = Posterior communicating artery
E = Anterior inferior cerebellar artery
F = Superior cerebellar artery
G = Posterior cerebral artery

H = Muscular branches
I = Posterior parietal branches
J = Calcarine artery

A. Lateral view

B. AP view

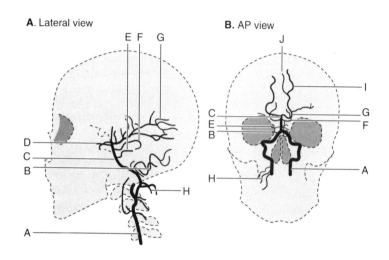

Identify the arteries in and around the circle of Willis on the following figure:

A = Basilar artery
B = Posterior cerebral artery
C = Thalamoperforators
D = Posterior communicating artery
E = Internal carotid artery
F = Middle cerebral artery
G = Anterior cerebral artery
H = Anterior communicating artery

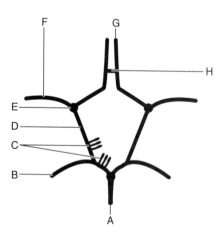

Which vessels supply the following brain territories?

A = Anterior cerebral artery
B = Middle cerebral artery
C = Posterior cerebral artery
D = Lenticulostriate arteries

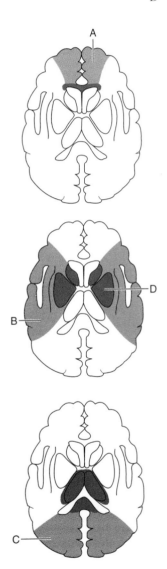

Identify the following structures comprising the venous drainage of the brain:

A = Basilar vein of Rosenthal
B = Septal vein
C = Thalamostriate vein
D = Superior sagittal sinus
E = Inferior sagittal sinus
F = Vein of Galen
G = Straight sinus
H = Torcula
I = Transverse sinus
J = Sigmoid sinus
K = Internal jugular vein

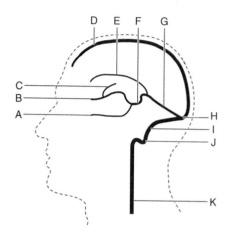

ORBIT ANATOMY

List the 3 major foramina of the orbit.

1. Optic canal
2. Superior orbital fissure
3. Inferior orbital fissure

What structures pass through each?

Canal: optic nerve; ophthalmic artery and vein
Superior orbital fissure: CN III, IV, V_1, and VI; superior ophthalmic vein
Inferior orbital fissure: CN V_2; infraorbital artery and vein; inferior ophthalmic vein

List the 3 anatomic compartments into which the orbit is partitioned by the rectus muscles.

1. Intraconal space
2. Conal space
3. Extraconal space
(Note: There is also a preseptal space that is part of the face and is separated from the postseptal space by the orbital septum.)

Name the 4 segments that radiologists divide the optic nerve into for clinical purposes.	1. Intraocular 2. Intraorbital 3. Intracanalicular 4. Intracranial

NECK ANATOMY

It is useful to divide the neck into 2 parts cephalad and caudal. At what structure are these parts separated?	The hyoid bone
What are these divisions called?	Suprahyoid neck and infrahyoid neck
What are the divisions of the pharynx?	Nasopharynx: Base of skull to soft palate Oropharynx: Soft palate to hyoid Hypopharynx: Hyoid bone to lower aspect of cricoid cartilage
What are the 3 major salivary glands?	Parotid, submandibular, sublingual
How are the parapharyngeal spaces divided?	Parotid space Masticator space Parapharyngeal space Pharyngeal mucosal space Carotid space Retropharyngeal space Prevertebral space
Name the 4 muscles of mastication.	1. Medial pterygoid 2. Lateral pterygoid 3. Masseter 4. Temporalis
These muscles constitute what anatomic space?	The masticator space
A lesion arising in this space would be expected to displace the parapharyngeal fat in which direction?	Posteromedially
The poststyloid parapharyngeal space is also known as what?	The carotid space

What 4 structures reside in this space?

1. Internal carotid artery
2. Internal jugular vein
3. Cranial nerves (IX, X, XI, XII)
4. Lymph nodes

What is present in the parapharyngeal space?

Internal maxillary artery
Ascending pharyngeal artery
Fat
Branches of CN V_3 branches
Pharyngeal venous plexus

Identify the following parts of the ostiomeatal complex (OMC) and its surroundings:

A = Cribriform plate
B = Infundibulum
C = Ethmoidal bulla
D = Maxillary sinus
E = Maxillary sinus ostium
F = Uncinate process
G = Middle turbinate
H = Middle meatus
I = Inferior turbinate
J = Nasal septum

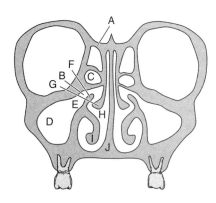

What are the 3 anatomic divisions of the larynx?

Supraglottis, glottis, and subglottis

The false vocal cords, arytenoids, epiglottis, and aryepiglottic folds are part of what level?

Supraglottis

The true vocal cords are part of what level?

Glottis

What junction or joint marks the level of the true vocal cords?

Cricoarytenoid joint

The complete ring visible just below the true cords is what?

The cricoid cartilage

Identify the following laryngeal structures:

A = Base of tongue
B = Pre-epiglottic fat
C = Hyoid bone
D = Laryngeal ventricle
E = Thyroid cartilage
F = True cord
G = Cricoid cartilage
H = Vallecula
I = Epiglottis
J = Aryepiglottic fold
K = False cord
L = Corniculate cartilage
M = Arytenoid cartilage
N = Cricothyroid ligament

A. Lateral view

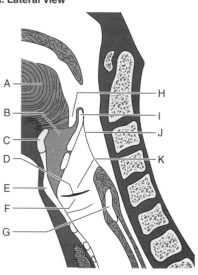

B. Anterior view   **C. Posterior view**

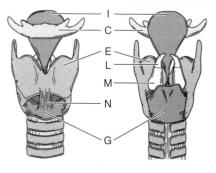

Identify the labeled structures on the following axial sections of the neck:

A = Nasal septum
B = Maxillary sinus
C = Medial pterygoid plate
D = Lateral pterygoid plate
E = Lateral pterygoid muscle
F = Nasopharynx
G = Torus tubarius
H = Eustachian tube

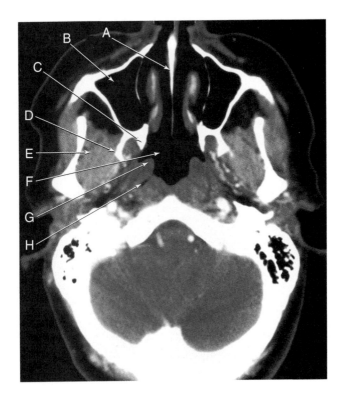

A = Maxilla
B = Masseter muscle
C = Ramus of the mandible
D = Parapharyngeal fat
E = Deep lobe of the parotid gland
F = Soft palate
G = Uvula
H = Oropharynx
I = Medial pterygoid muscle
J = Parotid gland

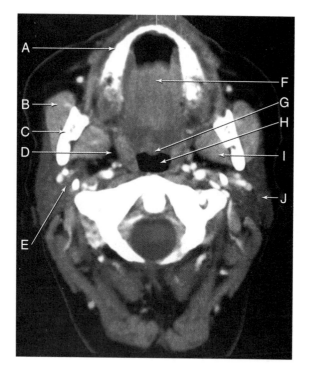

A = Mandible
B = Tongue
C = Submandibular gland
D = Parotid gland
E = Retromandibular vein
F = Oropharynx
G = Tonsil
H = Internal carotid artery
I = Internal jugular vein
J = Sternocleidomastoid muscle

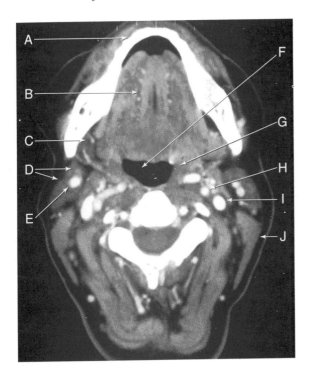

A = Mandible
B = Hyoid bone
C = Submandibular gland
D = Glossoepiglottic fold
E = Epiglottic tip
F = Common carotid artery
G = Internal jugular vein
H = Pre-epiglottic fat
I = Vallecula
J = External carotid artery
K = Internal carotid artery

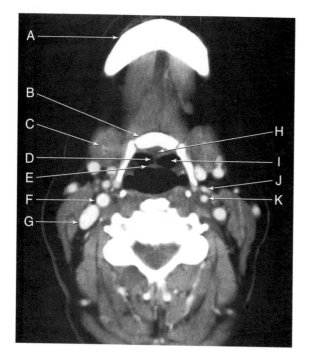

A = Pre-epiglottic fat
B = Strap muscles
C = Anterior jugular vein
D = Thyroid cartilage
E = Common carotid artery
F = Internal jugular vein
G = Aryepiglottic fold
H = Pyriform sinus
I = Sternocleidomastoid muscle

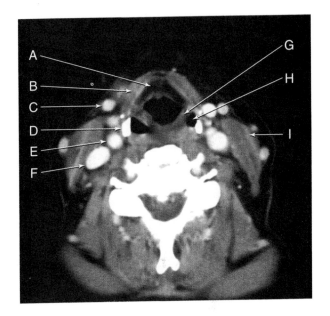

A = Anterior commissure
B = Anterior jugular vein
C = Cricoid cartilage
D = Common carotid artery
E = Internal jugular vein
F = True cords
G = Thyroid cartilage
H = External carotid artery
I = Sternocleidomastoid muscle

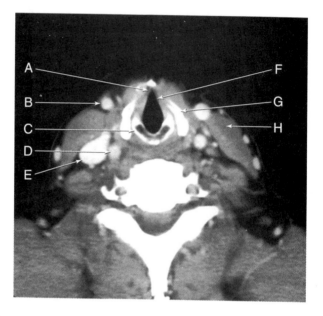

SPINAL ANATOMY (See Chapter 6, "Musculoskeletal Imaging")

IMAGING STUDIES

How is a head CT or MRI read?	Inside to outside or the reverse (be systematic)
What should you look for in each of the following areas?	
Ventricles and cisterns	Mass effect (symmetry is important; look for midline shift) Herniation (especially the effect on the quadrigeminal plate and suprasellar cisterns) Hydrocephalus Blood

Brain parenchyma	Hemorrhage Edema Contusion Masses Signs of stroke Enhancement
Periphery of the skull	Scalp contusions Skull fractures Extra-axial fluid collections (e.g., subdural or epidural hematoma)
What other areas need to be evaluated?	The sinuses, airway, globes, and scout image (i.e., the digital x-ray obtained for planning the study)
What characteristics are useful for determining if a lesion is intra-axial or extra-axial?	

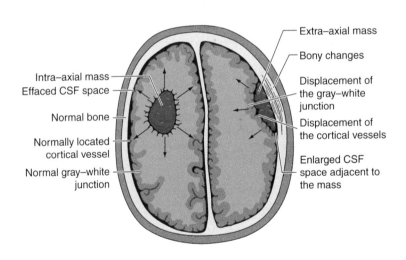

Intra–axial mass
Effaced CSF space
Normal bone
Normally located cortical vessel
Normal gray–white junction

Extra–axial mass
Bony changes
Displacement of the gray–white junction
Displacement of the cortical vessels
Enlarged CSF space adjacent to the mass

What are the imaging modalities of choice for evaluating the temporal bone?	CT and MRI
What tissue serves as a natural low-density "contrast" on CT?	Fat (the presence of a natural low-density "contrast" is especially useful in neck CT)

NEUROLOGIC DISORDERS

CEREBROVASCULAR DISORDERS

What is a stroke?
A clinical diagnosis of acute focal neurologic deficit

What is the imaging test of choice for a patient suspected of having had a stroke?
Noncontrast CT

Why is this done? (List 3 reasons)
To evaluate for hemorrhage, rule out stroke mimics, and find early signs of infarction

Cerebral infarct

What are the common changes seen on CT with acute infarct?
Loss of gray-white matter differentiation and swelling

What pathophysiologic process accounts for these changes?
Cytotoxic edema of the gray matter

How many days after an infarct does the edema increase to a maximum?
Approximately 3 days

How long after an infarct is cystic cavitation of brain tissue seen?
6–8 weeks

What is this cavitation called?
Encephalomalacia

What can be seen in a region of subacute ischemic infarct after the administration of intravenous contrast?
A ribbon of cortical gyral enhancement

If the infarct is accompanied by hemorrhage, how does the blood appear on noncontrast CT?
High CT density (i.e., blood is brighter than gray matter)

How does an acute infarct appear on:

    T_1-weighted MRI images?   Low-signal (edematous)

    T_2-weighted MRI images?   High-signal (edematous)

What is the most common cause of infarction?

Thromboembolic disease, usually as a result of atherosclerosis

What is the most common location for atherosclerosis in the carotid system?

At the bifurcation of the common carotid into the internal and external carotid arteries

What is the standard non-invasive screening test for detection of atherosclerosis at this location?

Duplex ultrasound scan

List 3 signs of significant stenosis on Doppler ultra-sound.

1. Increased flow velocity at stenosis
2. Turbulent flow
3. Luminal narrowing

What is the "gold standard" diagnostic procedure for carotid artery stenosis?

Carotid angiography

How can blood reach brain tissue distal to an occlusion?

Reconstitution of more distal small vessels; restoration of blood flow in a vessel distal to a lesion via inflow from collateral leptomeningeal vessels; circle of Willis

What is subclavian steal syndrome?

Symptoms from severe stenosis of the proximal subclavian artery with collateral blood flow developing through reversal of flow in the ipsilateral vertebral artery

Which condition is associated with a "string of beads" appearance of the cervical internal carotid artery on angiography?

Fibromuscular dysplasia (FMD)

What other condition can also mimic this appearance?

Arterial spasm

What is the usual cause of arterial spasm?

Stimulation of the vessel wall with a catheter or a wire

Intraparenchymal hemorrhage

What is the most common cause of intraparenchymal hemorrhage in adults?	Trauma
What is the most common underlying cause of spontaneous intraparenchymal hemorrhage in adults?	Hypertension
List 5 other causes of spontaneous intraparenchymal hemorrhage in adults.	1. Amyloidosis 2. Tumor 3. Coagulopathy 4. Venous infarct 5. Arteriovenous malformation (AVM)
List 4 sites where spontaneous intraparenchymal hemorrhages usually occur.	1. External capsule and basal ganglia 2. Thalamus 3. Pons 4. Cerebellum If there is hemorrhage at an atypical location, think of other causes.
What density is acute blood on CT?	Approximately 45 HU
How long does it take for an intracerebral hematoma to become less dense, matching the cerebrospinal fluid (CSF) in density?	2–3 months
On contrast CT, a ring of enhancement on a post-contrast image may become evident around a hemorrhage after what period of time?	7–10 days (subacute)
How long may this ring enhancement last?	3–4 months
List 9 other types of lesions associated with ring enhancement.	**MAGICAL DR** **M**etastasis **A**bscess **G**lioblastoma or high-grade glial neoplasm

m

Infarct
Contusion
AIDS (toxoplasmosis)
Lymphoma
Demyelination
Resolving hematoma

Characteristics of hemorrhage on MRI are complex and evolve with the age of the lesion. What signal intensity do acute, subacute, and chronic hemorrhages have on T_1- and T_2-weighted images?

Stage	Age of Lesion	Blood Component	T_1	T_2
Acute	1–7 days	Deoxyhemoglobin	– or ↓	↓↓
Subacute	1–4 weeks	Methemoglobin	↑↑	↑↑
Chronic	> weeks			
Center		Methemoglobin	↑	↑
Rim		Hemosidern	– or ↓	↓↓

Subarachnoid hemorrhage (SAH)

What are the 2 most common causes of SAH?

Trauma and rupture of a cerebral aneurysm

What are 5 other rare causes of SAH?

1. AVM (dural)
2. Neoplasm
3. Hypertension
4. Pituitary tumor hemorrhage (apoplexy)
5. Coagulopathy

What is the best imaging test when SAH is suspected?

Noncontrast head CT

What is seen?

High-density material (blood) in the basal cistern and cerebral sulci

What are the 5 most common locations of a congenital (berry) aneurysm?

1. Anterior communicating artery
2. Posterior communicating artery
3. Middle cerebral artery
4. Posterior inferior cerebellar artery
5. Basilar tip

Cerebral aneurysm

What imaging test is the "gold standard" for identifying cerebral aneurysms?	Angiography
What are the treatment options?	Endovascular occlusion of the aneurysm, surgical clipping, or proximal vessel occlusion
List 4 major causes of morbidity and mortality in aneurysm patients.	1. Rerupture 2. Hydrocephalus (1–2 weeks) 3. Vasospasm and infarction (1 week) 4. Herniation

Arteriovenous malformation (AVM)

What are the 2 most common clinical presentations of AVM?	Seizures and intraparenchymal hemorrhage
What does an AVM look like on noncontrast CT?	It may be difficult to see, but there can be a poorly defined area of mixed high- and low-density, often with occasional calcifications; little mass effect is seen.
What change is often seen in the brain parenchyma located near an AVM?	Atrophy
What is seen on MRI of an AVM?	Multiple low-signal flow voids with occasional hemorrhagic products
List 3 appropriate imaging tests for identifying an AVM.	Contrast-enhanced CT, MRI, angiography
What does an AVM look like on an angiogram?	Large artery (feeding), tangle of abnormal vessels (nidus), early draining vein (arteriovenous shunting)

Cerebral venous thrombosis

List 4 common causes of cerebral venous thrombosis.	Infection, trauma, hypercoagulable states (e.g., dehydration, pregnancy), congestive heart failure (CHF)
What is the delta sign?	The delta sign is a filling defect (i.e., absence of enhancement) in a dural venous sinus, which is seen on enhanced

CT and associated with thrombosis. This is not a sensitive sign, but it is specific.

What are diagnostic tests for venous thrombosis?

Contrast-enhanced CT
Magnetic resonance venography (MRV)
Angiography

BRAIN TUMORS

What is the imaging test of choice for evaluation of brain tumors?

MRI

Why do many tumors enhance?

There is no blood-brain barrier present within a high-grade glial tumor or metastasis, so intravascular contrast leaks into the extracellular space.

What are the typical signal characteristics of tumor on:

Noncontrast T_1-weighted MRI?

Low signal intensity

On T_2?

High signal intensity

What physiologic property of neoplastic brain tissue accounts for these signal characteristics?

Increased water content

Glial tumors

What percentage of newly diagnosed brain tumors in adults are of glial origin?

40%

What are the two most common types of glial tumors (i.e., gliomas)?

Glioblastoma multiforme (GBM) and astrocytoma

Name 2 other types of glial tumors.

Oligodendroglioma and ependymoma

In the adult, where do astrocytomas usually occur?

In the white matter of the cerebral hemispheres

How does a GBM appear on a post-contrast MRI?

As a thick, irregular, ring-enhancing lesion

Metastatic brain tumors

What percentage of newly discovered brain tumors in adults are metastatic?

35%

What 2 types of tumors account for 80% of metastatic brain lesions?

Lung and breast

Where are metastatic brain tumors usually located?

Along the gray-white junction

What will be seen on contrast-enhanced CT or MRI?

Multiple enhancing lesions

What 4 other lesions are in the differential diagnosis of multiple enhancing lesions?

Lymphoma, disseminated infection (septic emboli), multifocal infarction, and multiple sclerosis

Which brain metastases tend to present with intracranial hemorrhage?

MR CT
Melanoma
Renal cell carcinoma
Choriocarcinoma
Thyroid carcinoma

m

A cerebral metastasis is solitary in what percentage of cases?

As many as 50%

What is the treatment for a solitary metastasis?

Surgical excision

Meningioma

What is the most common extra-axial tumor?

Meningioma

What percentage of brain tumors are of mesodermal origin (e.g., meningioma)?

15%

What percentage of meningiomas are benign?

95%

What does a meningioma look like on:

    Noncontrast CT?

A homogeneous mass that has slightly higher attenuation (i.e., density) than

normal brain tissue, with or without
calcifications

On post-contrast CT?   A uniformly enhancing mass

What is a characteristic   Hyperostosis (i.e., thickening of skull)
change in the bone adjacent
to a meningioma?

What does a meningioma
look like on:

   T$_1$-weighted MRI?   A well-defined mass that is isointense to
the brain tissue in an extra-axial (i.e.,
extracerebral but intracranial) location

   Post-contrast T$_1$-weighted   Uniformly enhancing with resulting very
   MRI?   high signal

Pineal region tumors

List 7 diagnoses in the dif-   1. Germ cell tumor
ferential diagnosis of a   2. Pinealocytoma
pineal region tumor.   3. Pinealoblastoma
                                       4. Tectal glioma
                                       5. Meningioma
                                       6. Metastasis
                                       7. Aneurysm of the vein of Galen

What are the post-contrast   Isointense to brain tissue with uniform
characteristics of germ cell   enhancement
tumors on T$_1$-weighted and
T$_2$-weighted MRI?

What does a teratoma look   Heterogeneous mass with areas of
like on MRI?   calcification, fat, and cystic change

Pituitary tumors

Pituitary tumors account   5%
for what percentage of
cranial tumors?

List 10 diagnoses in the   1. Pituitary adenoma
differential diagnosis of a   2. Craniopharyngioma
sellar or parasellar mass.   3. Meningioma
                                       4. Metastasis
                                       5. Epidermoid
                                       6. Abscess

7. Aneurysm
8. Pituitary bleed
9. Pituitary sarcoid
10. Rathke cleft cyst

What is the most common tumor of the sella?

Pituitary adenoma

What is the preferred imaging modality for evaluation of this region?

MRI

What is an "empty" sella?

A defect in the diaphragma sella that allows CSF pulsations to flatten the pituitary gland, fill the sella with CSF, and often enlarge it. This is almost invariably of no clinical significance.

What is an epidermoid?

A congenital cyst lined with squamous epithelium

Cerebellar tumors

List 8 diagnoses in the differential diagnosis of a posterior fossa mass in an adult.

1. Metastasis
2. Hemangioblastoma
3. Astrocytoma
4. Medulloblastoma
5. Lymphoma
6. Extra-axial collection
7. Abscess
8. Infarct

Which of these diagnoses is most common?

Metastasis

What is the most common primary cerebellar tumor in adults?

Hemangioblastoma

What is the peak age of occurrence?

30 years

Ten percent of these tumors occur as part of what syndrome?

von Hippel-Lindau syndrome

List 7 disorders associated with von Hippel-Lindau

1. Renal cell cancer, renal cysts
2. Islet cell tumors

syndrome in addition to hemangioblastomas.

3. Pheochromocytomas
4. Pancreatic cystadenoma
5. Epididymal cysts
6. Liver cysts
7. Retinal angioma

What do hemangioblastomas look like on CT?

A cystic mass with an enhancing mural nodule

On MRI, what are characteristically seen in the mural nodular portions of these tumors?

Serpiginous low-signal intensity flow voids

What is the most common location for an extra-axial posterior fossa tumor in an adult?

Cerebellopontine angle

What 4 tumors account for nearly 95% of these lesions?

AMEN
Acoustic schwannoma
Meningioma
Epidermoid
Nonacoustic schwannoma

m

Acoustic schwannoma

What is an acoustic schwannoma?

A misnomer. The lesion is actually a schwannoma of the vestibular nerve.

Schwannomas of cranial nerves account for what percentage of primary intracranial tumors?

Approximately 3%

What is the most common cranial nerve involved?

CN VIII

Vestibular schwannomas usually arise from which branch of the vestibulocochlear nerve (CN VIII)?

The vestibular branch, superior division

This type of tumor in an adolescent could indicate what syndrome?

Neurofibromatosis type II (central)
    Multi-inherited schwannoma meningioma ependymoma (MISME) syndrome

What is the other type of neurofibromatosis and its characteristics?

Neurofibromatosis type I (Von Recklinghausen disease)
Characteristics include dermatologic

manifestations (café-au-lait spots) and neurofibromas of the peripheral nerves that tend toward malignancy

What is the imaging test of choice for acoustic schwannomas?

MRI with gadolinium enhancement

What is the signal characteristic of this tumor on enhanced T$_1$-weighted images?

Very high

What is the anatomic key for differentiating a schwannoma from a meningioma in this region with imaging?

The schwannoma arises in and enlarges the internal auditory canal. The meningioma usually does not.

What is Meckel's cave?

An invagination of dura posterolateral to the sella

What is in it?

The trigeminal nerve ganglion

Why is this important?

A schwannoma can arise here

Posterior fossa tumors

List 4 differential diagnoses of a posterior fossa mass in a child.

GAME
Glioma (brain stem)
Astrocytoma (juvenile pilocytic)
Medulloblastoma
Ependymoma

m

What does juvenile pilocytic astrocytoma look like on MRI?

Cyst (low intensity on T$_1$-weighted images and high intensity on T$_2$-weighted images) with mural nodule in cerebellar hemisphere

Where are juvenile pilocytic astrocytomas usually located?

In the hemisphere of the cerebellum

Do these tumors enhance?

Yes, the solid portions do but the cystic portions do not.

Are medulloblastomas aggressive, and do they exhibit rapid growth?	Yes.
What do they look like on MRI?	A midline mass in the area of the fourth ventricle
Do these tumors enhance?	Yes.
Where are ependymomas typically located?	Floor of the fourth ventricle
What is the classic appearance of an ependymoma on MRI?	"Toothpaste" squeezing through the fourth ventricle and out the foramina of Magendie and Luschka
Are these tumors aggressive (i.e., rapidly growing)?	Yes.
List 3 other tumors that occur within the ventricles.	Colloid cyst (third ventricle), choroid plexus papilloma (fourth ventricle), meningioma
Are brain stem gliomas highly malignant?	Yes.
In what part of the brain stem are these tumors most often found?	Pons
What is the appearance on CT or MRI?	An enlarged pons with occasional abnormal enhancement

CONGENITAL MALFORMATIONS AND PHAKOMATOSES

Name the 2 most common congenital malformations found in the nervous system.	Arnold-Chiari and Dandy-Walker deformities
List 4 possible components of the congenital Arnold-Chiari type I deformity.	1. Downward displacement of the cerebellar tonsils through the foramen magnum 2. Small fourth ventricle

3. Syringomyelia
4. Fusion of vertebra C1 with the cranium

List 11 possible components of Arnold-Chiari type II deformity.

1. Inferiorly displaced tentori
2. Small posterior fossa
3. Large foramen magnum
4. Myelomeningocele
5. Agenesis of the corpus callosum
6. Stenogyria (small but normal gyri)
7. Inferiorly displaced brain stem
8. Elongated and kinked medulla
9. Elongated fourth ventricle
10. Vermian peg (cerebellum displaced inferiorly)
11. Beaked tectum (brain stem)

List 6 possible components of the Dandy-Walker syndrome.

1. Enlarged fourth ventricle
2. Agenesis of the inferior vermis
3. Varying degrees of hypoplastic cerebellar hemispheres
4. Enlarged posterior fossa
5. High confluence of the dural sinuses (i.e., torcular inversion)
6. Absent falx cerebelli

What are the 5 most common phakomatoses?

1. Von Hippel-Lindau disease
2. Tuberous sclerosis
3. Neurofibromatosis
4. Sturge-Weber syndrome
5. Ataxia-telangiectasia

What tumor is associated with tuberous sclerosis?

Subependymal giant cell astrocytoma

List the 4 other characteristics of tuberous sclerosis.

1. Adenoma sebaceum (reddish brown facial papules)
2. Multiple hamartomas
3. Renal angiomyolipomas and cysts
4. Tubers (i.e., lesions with high T_2 signal in the cerebral hemisphere and calcified lesions along the ventricles)

Encephalofacial angiomatosis is also known as what?

Sturge-Weber syndrome

List 5 components of Sturge-Weber syndrome.

1. Vascular facial nevus
2. Vascular malformation involving the meninges

3. Calcification along the cerebral gyri
4. Cerebral atrophy
5. Glaucoma

HEAD TRAUMA

What is the preferred study for trauma patients in the acute setting?	Noncontrast head CT
How is this better than skull films?	CT shows traumatic effects to the brain and intracerebral fluid collections. It also assesses the need for treatment of increased intracerebral pressure. It is not as good for diagnosing skull fracture as skull films, but better at all the rest.
List 4 common post-traumatic CNS lesions.	SAH, cerebral contusion, shear injury, extra-axial hemorrhage
What are the 2 most common locations for contusion?	The inferior frontal lobe and the anterior-inferior temporal lobe
What does a contusion look like on CT?	Low density (edema) with irregular areas of high density (hemorrhage)
What is shear?	Shear is disruption of axons from the cell body caused by acceleration or deceleration forces. It is usually a devastating injury, and often occurs at the gray-white junction.
What is most commonly seen on CT with this type of injury?	Edema and occasionally, small intraparenchymal hemorrhage are seen on CT. The examination may appear normal. MRI is a better examination but is not feasible in the acute setting.
What percentage of axonal injury is associated with hemorrhages on CT?	20%

Subdural hematoma

What is the radiographic appearance of a subdural hematoma?	A crescent-shaped extra-axial fluid collection in a patient with a history of trauma

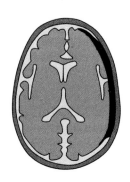

List the 3 groups into which subdural hematomas are classified, according to length of time since the injury.	1. Acute (1–7 days) 2. Subacute (7–21 days) 3. Chronic (> 21 days)
Describe the appearances of each on:	
CT	Acute = dense; subacute = isodense; chronic = hypodense
T$_1$-weighted MRI	Acute = isointense; subacute = hyperintense; chronic = hypointense
T$_2$-weighted MRI	Acute = hypointense; subacute = hyperintense; chronic = isointense
A collection of CSF in the subdural space is known as what?	Subdural hygroma or effusion
These lesions can look just like what on a CT scan?	A chronic subdural hematoma

Epidural hematoma

What is the radiographic appearance of an epidural hematoma?	A biconcave (lenticular) extra-axial fluid collection in a trauma patient

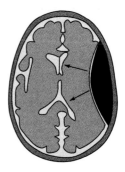

How is an epidural lesion treated?

With immediate surgical evacuation if the lesion is large or the patient exhibits progressive neurologic dysfunction

Cerebral herniation

Cerebral herniation can be a complication of what?

Extra-axial hemorrhage or any space-occupying intracerebral mass

Names 2 types of herniations seen on brain imaging.

1. Subfalcine
2. Transtentorial

What are the 2 types of transtentorial herniations?

Uncal (downward) and vermian (upward)

Which type of herniation is associated with:

Midline shift and distortion of the frontal horns of the lateral ventricles?

Subfalcine

Obliteration of the quadrigeminal plate cisterns with hydrocephalus via compression of the cerebral aqueduct?

Transtentorial

Skull fracture

Which is the more common lesion associated with a fracture—subdural or epidural hematoma?

Epidural hematoma

What are secondary signs of skull fracture on CT?	Fluid in the mastoid sinuses and intra-cranial air (from the sinus)
Skull fractures can result in air entering the CNS. What is this called?	Pneumocephalus
The key to determining a case of child abuse is noting injuries of differing ages. List 4 common CT findings in cases of child abuse.	1. SAH 2. Subdural hematoma (often located in the interhemispheric fissure) 3. Diffuse cerebral edema (secondary to anoxia or ischemia) 4. Skull fractures

INFLAMMATORY AND INFECTIOUS LESIONS

What is the most common form of CNS infection?	Meningitis

Meningitis

Noncontrast CNS imaging during the acute phase of meningitis usually shows what?	The examination may be completely normal.
Post-contrast CT may show what?	Leptomeningeal enhancement
List 9 differential diagnoses of gyriform enhancement.	1. AVM 2. Infarct 3. Cerebritis 4. Encephalitis 5. Cortical vein thrombosis 6. Meningeal carcinomatosis 7. Meningitis 8. Lymphoma 9. Sturge-Weber syndrome
What structures should be studied to evaluate for a possible underlying cause of meningitis?	The ethmoid, frontal, sphenoid, and mastoid sinuses
List 3 possible complications of meningitis.	Hydrocephalus, abscess, infarction

Brain abscess

What does a brain abscess look like on contrast CT?

A ring-enhancing lesion

A uniform ring that is slightly thinner on the medial side suggests what type of lesion?

Abscess

A thick, irregular ring suggests what?

Brain tumor

HIV infection

What is the most common finding in patients with HIV?

Generalized brain atrophy

This finding is usually caused by what condition?

HIV encephalitis

What are 3 other common CNS disorders in HIV-infected patients?

Lymphoma, toxoplasmosis, and progressive multifocal leukoencephalopathy

What is the most common CNS neoplastic disease in patients with HIV?

Non-Hodgkin's lymphoma

What is seen on MRI in HIV-positive patients with CNS lymphoma?

Variable high-signal abnormalities in the white matter on T_2-weighted images or ring-enhancing lesions

What is the most common CNS infection in patients with HIV?

Toxoplasmosis

What is the MRI appearance of toxoplasmosis?

Multiple or single ring-enhancing lesions

White matter lesions in the occipital region in an immunodeficient individual might be what?

Progressive multifocal leukoencephalopathy

Viral encephalitis

What is the most common viral encephalitis?

Herpes encephalitis

Who is at risk for herpes encephalitis?	Herpes encephalitis may be seen in otherwise healthy patients, but immunocompromised patients are at higher risk.
What is the typical MRI appearance of herpes encephalitis?	Abnormal signal on T_1- and T_2-weighted images in the frontal and temporal lobes with gyriform enhancement and occasional evidence of hemorrhage

Parasitic infections

What common parasites involve the CNS?	*Taenia solium* (cysticercosis) *Toxoplasma gondii* (toxoplasmosis) *Echinococcus multilocularis* (hydatidosis)
Which one is associated with spherical cystic lesions?	Cysticercosis
Which is associated with a large unilocular cystic lesion?	Hydatidosis

WHITE MATTER DISEASE

What is the most common demyelinating disease?	Multiple sclerosis
What is the most common location for lesions associated with this disease?	Periventricular white matter
What is the best imaging test?	MRI. T_2-weighted, fluid-attenuated inversion recovery (FLAIR) images are excellent.
What is seen on this sequence?	Multiple periventricular high-signal abnormalities perpendicular to the ventricles
High-signal T_2 abnormalities in the brain stem of a patient with a metabolic derangement might be what?	(Central pontine) osmotic myelinolysis

GENERALIZED DEGENERATIVE DISEASE

What is the major finding on neuroimaging in a patient with Alzheimer's disease?	Generalized brain atrophy, often involving the temporal lobes

What is the most common cause of cerebellar atrophy?	Alcoholism
What parts of the cerebellum are most commonly affected?	The anterior and superior vermis

MESIAL TEMPORAL SCLEROSIS

Mesial temporal sclerosis (gliosis of the hippocampus and parahippocampus) is often implicated in what type of disorders?	Complex seizure disorders
What is seen on MRI with this condition?	Abnormal high signal in the hippocampus on T_2-weighted images with accompanying volume loss

HYDROCEPHALUS

What are the 2 major categories of hydrocephalus?	Communicating and noncommunicating
List 4 common causes of communicating hydrocephalus.	Infection, postsubarachnoid hemorrhage, dural vein thrombosis, normal pressure hydrocephalus (uncommon)
List 3 common causes of noncommunicating hydrocephalus.	Aqueductal stenosis, masses (e.g., colloid cyst, meningioma), congenital abnormality
What tumor can make CSF, causing hydrocephalus by way of overproduction?	Choroid plexus papilloma
Hydrocephalus can be mimicked in appearance on neuroimaging in cases of generalized brain atrophy. What is this called?	Hydrocephalus ex vacuo
What is the major finding on neuroimaging in normal pressure hydrocephalus?	Ventricular enlargement (especially in the temporal horns of the lateral ventricles) out of proportion to cerebral volume loss; can also be normal

SPINAL DISORDERS

What are 2 major causes of back pain?	Disk herniation and spinal stenosis
What age-related change is seen in the intervertebral disk on T_2-weighted MRI?	Loss of signal intensity in the central portion of the disk owing to diminished water content and cartilage metaplasia

Intervertebral disk herniation

What are the two major components of an intervertebral disk?	The nucleus pulposus and annulus fibrosis
What is a Schmorl's node?	Herniation of the nucleus pulposus into an adjacent vertebral body
What are the 3 grades of disk abnormality?	Bulge, protrusion, extrusion
Does a bulge commonly compress nerve roots?	No.
What is a protrusion?	Incomplete, focal herniation of the nucleus through the annulus
What is an extrusion (herniation)?	Complete passage of the nuclear contents through the annulus
In what 2 parts of the spine do symptomatic herniations most commonly occur?	The lumbar spine (L4–L5 herniations are most common) and the cervical spine
What are the options for evaluation of these patients?	Plain CT, myelography and postmyelogram CT (invasive), and MRI
How does the sensitivity and specificity of MRI in the detection of disk herniation compare to that of CT myelography?	About the same
What are the 2 basic steps of myelography?	1. Introduction of contrast into the thecal sac through a needle 2. Acquisition of plain films, postcontrast CT

What does a herniation look like on myelography?
Deviation of the thecal sac away from the disk space with compression of the adjacent nerve roots

What does a herniation look like on CT?
Abnormal density in the extradural space at a disk level representing disk material with displacement of nerve roots

In what direction do disks usually herniate?
Posterolaterally

Lateral disk herniations can compromise the intervertebral neural foramina. What is the best imaging test for this?
MRI

Why?
MRI has multiplanar capabilities.

What is the term for persistent or recurrent symptoms following surgery for back pain?
Failed back syndrome (FBS)

In postoperative patients with FBS, the radiologist must commonly differentiate what two conditions?
Postoperative scar and recurrent disk herniation

Mass effect in the spinal canal suggests which diagnosis?
Herniation

Enhancement on post-contrast CT or MRI suggests which diagnosis?
Scar

The formation of adhesions within the arachnoid layer of dura (most often seen postoperatively) is known as what?
Arachnoiditis

What is seen on imaging with this condition?
Clumping of nerve roots

Spinal stenosis

What is spondylosis?	Spinal osteophyte formation caused by disk degeneration
What are 4 common findings of spinal degenerative disease seen on plain film?	Disk space narrowing, osteophyte formation, sclerosis, vacuum disk phenomenon
What are the 2 most common types of spinal stenosis?	Developmental and acquired (caused by facet joint disease or disk degeneration)
Which 3 spaces must a radiologist evaluate for adequacy in the setting of spinal degenerative disease?	Spinal canal, lateral recesses, intervertebral foramina
Narrowing of the lateral recesses or intervertebral foramina is known as what?	Lateral canal stenosis
What happens to the epidural fat that is normally present in these spaces in cases of stenosis?	It is obliterated or displaced.
Narrowing of the spinal canal is known as what?	Central stenosis
Anterior displacement of a superior vertebra in relation to the one below it is known as what?	Spondylolisthesis
At what level does congenital spondylolisthesis usually occur?	L5–S1
What is seen on axial CT or MRI with this condition?	Degeneration of L5–S1 facets or disruption (usually bilateral) at the level of the pars interarticularis; **must look for complete ring at each level**
What effect does this slippage have on the size of the L5 intervertebral foramen?	Decreases size

At what level does degenerative spondylolisthesis usually occur?	L4–L5
What is seen on axial CT or MRI?	Facet arthropathy and slippage without disruption of the pedicles

Spinal trauma (see Chapter 6, "Musculoskeletal Imaging")

Spinal tumors

What are the 2 most common tumor types in the vertebral column in the adult?	Metastatic tumors and myeloma
Tumors of the spine are divided into 4 categories according to anatomic location. List them.	Vertebral, extradural, intradural (extramedullary), spinal cord (intramedullary)
What type of tumor would produce each one of the following patterns?	A = Intradural extramedullary B = Extradural C = Intramedullary

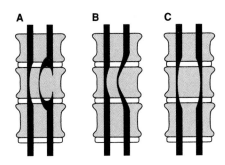

Displacement of the spinal cord away from the margins of the dural tube indicates that the lesion is in what location?	Intradural (extramedullary)
Enlargement of the spinal cord suggests what type of lesion?	Intramedullary

Vertebral tumors

Which portion of a vertebra do metastatic tumors most commonly involve?

The pedicle

What structural complication can occur in a vertebra that is involved with tumor?

Collapse

Patients with spinal tumors who were treated with radiation can be expected to have what change in their vertebral bodies on T_1-weighted MRI at follow-up?

Increased signal (caused by obliteration of the tumor and normal marrow with subsequent fatty change)

A purely osteolytic lesion in the vertebral body of a 50- to 70-year-old is most likely what tumor?

Myeloma

List 4 other primary bone tumors that occur in the vertebral column.

COAG
Chordoma (clivus, C2, sacrum)
Osteoblastoma
Aneurysmal bone cyst
Giant cell tumor

m

What is the cellular origin of chordoma?

Fetal notochord

Extradural tumors

List 8 differential diagnoses of an extradural lesion.

1. Herniated disc (most common)
2. Metastasis
3. Lymphoma
4. Meningioma
5. Nerve sheath tumor (e.g., schwannoma, neurofibroma)
6. Dermoid or epidermoid tumor
7. Lipoma
8. Epidural abscess

Multiple schwannomas can occur with what syndrome?

Neurofibromatosis type II

Can these lesions extend beyond the dura and through the intervertebral foramina?

Yes.

Extension of the lesion through the foramen is called what?	"Dumbbell" lesion
What are the signal characteristics of schwannomas on MRI?	Isointense to hypointense to the spinal cord on T_1-weighted images, hyperintense on T_2-weighted images

Intradural tumors

List 5 differential diagnoses of an intradural extramedullary lesion.	1. Meningioma 2. Nerve sheath tumor (e.g., neurofibroma, schwannoma) 3. Drop metastasis (i.e., from the brain) 4. Dermoid or epidermoid tumor 5. Lipoma
What is the most common spinal region for a meningioma?	Thoracic region
Are bone changes rarely associated with spinal meningioma?	Yes.
What are the signal characteristics of meningioma on MRI?	Isointense to the spinal cord on T_1- and T_2-weighted images with enhancement
List 4 types of intracranial tumors associated with "drop metastasis" to an intradural location.	1. Medulloblastoma 2. Ependymoma 3. Pineal dysgerminoma 4. Glioblastoma multiforme
What is the best imaging test for evaluating intradural metastasis?	MRI with contrast

Intramedullary tumors

List 12 differential diagnoses of an intramedullary lesion.	1. Ependymoma 2. Astrocytoma 3. Hemangioblastoma 4. Lipoma 5. Dermoid or epidermoid tumor 6. Hemangioblastoma 7. Metastasis 8. Syringomyelia 9. Hematoma

10. Inflammation (myelitis)
11. AVM
12. Infarct

What is the best imaging modality for evaluating these lesions?

T_1-weighted MRI with contrast

What percentage of intramedullary tumors are ependymomas?

60%

In what spinal region do they occur?

Lumbar or conus medullaris

What is the second most common type of intramedullary tumor?

Astrocytoma

Where do they occur most often?

Cervical cord

OTOLARYNGOLOGIC AND OPHTHALMOLOGIC DISORDERS

EAR DISORDERS

A soft tissue mass in the external auditory canal of an elderly patient with diabetes and purulent otorrhea probably represents what?

Malignant otitis externa

What is the most common malignant neoplasm of the external ear?

Squamous cell carcinoma

Opacification of the middle ear with thickening of the tympanic membrane but no bony erosion or mass effect suggests what diagnosis?

Otitis media

What is a common lesion of the middle ear that may erode the ossicles?

Cholesteatoma

Opacification of the mastoid air cells with or without bony destruction indicates what condition?

Mastoiditis

List 4 other masses that may involve the middle ear.

Glomus tympanicum tumor, aberrant internal carotid artery, lymphoma, rhabdomyosarcoma

What is a prominent clinical symptom of glomus tympanicum tumors?

Pulsatile tinnitus

What does a glomus tympanicum tumor look like on CT?

A small middle ear mass centered over the cochlear promontory

Are malignant middle ear lesions common?

No.

What are the common causes of sensorineural hearing loss?

Mondini malformation (cochlear hypoplasia), vestibular aqueduct enlargement, vestibular schwannoma

Increased density of the cochlea seen on the CT of a patient with a history of chronic ear infections is probably what?

Labyrinthitis ossificans

Bilateral lytic lesions (i.e., bony erosions) around the cochlea of a young or middle-aged woman likely represent what?

Otosclerosis (otospongiosis)

SINUS DISORDERS

What is the best imaging modality for evaluating the sinuses?

CT

Which sinuses are most commonly involved in sinusitis?

Ethmoid (anterior) sinuses

Sinusitis

An air-fluid level involving the sinuses suggests what condition? — Acute sinusitis

What are the 2 radiographic hallmarks associated with chronic sinusitis? — Mucosal thickening and bony sclerosis

What is the key area for evaluation in the patient with chronic sinusitis complaints? — The osteomeatal complex (OMC)

What is the name of the surgery that patients with OMC disease often undergo? — Functional endoscopic sinus surgery (FESS)

What are 3 common causes of a hyperdense sinus lesion? — Inspissated (i.e., dried up) secretions, fungal sinusitis, hemorrhage

Benign sinus lesions

List 4 benign lesions that affect the sinuses. — Mucous retention cyst, mucocele, osteoma, ossifying fibroma

What is a mucous retention cyst? — A benign cyst (often found incidentally) that forms in a sinus as a result of fluid collecting between layers of the submucosa owing to blockage of a mucous gland.

Where does a mucocele commonly arise? — The frontal sinuses more often than the ethmoid sinuses

Why does it form? — Occlusion of a sinus ostium leading to complete opacification of the sinus

What does it look like on CT? — A moderate density lesion arising in a completely opacified sinus, causing thinning and bowing of adjacent bone

Malignant sinus lesions

What is the most common malignant sinus tumor? — Squamous cell carcinoma

What percentage of these tumors occur in the maxillary sinus? — 80%

Do these tumors enhance?	Yes.
Is there bony destruction?	Yes.
These tumors usually spread from the sinuses to involve what space?	Parapharyngeal space (and many other spaces, too)
Sinonasal malignancies have what signal characteristic on T_2-weighted MRI?	Low. Obstructive secretions are very bright.
Name 2 other malignant neoplasms that are not uncommon in the sinonasal region.	Minor salivary gland tumor (usually adenoid cystic carcinoma) and melanoma
Do these tumors have similar radiographic characteristics to those of squamous cell cancer?	Yes.
What imaging studies are typically used to examine this region?	CT with contrast and MRI

PHARYNGEAL AND LARYNGEAL DISORDERS

What is the most common benign tumor of the nasopharynx?	Juvenile angiofibroma
What is the characteristic feature of this tumor on MRI?	A mass in the pterygopalatine fissure with flow voids
What type of tumor is the most common nasopharyngeal malignancy?	Squamous cell carcinoma
Why is unilateral serous otitis media in an adult a concerning presenting condition?	It could indicate obstruction of the eustachian tube by tumor.
What percentage of nasopharyngeal malignancies involve lymph nodes at the time of diagnosis?	80%

What nodes are most commonly involved?	The lateral retropharyngeal nodes (node of Rouvière)
What is the most common malignant tumor of the oropharyngeal region?	Squamous cell carcinoma
From what structure do these malignancies most commonly arise?	The tonsil
Name 2 other malignancies of the oropharynx and where they most commonly occur.	Lymphoma (tongue base) and adenoid cystic carcinoma (soft palate)
List 4 benign tumors that occur in the larynx.	Papilloma, hemangioma, neurofibroma, amyloidoma
What is the most common laryngeal malignancy?	Squamous cell carcinoma
What percentage of laryngeal squamous cell carcinomas are subglottic?	5%
Why is this important?	These are not always visible endoscopically.

LYMPH NODE DISORDERS

What is the study of choice for evaluating lymph nodes in the neck?	CT with intravenous contrast
Why is contrast given?	To help differentiate nodes from vessels and to evaluate the internal architecture of the node
What does an involved node look like?	An involved node is a nonenhancing, enlarged, rounded structure that often exhibits central necrosis. It may resemble a vessel on a single section. Contrast helps, as does putting the sections together.

What is the current size criterion for an abnormally large lymph node in a patient with squamous cell cancer of the larynx or pharynx?	11-mm short-axis diameter
List 5 inflammatory causes of cervical lymphadenopathy.	Tuberculosis, Castleman's disease (angiofollicular hyperplasia), mononucleosis, cat-scratch disease, sarcoidosis
What are the two major cervical malignancies associated with lymphadenopathy?	Squamous cell carcinoma and lymphoma
Name 2 types of lymphoma.	Hodgkin's and non-Hodgkin's
Which is the more common type in the neck?	Non-Hodgkin's (75% of cases)

SALIVARY GLAND DISORDERS

In which gland do calculi most commonly occur?	Submandibular gland
What imaging test is the most sensitive for this condition?	CT
Painless enlargement of the parotid glands is termed what?	Sialosis
What is sialadenitis?	Inflammation of the salivary gland
What is seen on CT with this condition?	Enlargement of the gland with an increase in density
What is the most common benign tumor of the parotid gland?	Pleomorphic adenoma or benign mixed tumor
What does it look like on CT?	A solid, round, soft-tissue density lesion
Does it enhance?	Yes.

Multiple bilateral parotid tumors in an adult with heterogeneous imaging characteristics are usually what?	Warthin's tumors
What percentage of parotid tumors are malignant?	20%
What are the most common parotid malignancies?	Mucoepidermoid carcinoma, adenoid cystic carcinoma, squamous cell carcinoma
What is the most common malignancy in the non-parotid salivary glands?	Adenoid cystic carcinoma
Can these lesions be differentiated from benign neoplasms radiographically?	No.

DISORDERS OF THE EXTRAMUCOSAL SPACES AND BASE OF THE SKULL

What are the most common odontogenic (tooth) masses?	Abscess and osteosarcoma
A septated, lytic lesion of the mandible could represent what benign bony tumor?	Ameloblastoma
Are carotid space tumors usually benign?	Yes.
Name the 2 most common benign tumors found in this space.	Schwannoma and glomus tumor
A low-density, round, well-defined mass that displaces the carotid artery anteriorly and enhances on CT is probably what?	Vagus nerve schwannoma
A dramatically enhancing tumor located at the carotid bifurcation is probably what?	Glomus tumor (paraganglioma, carotid body tumor)

What 5 conditions comprise the differential diagnosis of a jugular fossa mass?	1. Paraganglioma 2. Nerve sheath tumor 3. Metastasis 4. Chordoma 5. Chondrosarcoma
A well-defined, high-signal T_2 lesion located in the retropharyngeal space in a patient with a history of pharyngitis or tonsillitis likely represents what?	Retropharyngeal abscess
What is normally in the retropharyngeal space?	Fat and lymph nodes
What important neurologic structure is found in the paravertebral space?	The brachial plexus
This structure is sandwiched between which two muscles?	The anterior and middle scalene muscles
What are the 2 most common types of brachial plexus lesions that cause symptoms?	Lymphadenopathy (malignant) and trauma

Thyroid and parathyroid gland disorders

How is the thyroid gland imaged?	Nuclear medicine scanning provides functional information. Ultrasound can determine if the nodule is cystic or solid and can provide guidance for biopsy.
What is a thyroid uptake study, and when is it indicated?	A thyroid uptake study is a nuclear medicine study that measures the percentage of a dose of radioactive iodine taken up by the thyroid gland in a given period of time, usually 24 hours. It evaluates the physiologic process whereby the thyroid takes up iodine to manufacture thyroid hormone. The test is indicated when there is thyroid

disfunction, particularly hyperthyroidism.

What is the diagnosis of homogeneously increased uptake in an enlarged gland?

Grave's disease

What are the leading causes of decreased thyroid uptake?

Subacute thyroiditis: Inhomogeneous, decreased uptake in a mildly enlarged gland; patients report a painful, swollen gland

Multinodular goiter: Inhomogeneous, enlarged gland with focal areas of increased and decreased uptake; diagnosis may be confirmed by thyroid scan

Thyroid-blocking medication: These include propylthiouracil and a recent iodine load (e.g., intravenous iodinated contrast material from CT, IVP)

Exogenous thyroid hormone administration

Primary hypothyroidism

How is the thyroid gland imaged with nuclear medicine?

Thyroid scan with either technetium 99m (Tc-99m) or iodine 123 (I^{123}). For a scan only, Tc-99m is preferred. I^{123} is used for uptake studies.

What is the leading diagnosis for a focal area of increased uptake (i.e., a "hot" nodule)?

Thyroid adenoma, which is either under normal hormonal control or autonomous and has a less-than-1% chance of being malignant

What are 6 primary causes of a focal area of decreased uptake (i.e., a "cold" nodule)?

1. Colloid cyst
2. Adenoma
3. Thyroid malignancy (papillary, follicular, medullary, or anaplastic)
4. Thyroiditis (focal)
5. Parathyroid cyst or adenoma
6. Metastatic deposit or lymphoma

What is the risk of malignancy in a cold nodule, and how are cold nodules managed?

Approximately 10% are malignant. Nodules are generally biopsied. Ultrasound can be helpful for image-guided biopsy.

Name the 4 most common types of thyroid carcinomas.	1. Papillary (50%) 2. Follicular (20%) 3. Mixed (10%) 4. Medullary (7%)
Can these lesions be differentiated from adenomas by CT or MRI?	Usually not.
Medullary carcinoma of the thyroid is sometimes associated with what syndrome?	Multiple endocrine neoplasia (MEN) II
What is the significance of multiple hot and cold nodules?	These signs are consistent with a multi-nodular goiter. The risk of malignancy in the cold nodules, if they have been stable in size, is very low. Biopsy usually is not performed unless a nodule has suddenly enlarged.

DISORDERS OF THE EYE AND ORBIT

What is the best imaging test for evaluation of the orbit of most nontrauma patients?	MRI
What is the most common pediatric intraocular tumor?	Retinoblastoma
How often is this tumor either bilateral or multifocal in the same eye?	30%
What does this tumor look like on CT?	Calcification of the posterior globe with extension into the vitreous
What is the most common adult primary intraocular tumor?	Melanoma is the most common primary ocular tumor. Metastatic lesions are most common overall.
Orbital melanoma has a characteristic appearance on T_1- and T_2-weighted MRI. What is it?	T_1 = hyperintense; T_2 = hypointense

List 4 differential diagnoses of an adult ocular mass.

1. Metastasis (breast and lung)
2. Lymphoma
3. Melanoma
4. Choroidal hemangioma

List 6 differential diagnoses of an intraconal mass.

1. Glioma
2. Meningioma
3. Optic neuritis
4. Hemangioma
5. Orbital cellulitis
6. Varix

What is the average age of patients with optic nerve glioma?

8 years

Do these tumors grow slowly, and are they benign?

Yes.

What are the T_1 and T_2 characteristics of this tumor?

T_1 = isointense (to nerve); T_2 = hypointense

What is the average age of patients diagnosed with optic nerve sheath meningioma?

50 years

What percentage of these tumors calcify?

One-third

What are the T_1 and T_2 characteristics of this tumor?

T_1 = isointense; T_2 = hyperintense

Can the optic nerve often still be seen within this type of tumor?

Yes.

Post-contrast axial images of this tumor can have a characteristic appearance that is known as what?

The "tram-track" sign (hypointense nerve is flanked by enhancing tumor)

What disease is most often associated with optic neuritis?

Multiple sclerosis

List 4 differential diagnoses of an intraconal mass.	1. Thyrotoxic ophthalmopathy 2. Rhabdomyosarcoma 3. Orbital pseudotumor 4. Sarcoid
What does thyrotoxic orbitopathy look like on CT?	Extraocular muscle enlargement with proptosis
What happens to the orbital fat?	It is sometimes increased.
What age group gets orbital rhabdomyosarcoma?	Children
What can this tumor do to adjacent bone?	Destroy it.
Orbital pseudotumor commonly causes what 2 symptoms?	Unilateral exophthalmos and pain
List 5 orbital structures that can be affected by this process.	1. Sclera 2. Fat 3. Epidural tissue surrounding the optic nerve 4. Extraocular muscles 5. Lacrimal gland
What are the T_1 and T_2 characteristics of this lesion?	T_1 = high intensity; T_2 = low intensity
List 5 differential diagnoses of an extraconal mass.	1. Metastasis 2. Lacrimal gland lesion 3. Orbital cellulitis 4. Dermoid 5. Sinus lesion
What is the most common extraconal mass in children?	Dermoid
Where in the orbit do dermoids most commonly occur?	Superolaterally, near the lacrimal gland
What do they look like on CT?	A well-defined, low-density cystic lesion that displaces the globe

List 5 differential diagnoses of a unilateral lacrimal gland mass.

1. Pleomorphic adenoma
2. Malignant epithelial cell tumor
3. Adenoid cystic carcinoma
4. Orbital pseudotumor
5. Dacryadenitis (nonspecific inflammation)

What are the 3 differential diagnoses for bilateral involvement?

1. Lymphoma
2. Sarcoid
3. Collagen vascular disease

Index

References in *italics* indicate figures; those followed by "t" denote tables